D1520527

Immunology
of
Nude Mice

Author
Miroslav Holub
Head, Experimental Immunology Group
Institute for Clinical and Experimental Medicine
Prague, Czechoslovakia

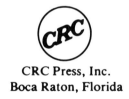

CRC Press, Inc.
Boca Raton, Florida

Library of Congress Cataloging-in-Publication Data

Holub, Miroslav, 1923-
   Immunology of nude mice.

   Includes bibliographies and index.
   1. Nude mouse—Immunology. I. Title.[DNLM:
1. Mice, Nude—immunology. 2. Mice, Nude—physiology.
QY 60.R6 H758i]
QR182.2.A54H65   1989   616.07′9′0724   88-7259
ISBN 0-8493-6662-3

International Standard Book Number 0-8493-6662-3
Library of Congress Card Number 88-7259
Printed in the United States

PREFACE

At the 1st International Workshop on Nude Mice held in Aarhus, Denmark in 1973, 36 papers were delivered, as judged from the proceedings published 1 year later. Of these, 92% were devoted to the breeding, biology, immunology, embryology, cytology, physiology, pathology, and reconstitution of the mouse itself, so to speak, of the mouse personally. Only three papers dealt with the application of this model for in vivo culture of xenografts.

At the 5th International Workshop held in Copenhagen, Denmark in 1985, 67 papers (and posters) dealing with nude mice were presented, as evident from the proceedings (*Immune-Deficient Animals in Biomedical Research*) published 2 years later. Of these, 21% were concerned with the nature (biology, immunology) of the mouse, 53 papers and posters addressed the use of the mouse as a living test tube.

The shift in the proportion of contributions on basic questions about the nu mutation from 92 to 21% is representative also for the situation in biomedical laboratories and journals in general. It looks as if the nude mutation is sufficiently known to be justly applied as a standard and routine tool. It is not, of course; not only are there some physiological problems that have failed to trigger enough attention, but many of the basic immunological and endocrinological studies have been performed on poorly defined animal material and with hardly comparable methods. The purpose of this book is to survey at least some areas of solid knowledge and to show how many questions regarding the nude mouse itself remain unanswered.

The scope of a single author must be, by definition, limited, but writing scientific monographs in this old-fashioned way has one advantage: there is less overlapping and less background noise than in a collection of chapters/articles by single specialists.

I am much indebted to the people at CRC Press for coping with the manuscript written in a nonmaternal language and in conditions where technological progress has to be supplemented by human effort and dedication. I am also deeply grateful to the Director and workers of the Institute for Clinical and Experimental Medicine in Prague.

Miroslav Holub

THE AUTHOR

Miroslav Holub, M.D., Ph.D., is a senior scientific worker at the Institute for Clinical and Experimental Medicine in Prague, Czechoslovakia. He heads the experimental unit of the Institute's Immunological Department.

Dr. Holub graduated and received the M.D. degree from the Charles IV. University, Prague, in 1953 and worked as a clinical pathologist. In 1954, he joined the newly formed immunological laboratory in the Biological (later Microbiological) Institute of the Czechoslovak Academy of Sciences and obtained the scientific degree, about equivalent to Ph.D. in 1958. He was engaged in the studies of cytological aspects of antibody formation and of the key role of the lymphocyte.

During 1965 to 1967, he worked in the immunological laboratory of the Public Health Research Institute of New York City and in 1968 to 1969 at the Max Planck Institute for Immunobiology in Freiburg, W. Germany. He was introduced to the nude mouse club by the late Dr. Berenice Kindred, and has stayed on as a faithful member for all years thereafter, with the main interest focused on the nature of thymic dysgenesis.

In 1972, he was transferred from the Academy to the Institute for Clinical and Experimental Medicine. He has published, so far, 130 scientific papers in immunology, one monograph (*Structure of the Immune System,* Prague 1979) and chapters in the *Modern Trends in Immunology 2,* London 1967 and in the *Grundriss der Immunbiologie,* Leipzig 1978 and 1988.

During 1968 to 1970 Dr. Holub was a member of the presidium of the Union of Czechoslovak Scientific Workers. He is also a known writer translated in most European countries, the U.S., India, China, and Japan. In 1985, he obtained an honorary degree from Oberlin College, Oberlin, Ohio, and is a member of the Bavarian Academy of Arts.

TABLE OF CONTENTS

Chapter 1

INTRODUCTION: THE CONTRADICTORY MOUSE

In a Czech fairy tale a smart mountaineer woman is charged by a man of power to come to see him "neither in the day nor at night, neither naked nor dressed, neither on foot nor riding". The clever girl solves the problem by coming at dawn, with a loosely woven sack on her body, with one shoe and one sock on her feet, sitting on a goat with her legs on the ground.

The athymic nude mouse reminds me of that viable mountain-girl-mutant; the mouse is not athymic, because it possesses at least one component of the normal mouse thymus; it is not nude, but it grows hair which is invisible most of the time. And lacking the key part of the immune defenses, it is not defenseless; on the contrary it may be better equipped to fight certain bacterial infections, at least in the early or acute phase, than a normal mouse. Lacking the key part of the "immune surveillance" system, it has no higher incidence of spontaneous tumors, at least not of solid epithelial tumors, and lives in a germ-free state or in perfect specific-pathogen-free (SPF) conditions for the same 1000 days as do normal mice of the given background, outliving even the immune surveillance theory in its original form.

The nude mutant may have been here since 1962, or indeed since 1850, when two hairless mice died in a zoologist's grape vase and the third one escaped. Even since 1962 or 1968, the year the immunological career of the nude mutant started, when it occurred to one of the nude mice pioneers to check what the nude mouse had inside, the nude mouse may have changed considerably due to nu gene transfer to different background strains and for different levels of backcrossing, and as a result of progressively improving housing conditions, breeding and husbandry, with consequent elimination of some known or unknown natural pathogens. It cannot be claimed that an SPF BALB/c(10th backcross)*nu/nu* mouse of 1987 is exactly the same as such a mouse from 1972. This is very good for the mouse which nowadays has litters from homozygous (*nu/nu* × *nu/nu*) matings in almost every breeding center — a rarity 15 years ago; but this is not good for the results or the comparability of immunological and physiological studies (Figure 1).

In any case, the nude mouse has been a tool for an impressive amount of work on the nature of T cells and on the interaction of T cells with MHC class I and class II antigens (or rather molecular complexes with processed exogenous antigen). The T-cell studies were motivated by the "athymic state" of the model, but the "athymic state" itself was not enough of a motive for deeper embryological investigation or manipulation to pin down the reason for the athymic state, which is as obscure today as it was in 1968. Hence, one may read in the discussion in a paper on nude mice that "the presence of thymus cells in the nude mouse is undoubtedly related to the presence of a thymus during the first 12 days of gestation...".

I wonder what would have happened to the poor nude mouse if it had first fallen into the hands of neurophysiologists — given its cortical and oligodendroglial deficits — or of endocrinologists — given its hypothalamic or even pineal body alterations and disturbed circadian rhythms — or of students of phagocytosis — given its impressive phagocytic capacities. Undoubtedly, thymic dysgenesis would have been discovered eventually, and it would have become the immunologically dominant trait, but the thinking would then not have been so thymus-monomanic. Not every single physiological alteration would have been attributed primarily to the athymia, which may, at best, affect the ontogeny from the 12th to 13th gestational day onwards, but also to something that may have gone wrong earlier, due to the *nu* gene.

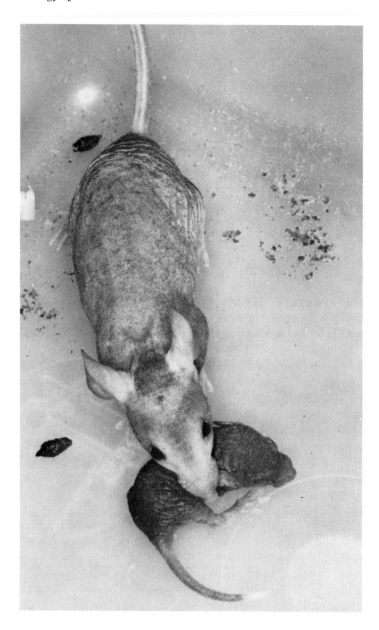

FIGURE 1.   C57Bl.10 LP female nude mouse, 3 months old, carrying her off-spring from a homozygous litter (*nu/nu* × *nu/nu*).

As Hans Grüüneberg wrote in 1948:[1]

On the morphological level, gene-controlled disturbances provide a unique material for the study of epigenetic relationships... Work of this kind has as its background the postulate of the unity of primary gene action. From this postulate it follows logicaly that the various effects of a gene on the morphological level, however ill-assorted they may appear at first glance, are causually connected as an epigenetic pattern... That the progress made in the analysis of these phenomena is so far slight has two main reasons. One is that one cannot usually penetrate to this level without breaking down a solid morphological crust which hides the more fundamental processes from view. The other is the comparatively untractable chemistry of these big molecules...

This monograph is based on the attempt not to ascribe too many phenomena within "the solid morphological crust" to athymia, but to try to penetrate back to the level of the possible

Table 1
PRINCIPAL PUBLICATIONS ON NUDE MICE

Proc. 1st Int. Workshop on Nude Mice, Rygaard, J. and Povlsen, C. O., Eds., G. Fischer, Stuttgart, 1974.
Proc. 2nd Int. Workshop on Nude Mice, Nomura, T., Ohsawa, N., Tamaoki, N., and Fujiwara, K., Eds., University of Tokyo Press, Tokyo, 1977 and G. Fischer, Stuttgart, 1977.
Proc. 3rd Int. Workshop on Nude Mice, Reed, N. D., Ed., G. Fischer, New York, 1982.
Immune-deficient Animals, Proc. 4th Int. Workshop on Immune Deficient Animals, Sordat, B., Ed., S. Karger, Basel, 1984.
Immune-deficient Animals in Biomedical Research, Proc. 5th Int. Workshop on Immune Deficient Animals, Rygaard, J., Brünner, N., Graem, N., and Spang-Thomsen, M., Eds., S. Karger, Basel, 1987.
Rygaard, J., *Thymus & Self, Immunobiology of the Mouse Mutant Nude,* F. A. D L. Copenhagen, 1973.
Bibliography of the Nude Mouse 1966—1976, Rygaard, J. and Povlsen, C. O. Eds., G. Fischer, Stuttgart, 1977.
Proc. Symp. on the Use of Athymic (Nude) Mice in Cancer Research, Houchens, O. P. and Ovejera, A. A., Eds., G. Fischer, Stuttgart, 1978.
The Nude Mouse in Experimental and Clinical Research, Vols. 1 and 2, Fogh, J. and Giovanella, B. C., Eds., Academic Press, New York, 1978, 1982.
Immunodeficient Animals in Cancer Research, Sparrow, S., Ed., Macmillan, London, 1980.
Thymusaplastic Nude Mice and Rats in Clinical Oncology, Bastert, G., Fortmeyer, H. P., and Schmidt-Matthiesen, H., Eds., G. Fischer, Stuttgart, 1981.
Fortmeyer, H. P., *Thymusaplastische Maus (nu/nu) Thymusaplastische Ratte* (rnu/rnu). *Haltung, Zucht, Versuchsmodelle,* Paul Parey, Berlin, 1981.
Kindred, B., Nude mice in immunology, *Prog. Allergy,* 26, 137, 1979.
Kindred, B., Deficient and sufficient immune systems in the nude mouse, in *Immunologic Defects in Laboratory Animals,* Vol. 1, Gerschwin, M. E. and Merchant, B. Eds., Plenum Press, New York, 1981, 215.

"primary gene action", at least by showing the multitude of alterations everywhere in the organism which has to survive the defect in one entire organ system.[2]

The alterations may affect other alterations, compensations may affect the defects and may themselves be altered by other compensations. Some of the alterations may be parallel, not consequent upon the thymic dysgenesis. In other words, the nu gene effect may well be operating before the first thymic epithelial cells assemble to the anlage. Absence of evidence is not evidence of absence of these ontogenic factors.

However, in view of the available monographs, special attention and discussion will be focused on the thymus problem proper which is a neglected orphan in all nude mouse literature, albeit an orphan blamed or made responsible for all of the nude mice.

This leaves little space for the favorite topics of nude mouse reconstitution, which were exhaustively surveyed by Kindred (Table 1) and no space to the applications of nude mice in experimental oncology, to which a special symposium and linearly increasing proportions of international workshops on nude mice and other immunodeficient animals (IWIDA) are devoted (Table 1).

A perfect introduction to the problems of nude mouse breeding and production is provided by Fortmeyer's monograph and by specialized chapters in the book edited by Fogh and Giovanella and in separate IWIDA proceedings (Table 1).

REFERENCES

1. **Grüneberg, H.,** Genes and pathological development in mammals, in *Growth in Relation to Differentiation and Morphogenesis,* Symposia of the Society for Experimental Biology No. 2, Cambridge University Press, Cambridge, 1948, 155.
2. **Rygaard, J.,** *Thymus & Self, Immunobiology of the Mouse Mutant Nude,* F. A. D. L., Copenhagen, 1973.

Chapter 2

THE NUDE MUTATION

What proved to be the nude mutant was introduced by Isaacson and Cattanach in a report in *Mouse News Letter* in 1962.[1] According to the first and timely monograph of Rygaard,[2] "Dr. N. R. Grist first saw the mutant, and one male without hair, a characteristic of the mutant, together with two phenotypically normal mice, male and female, were sent to the Institute of Animal Genetics in Edinburgh. The phenotypically normal mice were supposedly heterozygous for a recessive gene which was responsible for the mutation . . . "[2] It was good luck of the nude mutation, and of immunology, that this was the case and the two phenotypically normal mice became ancestors of all — or most — nude mice serving as experimental athymic models of immunology and test tubes for hybridomas and tumor biopsies all over the world. Flanagan[3] obtained segregation data from intercross and backcross matings; intercross matings of heterozygous mice produced the predictable proportion of nudes, 1349 out of 5239 mice, and matings of nu/nu males with heterozygous females produced 14 nudes from 30 mice. Linkage tests have shown that Rex and Trembler marker genes — in the linkage group VII — segregated with the *nu* gene with a recombination frequency of 13 and 9%, respectively.[3]

Gene transfers to BALB/c and other inbred strains were initiated by Rygaard and Friis in PAI, Kommunehospitalet, Copenhagen and at Gl. Bomholtgaard facilities in Ry, Denmark, respectively, in 1969.[2] The aim was congeneic strains differing from the original inbred in 0.4% of the genetic constitution.[4]

Rygaard recorded that 200 random matings of *nu/nu* males with heterozygous females yielded 1721 offspring, 870 *nu/nu* and 851 *nu/ +*.[2] In individual litters of BALB/c, B10.LP and B10 ScSn mice used for nu gene transfer in our laboratory, we observed that in litters of *nu/nu* males to *nu/ +* mothers, *nu/ +* offsprings tend to prevail, while in reversed matings of *nu/ +* males to *nu/nu* females — which are successful in the improved breeding and husbandry conditions — the majority of offspring are *nu/nu*. The breeding results are affected, of course, by increased *nu/nu* mortality at weaning. The observation made mostly in utero is mentioned only to remind us of the multitude of factors which may influence the occurrence and establishment of a viable, but immunologically and physiologically altered mutant in natural populations. In laboratory conditions, the mutant has been successfully transferred into most common or interesting laboratory strains. Eleven different strains in eleven breeding centers are listed in 1974.[5] In 1978 Hansen alone reports the introduction of the nu gene into 21 strains representing a broad spectrum of different immune system characteristics.[6]

The reason of natural occurrence of mutants of this kind is unknown. Medawar stated in 1952: . . . "There is a constant feeble pressure to introduce new variants of hereditary factors into a natural population. For 'mutation', as it is called, is a recurrent process. Very often such factors lower the fertility or viability of the organism in which they make their effects apparent; but it is arguable that if only they make them apparent late enough, the force of selection will be too attenuated to oppose their establishment and spread. We only know of their existence through domestication; small wonder if they have no effect on the well-being of mouse populations in the wild" . . . [7]. These affections make themselves apparent at ages which wild mice seldom reach, i.e., after 100 days of life in a natural environment with all the strains and dangers. The nude mutant affects the phenotype and main physiological parameters of the mouse already in utero, however, they do not lead in most individuals to a deep deterioration of the condition before the 4th month of life even in very "conventional" conditions, provided we do not infest them artificially with mouse hepatitis virus or toxoplasma.

In terms of population genetics, it may be remembered that " . . . many geneticists feel that populations still maintain too much variation for selective control. If they are right . . . , then we must face the possibility that many genes remain in populations because selection cannot "see" them, and therefore cannot either mark them for elimination or remove other variants by favoring them. In other words, many genes may be neutral. They may be invisible to natural selection and their increase or decrease may be a result of chance alone."[8]

Consequently, it is no surprise that David could include into his histological classification so many hairless mutants in so many mammalian species in 1932[9] and that in a 1987 *Mouse News Letter*[10] 72 mutant genes are listed as having a phenotypic effect on mouse skin and hair and 89 genes as affecting the immune reactivity. One may have the impression that the hairlessness and immune deviation are especially numerous, but the numbers have to be compared with 95 mouse genes affecting the skeleton.[10] What is less common is a disclosed combination of the hair and immune defects and Rigdon in 1975 felt that " . . . it is difficult to visualize one chromosomal defect to account for hairlessness and an absence of the thymus in one mouse, hairlessness and an absence of mammary tissue in another mouse, and complete hairlessness in another mouse."[11]

Yet the nude mutation is due to one gene[6,10] and it is likely that the gene affects some key protein factor which lies deep in the ontogeny of many, if not all, cellular and tissue systems.

It is hard to judge how true this is for other mutations with a phenotypic effect on the hair and skin; the immunological parameters are, with the exception of *hr*, *me*, and a few others,[12] unknown (Table 1).

In view of the antigenic similarities between skin and thymic epithelia (see Chapter 3), it would be most useful to perform a deeper comparative analysis of the thymic markers and ultrastructural traits in many, if not most, of the mutants listed (Table 1).

Table 1
LIST OF MOUSE MUTANTS WITH HAIR AND SKIN DEFECTS[10,13]

Gene	Mutation	Chromosome	Dermatological	Immunological effect	Endocrine
ab — asebia	Spont. in a BALB/c strain	19	Progressive alopecia, sebaceous glands abnormal, defect in esterified sterols and waxes, collagen alteration	Unknown	Female fertility reduced
Al — alopecia	Spont. in an outcross	11	Progressive hair loss, more pronounced in *Al/Al*	Unknown	Unknown
ao — apampischo	Spont. in agouti mice	—	Recurring hair loss, females lose hair repeatedly with pregnancies, males lose the regrown hair after 1 year of age	Unknown	Unknown
ap — alopecia periodica	Spont. in an inbred	—	Recurring complete hair loss, altered keratinization of skin	Unknown	Unknown
at — atrichosis	Spont. in a DBA strain	10	Sparse hair on the trunk, especially	Unknown	Sterility, small gonads with few germ cells
ba — bare	Spont. in a Swiss albino strain	—	Delayed hair growth waves and recurring loss of hair, hairless at 6 months; abnormal keratinization in the follicles	Unknown	Unknown
bal — balding	Spont. in a C57Bl strain		Progressive hair loss in patches	Unknown	Small growth
Bpa — barepatches	Radiation induced	X	Bare stripes in female heterozygotes	Unknown	Unknown
Bsk[14] — bareskin	Chemically induced	—	Progressive thinning of the coat, adults bare; thick skin in folds; corneal opacities	Unknown	Unknown
cr — crinkled	Chemically induced	13	Thin, abnormal hair coat, bald spots, absence of Meibomian glands, abnormalities in other exocrine glands, abnormal teeth	Unknown	Poor breeding performance, reduced viability
crh — cryptothrix	Spont. in a non-inbred line	--	Short fuzzy hair, most hairs disintegrate at the level of sebaceous glands	Unknown	Unknown
cw[thd] — curly whiskers-tail hair depletion	Spont. in the SJL/J strain	9	Hair depletion in some areas	Abnormal response to polysaccharide antigens, accept tail skin grafts from normal mice	Unknown
dep — depilitated	Spont. in a stock carrying T, tf	4	Hair loss at 3 weeks in some individuals, derangement of hair follicles	Unknown	Unknown
dl — downless	Spont. in the A/H strain	10	Thin, abnormal hair, bald spots like *cr/cr*, incl. teeth abnormality	Unknown	Unknown
Dl[slk15] — sleek	Spont.	10	Delayed, thin, untidy coat, baldspots like *cr/cr*; only one type of hair; incisors abnormal or absent	Unknown	Unknown

Table 1 (continued)
LIST OF MOUSE MUTANTS WITH HAIR AND SKIN DEFECTS[10,13]

Er — repeated epilation	Semidominant, radiation-induced	4	Recurrent hair loss; defective differentiation of the epidermis; homozygotes die — closed oral, anal, and urogenital orifices	Unknown	Unknown
exf — exfoliative	Spont. in the A^y viable-yellow inbred	—	Recurring hair loss and exfoliation in epidermis from 4th week; recurrent conjunctivitis	Recurrent bacteriemia-phagocytosis defect?	Unknown
fd — fur deficient	Spont. in the CBA/2J strain	9	Sparse underfur	Unknown	Unknown
fr — frizzy	Spont. in an outbred	7	Curly vibrissae, short and thin coat in older animals	Unknown	Unknown
Frl — furloss	Spont. in a stock carrying d and se; an allelic series Frl^a, Frl^b Frl^c		Wrinkled skin, progressive hair loss and regrowth, complete hair loss at 4 months	Unknown	Unknown
fs — furless	Spont. in an outbred	13	Recurring loss of hair, complete hair loss in some adults	Unknown	Unknown
fz — fuzzy	Spont. in the CFW stock		Thin vibrissae, hair coat uneven, curly; abnormal epidermal hair bulb	Unknown	Unknown
hl — hair-loss	Spont.	15	Progressive degeneration of hair follicles, complete loss of hair and wrinkled skin in some individuals after 1 month	Unknown	Low calcium requirement, fragile bones in hl/+ offspring of hl/hl females
hr — hairless	Spont., found in the wild	14	Hyperkeratosis in the hair canal from day 14 on, recurring complete hair loss from the follicle, foll. cyst formation; hr^{ba} and hr^{rh} are spont. mutations without hair regeneration, with extensive hyperkeratosis	Depression of B-cell proliferation and responses, defect of Lyl 1 cell differentiation, may be due to a suppressive effect of macrophages;[16,17] in hr^{rh}Y/hr^{rh}Y immunocomplex disease and loss of cortical thymocytes;[18] incidence of thymic lymphoma	Unknown
Hr^n — near naked	Spont. in a stock derived from irradiated mice	14	Thin and slick skin short curly vibrissae, a thin coat of fur in heterozygotes, complete loss of hair in homozygotes[20]	Unknown	Unknown

Table 1 (continued)
LIST OF MOUSE MUTANTS WITH HAIR AND SKIN DEFECTS[10,13]

ic — ichthyosis	Spont. in a sibmated stock	1	Short, thin hair, some individuals hairless, skin develops hard scales; epidermal disorder	Abnormal nuclear morphology in leukocytes, increased DNA content in all nuclei/immunocomplex disease?	Reduced fertility
me — moth-eaten	Spont. in the C57B1/6J strain	6	Skin abscesses immediately after birth, subepidermal lesions disrupting hair follicles	Severe immune defect; impaired B-cell proliferation and responses, lack of cytotoxic T cells and NK cells; autoimmunity, Ig hyperproduction[17]; macrophages with increased proliferative capacity	Unknown
N — naked	Semidominant, spont. mutation in a lab. stock	15	Progressive cyclic hair loss in patches, more pronounced in homozygotes; incomplete keratinization in the follicle, hair is deficient in a protein fraction (HG) with a high glycine and tyrosine[21]	Unknown	Unknown
Ng — nacking	Semidominant, spont. in the NMRI strain		Sparse hair coat, homozygotes completely hairless; interfollicular epidermis in *Ng/Ng* hyperplastic, with hyperkeratosis, lower part of follicles reduced	Unknown	Unknown
nu — nude	Spont. in a closed stock of albino mice	11	Faulty keratinization in hair follicles from birth on, hairless with occasional thin hair patches	Thymic dysgenesis, delayed and defective development of T-cell systems and cell-mediated reactions; low responses to T-dependent antigens	Hypothalamic-pituitary derangement, mild hypothyroidism and delayed ovarian functions
NY[22] — progr. fur loss	Spont. on A2Q background	—	Progressive loss of hair, the front half bald at 5 weeks[23]	Thymus enlarged	Unknown
olt — oligotriche	Spont. in the C3H/HeOrl strains	—	Retarded growth of ventral hair coat, sparse coat, especially in adult females	Unknown	Males sterile, abortive spermatogenesis
pf -- pupoid fetus	Radiation induced, homozygotes die at birth	4	Abnormally keratinized epidermis; in $11\frac{1}{2}$-day embryos — confusion of the epidermal-mesenchymal boundary at the sites where peripheral nerves grow into the epidermis, naked nerve fibers on the surface of the embryo, plaque formation	Unknown	Unknown

Table 1 (continued)
LIST OF MOUSE MUTANTS WITH HAIR AND SKIN DEFECTS[10,13]

pk — plucked	Spont. in the DBA/ 2J strain	—	Thickened skin, delay in hair growth waves, disorders in hair structure and sebaceous glands, disruption of the passage of the hair shaft up the follicle	Unknown	Unknown
Ra — ragged	Semidominant, spont. in a crossbred stock	2	Homozygotes naked, heterozygotes with only partial development of some hair types; low viability	Alteration in lymph flow, edema and ascites formation	Unknown
*Re*den — denuded (rex)	Spont. in a congeneic strain	11	Hair loss after 6 weeks of life, all *Re* mutants have irregular hair shaft and a defect in the internal root sheath which does not support the shaft	Unknown	Unknown
sch — scant hair	Spont. in the C57Bl/ KS db strain	9	Cessation of hair growth at 7—8 days resulting in complete nakedness in some homozygotes	Unknown	Unknown
Sha — shaven	Semidominant, spont., closely linked to N	15	Cyclic growth and loss of hair coat in homozygotes; hair thin and uneven, keratinization defective	Unknown	Unknown
Sk — scaly	Semidominant, spont.	—	In extreme cases scaly skin on the back with sparse hair growth	Unknown	Unknown
spc — sparse coat	Spont. in a stock carrying jg and bf	14	Sparse and patchy hair coat	Unknown	Fertility reduced
spf — sparse fur	Incompl. recessive, radiation induced	X	Sparse hair, some individuals hairless, with wrinkled skin	Unknown	Hairless individuals, dwarfed, metabolic disorders
Str — striated	Semidominant, radiation-induced	X	Coat defective in some hair types, in stripes; due to an epidermal alteration	Unknown	Unknown
Ta — tabby	Semidominant, spont.	X	Abnormal hair, bald spots, defect in some exocrine glands and in teeth ; defects caused by a deviation of epithelial proliferation in embryogenesis in *Ta/Ta* females and hemizygous males	Unknown	Ta/Ta females sterile
tf — tufted	Spont.	17	Repeated hair loss and regrowth in antero-posterior waves	Unknown	Unknown
thf — thin fur	Spont. in a moderately inbred strain	17	Sparse hair after the first molt	Unknown	Unknown

Table 1 (continued)
LIST OF MOUSE MUTANTS WITH HAIR AND SKIN DEFECTS[10,13]

wal^{21} — waved alopecia	Spont. in a BALB/c strain	14	Long waved fasciculated hair, progressive thinning of the coat after 1 month of life especially in females, hairless after 2 months; irregular distribution of hair follicles, degeneration of follicles, dermal cysts	Unknown	Unknown

REFERENCES

1. **Isaacson, J. H. and Cattanach, B. M.**, *Mouse News Lett.*, 27, 31, 1962.
2. **Rygaard, J.**, *Thymus & Self, Immunobiology of the Mouse Mutant Nude*, F. A. D. L., Copenhagen, 1973.
3. **Flanagan, S. P.**, 'Nude', a new hairless gene with pleiotropic effects in the mouse, *Genet. Res.*, 8, 295, 1966.
4. **Snell, G. D.**, Methods for the study of histocompatibility genes, *J. Genet.*, 49, 87, 1948.
5. *Proc. 1st Int. Workshop on Nude Mice*, Rygaard, J. and Povlsen, C. O., Eds., G. Fischer, Stuttgardt, 1974, 297.
6. **Hansen, C. T.**, The nude gene and its effects, in *The Nude Mouse in Experimental and Clinical Research*, Fogh, J. and Giovanella, B. C., Eds., Academic Press, New York, 1978, 1.
7. **Medawar, P. B.**, *The Uniqueness of the Individual*, Dover, New York, 1981, 47.
8. **Gould, S. J.**, Hen's Teeth and Horse's Toes, Norton, New York, 1983, 335.
9. **David, L. T.**, The external expression and comparative dermal histology of hereditary hairlessness in mammals, *Z. Zellforsch. Mikrosk. Anat.*, 14(Part B), 616, 1931/32.
10. **Peters, J., Ed.**, *Mouse News Lett.*, 77, 9, 1987.
11. **Rigdon, R. H.**, Hairlessness in *Mus musculus*, *Arch. Pathol.*, 99, 318, 1975.
12. **Smith, S. M., Forbes, P. D., and Linna, T. J.**, Immune responses in nonhaired mice, *Int. Arch. Allergy Appl. Immunol.*, 67, 254, 1982.
13. **Green, M. C.**, Catalog of mutant genes and polymorphic loci, in *Genetic Variants and Strains of the Laboratory Mouse*, Green, M. C., Ed., G., Fischer, Stuttgart, 1981, 8.
14. **Peters, J., Ed.**, *Mouse News Lett.*, 74, 96, 1986.
15. **Crocker, M. and Cattanach, B.**, The genetics of Sleek: a possible regulatory mutation of the tabby-crinkled-downless syndrome, *Genet. Res.*, 34, 231, 1979.
16. **Vogel, S. N., Weinblatt, A. C., and Rosenstreich, D. L.**, Inherent macrophage defects in mice, in *Immunologic Defects in Laboratory Animals*, Vol. 1, Gershwin, M. E. and Merchant, B., Eds., Plenum Press, New York, 1981, 327.
17. **Shultz, L. D. and Roths, J. B.**, Euthymic murine models for immunologic dysfunction, in *Immune-Deficient Animals in Biomedical Research, Proc. 5th IWIDA*, Rygaard, J. et al., Eds., S. Karger, Basel, 1987, 1.
18. **Peters, J., Ed.**, *Mouse News Lett.*, 73, 24, 1985.
19. **Reske-Kunz, A. B., Scheid, M. D., de Sousa, M., and Boyse, E. A.**, Correlation of immunogenetic and histological changes in immunodeficient mutant hr/hr mice, in *Function and Structure of the Immune System*, Müller-Ruchholz, W. and Müller-Hermelink, H. K., Eds., Plenum Press, New York, 1979, 55.
20. **Stelzner, K. F.**, Four dominant autosomal mutations affecting skin and hair development in the mouse, *J. Heredity*, 74, 193, 1983.
21. **Tenenhouse, H. S., Gold, R. J. M., Kachra, Z., and Fraser, F. C.**, Biochemical marker in dominantly inherited ectodermal malformation, *Nature*, 251, 431, 1974.
22. **Peters, J., Ed.**, *Mouse News Lett.*, 73, 14, 1985.
23. **Füchtbauer, E.-M. and Jockusch, H.**, personal communication.
24. **Peters, J., Ed.**, *Mouse News Lett.*, 73, 22, 1985.

Chapter 3

THE THYMIC DEFECT

I. INTRODUCTION

The thymic defect, which we refer to as "thymic dysgenesis", is the main reason for the laboratory existence of the nude mouse. The defect was discovered in 1968 when the concept of two basically different lymphocyte populations was emerging and led to an explosive proliferation of cellular immunology. The nude mouse, more fundamentally "thymusless" than the thymectomized model, immediately became part of the game.[1] Interestingly, most animal work performed in cellular immunology was concerned with the meanings and functions of thymus-dependent, thymus-derived, or thymus-processed cells on the periphery.[2] The bulk of the progress in the knowledge of the organ (thymus) itself came from human material.[3]

In view of the number of unsettled problems of thymus ontogeny and its deviations, we will survey the data on thymic dysgenesis by first outlining the normal thymic genesis and then proceeding to the peculiar nude mouse defect which is one of the least safe grounds in the life history of the poor nude mouse. Paradoxes are essential not only for the good functioning of the human mind.

II. THE DERIVATION OF THE EPITHELIAL STROMA

The nature of the thymus is one of the most romantic chapters of morphology and physiology. Since the beginning of the 19th century comparative anatomy led to a number of both meticulous and conflicting descriptions of the embryonic development of the thymus in different vertebrate species. Limited knowledge of the physiological role of the thymus permitted very liberal concepts about the ontogeny of the essential thymic component, the epithelial stroma. Born described in 1883 the endodermal derivation of the thymus anlage from the third pharyngeal pouch in the pig,[4] Schaffer and Rabl found in 1909 the mole thymus to be "purely ectodermal",[4] and in 1911 Zotterman felt free to conclude that there were three different genetic types of thymus: a purely endodermal, a purely ectodermal, and a mixed ecto-endodermal thymus.[4] The derivation of the thymic epithelial stroma from both the ectoderm (mainly in the cranial part, caput thymi) and endoderm gained more support in the last 50 years,[5,6] especially by the classical and much-quoted description of the embryonic development of the thymus in the mouse.[7] However, only recent results obtained with the use of cellular differentiation markers and stimulated in part by the revived interest in thymic dysgenesis provided decisive data.

One of the major human amnion antigens has been identified in the human embryonic thymus, namely in Hassall's corpuscles of normal, but not of immunodeficient children.[8,9] In other words, the amniotic epithelium which contains "some of the most biologically interesting growth-promoting substances" may have a decisive influence on the thymic organogenesis.[9] Amniotic epithelial cells appear to give rise both to the embryonic and to the extraembryonic ectoderm. A pocket of ectoderm which Faulk and McIntire denote as amniotic extraembryonic, is juxtaposed against the endodermal branchial pouches around the time when the endodermal thymic anlage migrates cranially.[9] The ectodermal cell layer of the third branchial cleft covers (at least in the mouse) the endodermal portion of the anlage.[10] At this point, ectodermal cells exert their inductive effect which produces the regular thymic differentiation of the mainly endodermal medulla surrounded by the mainly ectodermal cortex.[7]

The ectodermal component is derived exclusively from the third branchial cleft which undergoes intensive proliferation on the 11th day of gestation in the mouse[10] and at 4 to 5 weeks in man.[5,6]

Thus, it can be inferred that the epithelial stromal cells of a normal thymus are basically heterogeneous: the cortical (stellar) epithelial cells are ectodermal, the medullary epithelial cells, other than those cells which form Hassall's corpuscles, are endodermal.[6,10]

However, monoclonal antibodies identifying human endocrine epithelial cells in the thymus subcapsular cortex and medulla labeled epithelial cells in the thymic rudiment of a 7-week fetus; between 9 and 13 weeks the positive epithelial cells were arranged in lobulated zones, and by 15 weeks they compartmentalized into subcapsular cortical and medullary areas.[11] A monoclonal antibody defining one of the antigens of the endocrine epithelium first labeled cells of dendritic morphology at 12 to 15 weeks only. Positive cells were confined to the subcapsular region. At 4 months postpartum the positive cells formed a linear subcapsular lining of all lobules and occasional positive cells appeared in the cortex and in the medulla; the medullary positive cells became numerous at 30 months postpartum.[11]

Since the applied monoclonals label also the epidermal cells (keratinocytes) in the basal stratum of the skin and of other squamous epithelial linings[11] it may be suggested that the endocrine epithelial thymic cells are of ectodermal origin and that they migrate into the endodermal thymic anlage at different times of organ development. Haynes[11] proposes a similar maturation pathway for human thymic epithelial cells and keratinocytes: in addition to the shared surface antigens both contain keratin and have similar growth requirements in vitro. Thymic medullary epithelial cells forming Hassall's corpuscles undergo the same surface antigen changes with basal keratinocytes maturing into stratum granulosum and stratum spinosum cells. This agrees also with the morphological suggestions that medullary thymic epithelial cells have a potential for differentiation similar to skin epithelial cells.[12]

It must be noted that the typical cystic medullary epithelial cell described in the electron microscope[12,13] may not be identical with the endocrine medullary cell sharing in luminiscent microscopy the surface markers with the subcapsular cortical epithelial cell. The cystic medullary cells develop poorly in tissue culture conditions and upon implantation of fetal thymuses beneath the kidney capsule in mice.[12] The grafts, nevertheless, differentiate in normal thymic tissue with typical cortical epithelial cells. It may be inferred that the cystic medullary epithelial cell — possibly of endodermal origin — may have functions other than synthesis or storage of the known thymic hormones and may be dependent on normal lymphoid cell traffic through the medulla.

So far, it can be concluded that the thymic epithelial stroma derives basically from both endoderm and ectoderm: the medullary endocrine cells and the Hassall's corpuscle-forming cells may be ectodermal in nature, but migrate into the endodermal part of the thymic anlage.

The cortical epithelial cell, including the respective endocrine cells in the subcapsular area, have a typical ultrastructural appearance, they are stellate, with slender lamelliform processes connecting to the processes of neighboring cells by desmosomes and the cytoplasm contains characteristic vacuoles filled with osmiophilic granules and vesicles (possibly secretion or storage vacuoles). Tumors derived from these epithelial cells, when grown in tissue culture, do indeed secrete factors which can exert the thymic hormone effect on postthymic lymphocytes in the rat system, but with no species specificity.

Cortical epithelial cells in the obviously specialized subcapsular area contain keratin and the thymic hormones thymopoietin, thymosin α1, β3, and β4.[11] The latter two polypeptides are missing in medullary endocrine cells. Also, another thymic hormone, the FTS of French workers, seems to be associated with keratin-positive epithelial cells in the murine thymic cell cultures.[15] Human subcapsular epithelial cells, forming a dense mesh, express neuronal gangliosides on their surface; they may be derived from the neural crest and they belong to a family of neuroendocrine cells found in many organs[11] and in all species, including mice

(Section V). It cannot be excluded that neural crest mesenchyme (ectomesenchyme), also suggested as playing an inductive role in the epithelial anlage differentiation, may be directly involved in the subcapsular area. Thy-1-positive cells of epithelial appearance have been described in this layer[11] where Thy-1-positive immature, large lymphoid cells are stuffed among the epithelial cell processes.[13] Thy 1 antigen was suggested as triggering cell-stroma adhesions and interactions.[16,17] Almost all mouse, rat, or human thymic epithelial cells exhibiting tonofilaments and growing in culture can be shown to express Thy-1 or Thy-1-analogous antigens.[18,19]

Subcapsular lymphoid cells were shown to give rise to both cortical and medullary thymocytes.[20] The site of entry of lymphoid precursors is, however, the vascular cortico-medullary junction. Cortical thymocytes may not be immediate precursors of the mature, competent medullary thymocytes[21,22] and most die *in situ*.[23] It is possible that the clonal deletion, one of the most tricky thymic events, occurs here and some cortical epithelia sharing an interleukin receptor with cortical thymocytes prevent their survival. Only a small subset of cortical lymphocytes equipped with a lymphocyte homing receptor exists in the cortex.[24] Cortical thymocytes bearing simultaneously both the helper cell marker (L3T4) and the suppressor cell marker (Lyt 2) may represent a dead-end pathway.[25] Only the blast cells found in the outer cortex and negative for both these markers may be the immature precursors of functional T cells.[26] A pivotal intercellular event must take place between these cells and stromal, possibly epithelial cells in the outer cortex. Thymic nurse cells[27] derived from cortical epithelial cells represent such an event most dramatically: they engulf 20 to 40 viable small lymphocytes, some in mitosis; upon isolation the lymphocytes are completely sequestered within the caveolae of the nurse cells and caveolar membranes display groupings of invaginations of endocytic or exocytic character.[27] In vivo, the nurse cells are found in the subcapsular cortex both in mouse and man.[16,27,28] Most intranurse-cell thymocytes are nonfunctional and have a high cloning efficiency; a few may be of the helper-cell lineage.[29]

Since major histocompatibility complex (MHC) antigens are believed to play the key role in thymic interactions between lymphoid cells (equipped with the ''somatic mutagen'' terminal deoxynucleotidyl transferase) and stromal epithelial and/or mesenchymal elements, it is gratifying that both class I and class II antigens have been found on subcapsular cortical cells including nurse cells, on deep cortical and medullary epithelial cells both in mouse and man.[30-32] All endocrine cells seem to be positive for these markers.[11] In the mouse, monoclonal antibodies seem to produce evidence for antigenic differences between cortical and medullary epithelial cells.[33]

However, thymus seems to dictate the self-recognition of class II antigens only, self-recognition of class I antigen is not restricted to the normal thymic processing[34-36] and consequently may not be so deeply affected in the athymic model. Depletion of nonepithelial cells from normal thymus by deoxyguanoside (which affects mesenchymal interdigitating cells and macrophages) leads to the impairment of self-tolerance in T cells whereas the H 2 restriction of T cells trafficking through the thymus is preserved.[37] It was suggested that receptor-bearing thymocytes make an initial contact with H 2 determinants on epithelial cells in the thymic cortex and ''learn'' the self-restricted specificity, migrate further to the cortico-medullary border and contact the interdigitating cells here; this contact deletes T cells with high affinity for self H 2 determinants.[37]

Thymic epithelial cells exhibit thick bundles of tonofibrils; they seem to be more abundant in medullary epithelial cells[13] and are reminiscent of the cytoskeleton of squamous epithelia transmitting mechanical tension from the intercellular junctions (desmosomes) to the cell cytoplasm. However, isolated thymic medullary and cortical epithelial cells develop my-ofibrils and the resulting ''myoid cells'' represent a 100-year-old enigma of thymic cytology. In mammals, the myoid cells appear in greater numbers in fetal and perinatal stages.[38] Fully developed myoid cells exhibit a fiber pattern typical for striated muscle,[38] however, only smooth myofibrils were described in "myoepithelial cells" in thymuses of children up to 1 year of age.[39] The differentation of myoid cells from precursor cells was observed in tissue cultures of mouse thymuses and expression of acetylcholine receptors noted after fusion of myotubes, but not in mature myotubes.[40] It is intriguing that myoepithelial cells have been described in the thymic subcortical area where they form a continuous layer[39] and may be mixed with the endocrine epithelial cells. Other myoepithelial cells in human infant thymuses were seen in the medulla as unicellular Hassall's corpuscles and in multilayered Hassall's corpuscles. One of the possible explanations for the conservation of thymic myoid and/or myoepithelial cells through mammalian phylogeny may be related to extreme cellular condensations in the thymic cortex; cellular movements from the outer cortex to the deeper cortex and within the medulla must be ensured.

In general, it seems that ectodermal epithelial cells provide the inductive influence on endodermal epithelial material during organogenesis and are the source of the specific endocrine elements in the functioning thymus. The essential step of the thymic interaction between epithelial cells and lymphoid cells occurs in the subcapsular cortical area where the epithelial reticulum expresses both classes of MHC antigens and other surface markers, such as neuronal gangliosides; also keratinocyte surface markers and those of myoid cells may be confronted by the lymphoid cells on their passage into the deeper portions of the thymus.

III. THYMIC CYSTS AND BROWN FAT

Description of intrathymic cyst formation also has a 100-year-old history; the interpretation of this phenomenon ranged from degenerative sequestration within the lymphatic tissue or an accessory endocrine gland to a normal component of the organ at all developmental stages, in all vertebrate species studied.[41] Arnesen described the mouse thymic cyst formation with "alveoli and tubuli" as secretory units endowed with three types of epithelium: ciliated, mucous, and pseudostratified.[42]

A clear and systematic analysis of Groscurth et al.[43] on the cyst system in the hybrid *nu/*+ mouse provides an image which may be valid also for homozygous (+/+) mice of different inbred strains[44] as well. The first type occurs at different places in the medulla and cortex as cystic formations, always isolated and lined by cubic epithelia. These "intrathymic cysts"[43] contain cellular debris of epithelial and lymphoid cells (Figure 1).

The second type has a definite anatomic location at the dorso-medial aspect of both thymic lobes.[43] In the neonatal mouse it looks like a single flat epithelial duct lined by flattened endothelia in the ventro-lateral wall, and by high columnar epithelia at the dorsal wall, which is in direct contact with the connective tissue of the thymic capsule. During the first 2 postnatal weeks, the duct grows along the connective tissue septum of the thymic lobuli, its lumen widens and branching lateral ductuli are formed. The epithelial lining neighboring connective tissue differentiates, in part, into mucous and ciliated cells. From the 3rd week on, epithelial acini are formed in the close vicinity of the duct. Mucous and serous cells can be discerned in the acini. Fat cells appear in the connective tissue adjacent to the duct lining. In animals aged 9 and 12 weeks the whole duct and acinar system becomes embedded in a narrow rim of adipose tissue.

It is feasible to accept the derivation of this duct system from the material of the ectodermal vesicula cervicalis and dorsal diverticle of the third branchial pouch[43] which is chiefly endodermal and forms the caput thymi. The body of the thymus develops from the ventral diverticle. The development of the cranial part of the thymus anlage, the cervical vesicle and caput thymi, may result after the 15th embryonic day exclusively in the formation of the purely epithelial duct and acinar formation.[43] Consequently, this formation represents a normal component of the mouse thymus.

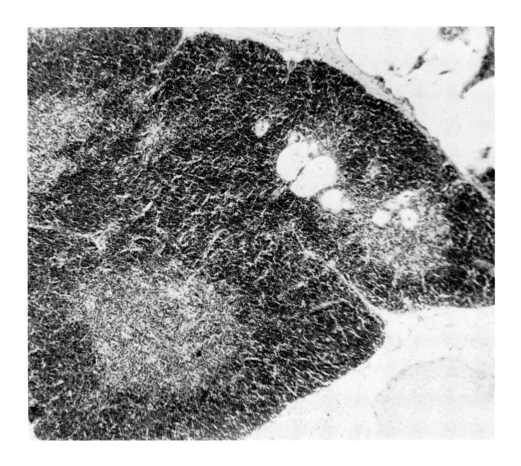

FIGURE 1.   Intrathymic cysts of a CBA/J male (+ / +), aged 2 months. (Hem.-eos.; magnification × 150.)

We have found this formation in most carefully sectioned mouse thymuses, in all *nu/ +*
and in 25 out of 29 + / + mice of the BALB/c, C3H, C57Bl/10 ScSn, C57Bl/10.LP or
CBA/J background.[44] In all animals under 2 months of age the duct and acinar systems were
well isolated in the subcapsular area of the cranial dorsomedial aspect of both thymic lobes
and lined by cylindrical or cuboid epithelia largely of a serous character. In the main duct,
the epithelia display long cilia and signs of both secretory or resorptive activity. In three
CBA/J mice the duct and acinar system was found embedded in adipose tissue and apposed
to the thymic capsule from the outside. In this case, the appearance was almost identical to
the nude mouse "polycystic organ": it was only smaller and lense-shaped in the transversal
section, ovoid in the frontal or sagittal sections; the acinar component was less developed[44]
(Figure 2).

In mice more then 2 months old the lateral ducts enlarged into cysts lined by cuboid or
squamous epithelia; only the epithelial lining adjacent to the adipose tissue and the thymic
capsule had cylindrical ciliated epithelia which suggests their continued activity.[44] In mice
more than 4 months old the duct system came into the vicinity of large intrathymic cysts
which are known to increase in numbers and enlarge during all kinds of thymic involution.[41]

In the rat, the ultrastructural appearance of intrathymic cyst is identical with the mouse
cysts and again very close to the nude mouse dysgenetic thymus structures.[45] The cystic
formations are under clear influence of estrogens[45,46] and thyroxine.[45] They display sexual
diformism in the rat[45] which has not been so far observed or looked for in mice and in nude
mice.

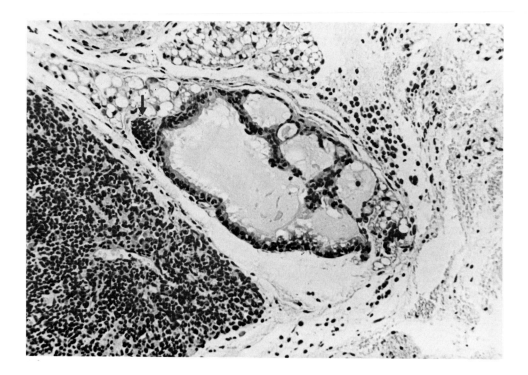

FIGURE 2.   Duct and cyst formation located dorsolaterally to the right thymic lobe of a CBA/J male (+/+), aged 2 months. The cysts are lined by high ciliated epithelia and flat cells; they contain a secretory product of the cylindrical cells. A condensed epithelial acinus is marked by arrow. (Hem.-eos.; magnification × 230) (Compare with Figure 13).

During these processes the intrathymic adipose tissue spreads from perivascular spaces where single undifferentiated mesenchymal cells are believed to turn into fat cells.[41] It is important to note a tendency towards brown (multilocular) fat-cell development in the rodents.[41,47] During hibernation the whole organ may be embedded into a brown fat body. In mice and rats undergoing stress, perivascular brown fat cells and, eventually, tissue develops, possibly in relation to the lowering of body temperature during stress and the need for increased nonshivering thermogenesis[47] (Chapter 10, Section II).

In conclusion, it is clear that the mouse thymus also has a purely epithelial component derived from the vesicula cervicalis and caput thymi anlage, endowed with a secretory activity more or less independent of the functioning thymic epithelial stroma. Intrathymic and perithymic adipose tissue, including brown fat tissue, develops reciprocally with the dense thymic lymphatic tissue.

IV. THE MESENCHYMAL COMPONENT

If the derivation of the epithelial thymic stroma was a past arena of conflicting theories, the mesenchymal-mesodermal component of the thymus has been a battlefield since 1879, when Kolliker formulated the first transformation theory. It was this field which prompted Beard to write in *Zoologische Jahrbücher* in Jena in 1902: '' . . . has it yet fallen to the lot of any writer upon the thymus to write the truth and be believed . . . ''.

The problem is threefold: the origin of thymic lymphocytes, the origin, or existence, of the mesenchymal (not necessarily mesodermal) thymic reticulum, and the origin of the thymic connective and, at least in some species, hematopoietic tissue of mesodermal derivation.

Even today, morphological evidence cannot disprove the possibility predicted by the transformation theory, namely, that thymic epithelial cells can differentiate in thymic lymph-oid cells. It is hard to dismiss the occurrence of desmosomes, i.e., sites of very strong attachment developing, usually, between epithelial cells of one kind, which have been found electron microscopically between mouse thymic epithelial cells and lymphoblasts and be-tween lymphoblasts, prior to vascularization of the thymus anlage.[48] Without evidence provided by surface markers one must assume that there may be some stroma-derived cell in the mouse and chick thymus which has the ultrastructure of an immature lymphoid cell and may or may not be the precursor of lymphocytes as defined by immunological functions and markers. Such a possibility complicates, of course, the problem of the nude mouse thymic dysgenesis.

The leading theory stemming from the morphological grand masters, Hammar[49] and Maximow,[50] maintains that the epithelial anlage is infiltrated by migrating lymphoid cells derived from primitive mesenchymal cells of the connective tissue adjacent to the epithelial anlage. This substitution theory gained decisive support from relatively recent experiments. Moore and Owen,[51] noting a ''remarkable similarity'' between ontogeny of the avian (chick) and mammalian (mouse) thymus, described the presence of wandering basophilic cells, presumably prelymphoid cells, in the epithlial anlage of the mouse thymus at gestational day 11 and of the chicken thymus at day 7. In both cases the cells were found before the vascularization of the anlage. Moore and Owen could show, in parabiosed chick embryos and by grafting of the thymic rudiment on the chorionallantoic membrane, using chromosomal markers for donor and host cells, that the basophilic cells colonizing the epithelial thymic anlage are blood borne. The blood-borne basophil prelymphoid cells were observed, when labeled, in the mesenchyme surrounding the anlage; from the mesenchyme they must have crossed the basement membrane of the anlage and settled among the epithelial cells.[52] One to two days after entry they seemed to turn into smaller lymphoid cells. Assuming that all ''basophilic cells'' are lymphoid precursors and that there are about 200 of these cells in the 12-day-old mouse fetal thymus and about 100 in the surrounding mesenchyme, ready to cross into the anlage, then each of these cells must have the capacity to produce 10^4 small lymphocytes (after 13 to 14 divisions) since the anlage would produce in organ culture or on the chorioallantoic membrane about 2×10^5 to 10^6 lymphocytes.[52]

The influx of what became ''the lymphoid stem cell'' into the epithelial anlage was accepted as the unique source of thymic lymphocytes: the lymphoid blast cell was shown to have a restricted period of proliferation in tissue culture, but 2-week-old cultures of mouse 12th day fetal thymuses would still produce upon implantation into thymectomized syngeneic mice up to 50 mg of typical thymic tissue in 6 to 10 weeks.[53] The influx of lymphoid stem cells continues apparently throughout life, as it has been shown in parabiosed mice[54] or in the irradiated mouse model.[55] The prethymic cells entering the ''empty'' thymic stroma on embryonal day 11 express Thy 1 and begin their rapid proliferation almost immediately.[55,56] The lymphoid stem cells from a 14-day-old mouse fetal thymus can be induced to express the Thy 1 marker also in vitro[57] and within days they display Lyt markers of mature T-cell subsets.[56] Also, interleukin 2 receptors develop on the thymus-seeded lymphoid cells before the 15th embryonic day.[58] Positive cells appear in the areas of lymphoid stem cell first localization, the subcapsular area and corticomedullary junction and the proliferation and differentiation is obviously triggered also by the IL 2 mechanism[58] which is in the adult thymus replaced to a high degree by another mitogenic factor.[59]

The lymphoid stem cell influx could be observed also in the experimental model of avian interspecific chimeras.[60] Here, the influx seemed to be induced by some attractant (''thy-motaxin'') from the epithelial anlage in a short period during fetal life (6.5 to 8 days for the chick) and in a second wave, replacing the progeny of the first one, around hatching. Here, too, it was concluded that the lymphocyte precursor comes from a distant hemopoietic site, not from the adjacent mesenchyme which may have another important role, namely the preparation of the thymic microenvironment for the lymphoid differentiation. This latter type of mesenchymal effect, not only the availability of lymphoid stem cells[61] and other bone marrow-derived mesenchymal precursor cells, may be missing in the nude mouse thymus.

The normal development of the thymic stroma is strictly dependent on the interaction of the epithelial cells with mesenchymal material. The invasion of the epithelial anlage by mesenchymal cells initiates proliferation and maturation of the ectodermal and endodermal epithelium as the basis of thymic histogenesis. In the classical experiments of Auerbach[62] using isolated epithelium from mouse 12-day embryos combined with mesenchyme from different sites, it was established that the epithelial morphogenesis requires undifferentiated mesenchyme, but different mesenchymal material induced a characteristic morphogenetic pattern of the epithelium. In accordance with Le Douarin's results on avian thymus[60,63] the cephalic mesenchyme was superior to mesenchyme from other sources. It was known from amphibian embryos that cephalic neural crest gives rise to mesenchymal cells which migrate ventrally into the branchial arches. Interspecific grafts of the neural tube with the neural crest between avian embryos provided evidence that in higher vertebrates as well the mesenchyme in the branchial arches is derived entirely, except for the muscle plates, from the cephalic neural crest.[60,64]

The same was established directly by an elegant experiment on the chicken thymus:[64] limited areas of the cephalic neural crest of chick embryos after 30 hr of incubation, before any migration of originally epithelial, later mesenchymal cells into the pharyngeal area could occur, were removed; marked reduction of thymic size with delayed development, in some embryos agenesis of thymus resulted, although there was no interference with the ecto- and endodermal pharyngeal pouch and cleft material. Consequently, a direct interaction of ectomesenchymal derivatives of the neural crest with pharyngeal epithelial mass may be the essential step of thymus development.

The interaction may be mediated at first by some humoral factors traversing the basement membrane of the epithelial anlage or, in experimental conditions, a thin millipore filter.[65] Later, the mesenchymal material penetrates the epithelial cords[60] and the mesenchymal cells surround the vessels in the anlage. As shown by monoclonal antibodies identifying the mesenchymal cells in the human thymus, these cells invaginate into the epithelial anlage at about the 7th gestational week and they never acquire the MHC class II (Ia-like) antigens and are weakly positive for MHC class I antigens.[11] These antigens are expressed mainly by the epithelial reticulum which bears the surface markers of endocrine epithelial thymic cells.

The mesenchymal invasion occurs in the mouse around fetal day 12 and before day 15 in the rat. Here again the mesenchymal cells do not bear the MHC-class II antigens (Ia) which are expressed first on epithelial cells (day 14 in the mouse,[66] day 16 in the rat[67]) and/or on blood-borne (mesodermal) macrophage and interdigitating cell precursors.[68] Interdigitating cell precursors were, in addition, found entering the epithelial anlage directly from the connective tissue strands.[31,69,70] The entrance of Ia$^+$ macrophages and interdigitating cell precursors or the expression of Ia surface marker may be dependent on the cells bearing the first traces of Thy 1 antigens;[67] these cells may or may not be lymphoid.

The first interconnected mesh of Ia$^+$ stromal cells is epithelial (gestational day 17 in the rat) and becomes complemented in the medulla by the mesenchymal (possibly mesodermal) Ia$^+$ network of interdigitating cells (day 19 in the rat).[67] The interdigitating cells of mesenchymal-mesodermal derivation increase in numbers after birth; in rat, a sharp increase was noted after the 1st postnatal month and the increase of interdigitating cells was concomitant to a decrease of numbers of medullary epithelial cells.[71] The expanding interdigitating cell reticulum may be connected with the presence and reentry of specifically sensitized effector T lymphocytes into the thymus[72] and of homing of splenic immature T cells into the thymus.[72a]

Strong evidence for the importance of the Ia-positive reticulum of possible mesenchymal derivation has been obtained by Kruisbeek et al. who claim that neonatal treatment of normal mice with anti-Ia monoclonal antibody results in a selective depletion of helper (L3T4[+]) lymphocytes in the peripheral lymphatic tissues and in a selective depletion of Ia[+] antigen-presenting cells within the thymus of adults.[73]

In the adult thymus, "nonepithelial phagocytic cells" can be readily obtained from thymic fragments; in secondary cultures these cells assume a dendritic morphology, display vacuoles, sometimes reminiscent of the specific vacuoles of the cortical epithelial cells, without a demonstrable "thymus factor" content, and some of them express Ia antigens.[74] They produce interleukin 1[74] and may be identical to the "macrophages" modulating in vitro the T-cell differentiation.[75]

There is strong evidence that the bone marrow-derived Ia[+] interdigitating cells of the thymic medulla have an important position in the generation of self-recognition repertoire.[76,77] The capacity to recognize self-MHC antigens is present already at the prethymocyte level.[78,79] Nude mice and rats may also be lacking in their dysgenetic thymus this essential population of interdigitating mesenchymal cells, but do have, on the other hand, precursors of these cells since they can repopulate implanted epithelial thymic fragments.[36,80,81]

The assumptions of the immunological functions of the cortical epithelial cells and of the mesenchymal cells may not be mutually exclusive. Their roles may be interconnected. As evidenced on fetal thymic explants, entry of macrophage precursors dramatically increases the Ia expression on presumed epithelial cells;[81a] On the other hand, cloned cells with the phenotype of subcapsular epithelial cells (human) were found to express not only T-cell binding sites, but also macrophage colony stimulating factor[82a] which may have a short- and long-range effect. These epithelial cells also synergize with macrophages in the production of interleukin 1.[82a] The production of the macrophage colony stimulating factor appears to be an important cue for the elucidation of the degree of dysgenesis of the thymus in the nude mouse. (Section V).

The thymus microenvironment does not exclude myeloid, and to some extent, erythroid hematopoiesis which has been thoroughly documented by past morphologists in almost all vertebrate species and also by advanced histochemical techniques in human thymuses.[82,83] Nonlymphoid hematopoiesis in the thymus is not restricted to early fetal life and can be followed well into the stage of thymic involution.[83] Resulting neutrophils, eosinophils, and basophils may have some local function. Extensive cyclical erythropoiesis found in the thymuses of birds and rodents[84,85] may contribute to the circulating erythrocyte pool. The localization of hematopoietic foci in the thymus does not suggest direct hematogenic derivation; myelopoiesis occurs in human thymuses in the connective tissue septa, but interestingly, also in the subcapsular cortex and at the cortico-medullary border.[82] The unbroken layer of precursor cells in the subcapsular area[82] — the crucial site of triggering the lymphoid cell differentiation — shows the extremely complicated and as yet unexplained cellular relations in the ectodermal-mesenchymal and mesodermal-mesenchymal domain; the concept of the precommitted lymphoid stem cell may not be altogether correct; other precursor cells are attracted into the thymus anlage.

On the whole, there are obviously three essential mesenchyme-dependent steps in thymus evolution: (1) humoral induction of the epithelial anlage, (2) direct penetration of mesenchymal cells into the anlage and influx of mesenchymal precursor cells from the bone marrow providing an interdigitating mesh with a high expression of class II MHC antigens and situated mainly in the medulla, and (3) the passage and directed differentiation of lymphoid stem cells. These three steps are strictly coordinalted in time and any deviation may cause some of the numerous thymic dysgenetic events.

V. THE ESSENTIAL DEFECT IN THE DYSGENETIC THYMUS

The history of the mouse dysgenetic thymus is comparatively short, but we managed to produce a good number of contradictions in the explanation of what is really missing. Six years after the mutation nude was first seen, it was found that the thymus is absent,[86] more exactly vestigial,[87] or replaced by epithelial acini and an epithelium-lined system of cysts and ducts.[1,88-91] This epithelial organ was thought to be something different from thymus, a derivate of ultimobranchial bodies or of parathyroids;[88] initially it was not even found in all nude mice.[1]

Since 1974, systematic studies of the thymic area of the nude mouse have led to a general agreement that this formation which we called "polycystic organ"[44] occurs in all nude mice of all ages and that it represents the final stage of a deviant development of the epithelial thymic anlage after the 11th day of gestation.[89-92]

The crucial steps of that deviant development were elucidated by detailed embryological analyses of Groscurth and Kistler[92] and Cordier and Haumont.[10] On the 9th day of gestation, the third pharyngeal pouch is shaped like a blind fistula with the distal end stretching to the third ectodermal cleft: the endodermal and ectodermal epithelia are placed back to back. A half-day later the ectoderm thickens and protrudes into the endodermal material, both layers blending together.[10] By the 10th day the endoderm forms a dorsal and ventral diverticle, the latter surrounded by mesenchyme, the former fusing with the cleft ectoderm.[92] The ectoderm of the dorsal part of the fourth branchial arch protrudes into the mesenchyme and forms an oval pouch, the cervical vesicle, by 10 1/2 days. Initially, the cervical vesicle has no "extensive contact" with the dorsal diverticle. However, on the 11th day, the cervical vesicle rotates and attaches itself to the endoderm.[10,92] At the same time, the proliferating ectoderm of the third cleft covers in euthymic mice the distal edge and a small part of the cranial and caudal walls of the third pouch.[10] By 11 1/2 days, after a double rotation of the entire complex which brings the main axis into the frontal plane, the ectodermal covering of the ventral and caudal part of the endodermal pouch thickens considerably and the complex detaches itself from the pharyngeal endoderm and external (peripheral) ectoderm.[91] At this stage, the well-developed endodermal pouch of the nude embryo is only partly covered by the ectoderm which did not proliferate. This is the first major difference beginning the divergence of normal and dysgenetic development.[10] The cervical vesicle, however, is also well formed in the nude embryo (Figure 3).

By the 12th day the ventral diverticle grows caudally and forms the corpus thymi in euthymic embryos;[10,92] the ventral and external surfaces, down to the caudal pole, are covered by ectoderm, in some embryos the vesicula cervicalis fuses with the ectoderm of the caput thymi which is formed from the dorsal diverticle; in some normal embryos and in all nude embryos vesicula cervicalis remains an isolated ectodermal nodule.[10] In nude embryos the endoderm is covered by ectoderm only in the midportion, while the caudal region stays exclusively endodermal.[10]

By 12 1/2 days the whole thymus of euthymic embryos is covered by ectoderm, the central cavity of the original pouch disappears and the epithelial tissue is invaded by vessels with accompanying mesenchymal cells and by isolated lymphoid cells; in the nude embryo the ectodermal material is limited to the cranial portion and to the persisting vesicula cervicalis and there is no mesenchymal invasion.[10,92]

On the 13th day the inner part of the corpus thymi has a looser reticular arrangement of the epithelial cells: in the nude embryo the corpus is visibly narrower and displays central necroses; the vesicula cervicalis is comparatively larger. Capillaries from the adjacent mesenchyma, though in abundance, have no tendency to enter the anlage.[92] Epithelial cells of the anlage are interconnected by desmosomes[93] which indicate their common origin.

The vascularization and reticulization of the central part of the normal thymus proceeds

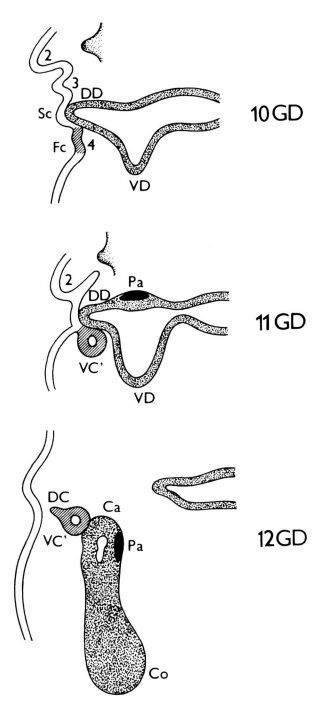

FIGURE 3. Schematic outline of normal thymic ontogenesis at
10th, 11th, and 12th gestation day. 2-4 — branchial arches, III —
third pharyngeal pouch, Sc — sinus cervicalis, Fc — fundus cervicalis, DD — dorsal diverticle, VC — vesicula cervicalis, Pa —
parathyroid anlage, DC — ductus cervicalis, Ca, Co — caput and
corpus thymi. (From Groscurth, P. and Kistler, G., *Beitr. Pathol.*,
156, 359, 1975. With permission.)

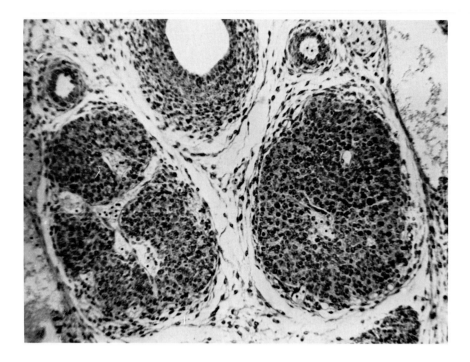

FIGURE 4.   Thymus of a normal BALB/c fetus, (+ / +), gestation day 15, transversal section. (Hem.-eos.; magnification × 300.)

on day 14; a tight epithelial nodule is present only in the caput. The nodule has a central lumen and connects with the vesicula cervicalis. The nude thymus consist of two to three compact epithelial layers and the inner layer is subdivided by lumina resulting from necrotic foci. Vesicula cervicalis is separated from the thymus epithelial layers by a basal membrane.[92]

The difference in the growth of the normal and dysgenetic thymus is striking in this period. In the normal embryo the thymic volume increases ten times between days 12 and 14; in the nude embryo the volume increases only twice and does not grow further until day 16.[10]

On the 15th day the epithelial reticulum in the normal thymus is filled with lymphoid cells (from blasts to small lymphocytes) and mesenchymal septa divide the organ into primordial lobules (Figure 4). Vesicula cervicalis now seems to be fused with the caput thymi epithelia in all embryos. Caput thymi forms a duct with a single layer of epithelial lining.[92] In the nu/nu embryo the whole dysgenetic thymus (without comparable vascular-izaton and mesenchymal invasion) is represented by a cranio-caudal duct which is situated in the area of the caput and upper portion of the corpus of the normal thymus. This duct has a single or multiple epithelial lining and forms multiple compact or duct-like epithelial branches at its cranial pole.[92]

It is important to note that, from this stage on, the dysgenetic thymus is similar to an enlarging duct system in the cranial dorsomedial part of the normal thymus. The cells in both organs contain cysts filled with a sulfated polysachharide product which also accu-mulates in the duct lumina and cystic expansions.[44,93,94]

In electron microscopical studies of the dysgenetic development of the nude mouse thymus it was noted that undifferentiated epithelial cells with no traces of secretory activity are found on the 12th and 13th gestational day.[95] The cells are ovoid and connected by inter-digitations and only occasional desmosomes; they are separated by basal lamina from the mesenchyme in the vicinity of the anlage. No vessels and no mesenchymal cells enter the epithelial mass which already has a central lumen with a few cell debris.[95] Some of these

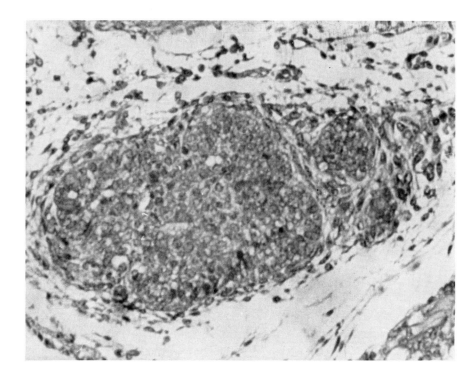

FIGURE 5. Dysgenetic thymus of a B 10.LP *nu/nu* fetus, gestation day 16, transversal section. A few dark lymphoid cells are present. (Hem.-eos.; magnification × 300.)

primitive epithelial cells contain abundant glycogen granules and many have distended rough endoplasmic reticulum cisternae.[96] In the same period the normal thymic anlage contains a lighter and darker undifferentiated epithelial cell type, the latter only in the central part, the former forming a dense layer under the demarcating basal lamina.[95] ''Lymphoblasts'' are found in the surrounding mesenchyme around both nude and normal mouse thymic anlage on day 12, but inside the thymus anlage only in normal thymuses. These lymphoblasts disappear from the mesenchyme of the nude mouse thymic area by day 13.[95] However, blasts, presumably lymphoid elements, were described in the dysgenetic thymus on gestational days 15 to 189; they did not proliferate and gradually disappeared[96] (Figures 5 to 7).

The undifferentiated epithelial cells of the dysgenetic thymus anlage do not proceed into the tonofilament-rich stellate epithelial cells found in normal thymus anlage, but undergo little change until gestational day 18.[96] The thymus-specific cortical epithelial cells containing vacuoles with flocculated material, medullary cystic epithelial cells, and myoid cells never appear,[44,89,91,93,95,96] or, to be more exact, cells phenotypically and morphologically identical with these types have not been found.

However, a detailed study of secretory granules of thymic epithelial cells[97] established that in 14-day-old nude mouse embryos (from homozygous matings) single membrane-bound secretory vesicles (230 nm in diameter) with a dense core and clear peripheral halo are present together with prosecretion vesicles of the Golgi area in the peripheral epithelia of the anlage. These secretory cells are identical to cells found in the normal thymus anlage of BALB/c mice (as well as of 35-day-old sheep fetuses) in the peripheral, condensed epithelial mass. Another type of secretory cells equipped with larger (250 nm) secretory vesicles with a conspicuous, wide peripheral halo was found in the central area of the normal thymus anlage only, not in the dysgenetic thymus. This type may be a predecessor of some medullary epithelial cells in the postnatal normal thymus. Interestingly, the secretory cells

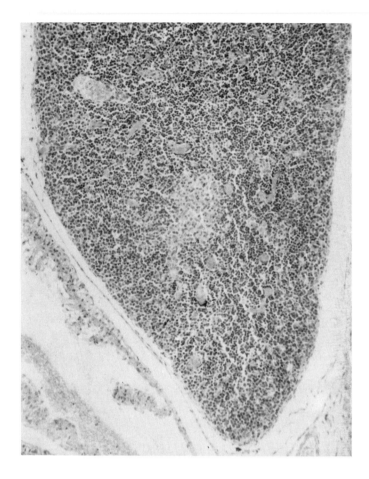

FIGURE 6.   Thymus of a normal BALB/c fetus (+ / +), gestation day 18 to 19,
sagittal section. Demarcation of cortex and medulla. (Hem.-eos.; magnification
× 100.)

present in the nude thymus anlage had ten times more secretion and prosecretion granules
and in 13-day-old embryos were more abundant than the respective cells in normal embryonic
thymuses.[97] This suggests that the secretory activity of these cells is dependent on the presence
of the lymphoid cells which use up the content of the secretory granules; alternatively, the
epithelial cells may compensate for the absence of the lymphoid target cells by increasing
their activity. In any case, it must be recognized that one type of secretory granules may
be identical both in the normal and dysgenetic thymus anlage.

On gestational days 17 to 19, normal thymus becomes dominated by lymphocytes with
islands of epithelial cells present in the deeper cortex and emerging medullary region (Figure
6). The dysgenetic thymus is at this stage considerably smaller, divided into single duct
systems displaying a few empty lumina and acinar epithelial components. Pycnotic lymphoid
cells can be found in some cases among the epithelia (Figure 7).

The postnatal development of the nude mouse dysgenetic thymus is due to the proliferation
of the epithelial cells lining the ducts and forming small acini in the surrounding loose
connective tissue.[43,44] The acinar cells which have, in part, the appearance of mucous cells
are situated at the dead ends of the branching central duct.[43] They discharge their product(s)
into the lumen. The branching ducts expand and form cyst-like structures. The onset of the
process is discernible in about 2-week-old animals. By this time the duct-lining cells dif-

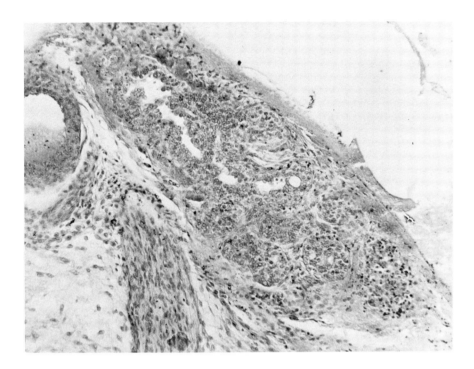

FIGURE 7.   Dysgenetic thymus of a B10.LP nu/nu fetus, gestation day 19, transversal section. Epithelial acini and ducts with small lamina. (Hem.-eos.; magnification × 140.)

ferentiate into mucous and ciliated types. At 1 month of age the growth of the paired polycystic organ still proceeds and the maximala dimensions are found after the 3rd month;[44] thereafter, the increase of size occurs only in some individuals and is due chiefly to the dilatation of cysts filled by the glycoprotein product. During growth, the acini of mucous cells become associated and incorporated into the walls of the enlarging duct and cyst systems, however, a few mucous cell acini enlarge and persist.

The largest cysts eventually lose their epithelial lining and are demarcated by the denuded basal lamina and connective tissue.

Ultrastructurally, there is an obvious differentiation of the epithelial cells turning into the cyst lining system: they form cylindrical (mostly at the cranial pole, in small cysts), cuboid, or pseudostratified epithelial lining connected by fine interdigitations and desmosomes at their apical surface. They display microvilli; in some cysts and ducts individual cells have well-developed cilia;[91,98] such ciliated epithelia are well known from normal thymuses and other derivates of the pharyngeal endoderm.[98]

Ciliated cells are undeniably a final stage of the epithelial cells of the polycystic organ.

The majority of cyst-lining cells is, in our experience, of a less differentiated type, frequently with a dark cytoplasmic matrix, few smooth endoplasmic reticulum profiles, and a very characteristic accumulation of oval or elongated mitochondria[99] both in the basal and the apical portion of the cell. Their interdigitations at the basal pole are extremely complex and sometimes loose; the basal lamina is irregular in most cysts lined by these undifferentiated epithelia (Figure 8). Undifferentiated epithelial cells with labyrinthine interdigitation persist in most acinar components (Figure 9).

A third type of epithelial cells are flattened cells with long processes extending on the basal lamina and with a conspicuous dark cytoplasmic matrix which resembles the thymic "dark epithelial cells".[100] These dark epithelial cells of the polycystic organ are sometimes

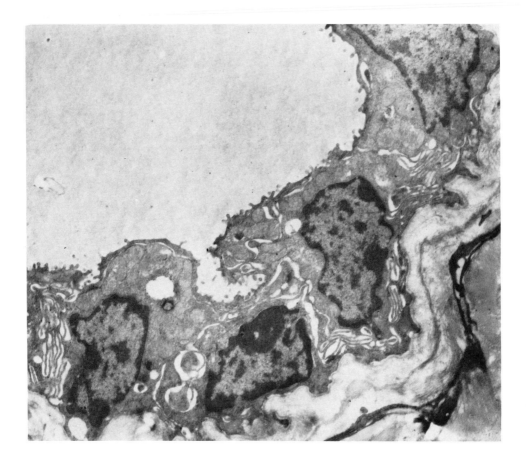

FIGURE 8.   Cyst lining epithelia in the dysgenetic thymus of a female BALB/c *nu/nu* mouse, aged 2 months, treated with six doses of cyclosporin A which induced temporary hair formation (Chapter 9, Section I). The lining epithelia show abundant interdigitations, also with slender cellular processes on the basal lamina. There is a marked widening of connective tissue space under the epithelial lining and dark (keratinized) cell processes are embedded in the collagen bundles. (Transmission electron microscope; magnification × 7500.)

found embedding single lymphoid cells (Figure 10). The lymphoid cells appear in optical microscopy as "distributed between the mesenchymal and epithelial cells" of the polycystic organ;[101] Groscurth's group reports the lymphoid cells being positioned outside the basal lamina (Figure 11) and occasionaly "inside", i.e., between the basal lamina and the epithelial cells.[99] To say the least, the cystic structures are not alymphocytic; the dark epithelial cells associated with the lymphoid elements are very close to the respective cells in the normal thymus epithelial reticulum.[100]

Four types of "glandular cells" were described in the polycystic organ by Cordier;[91] they could be distinquished by the size and shape of secretory granules ranging from 100 to 500 nm. Some of these endocrine cells may be identical to the cells equipped with the dense core-clear peripheral halo secretory vesicles found in embryos by Jordan.[97] The occurrence of the glandular cells seems to vary from cyst to cyst. In general, they are less numerous than the undifferentiated cells and some of them are argyrophilic[99] as are, in our experience, occasional epithelia in the medulla of a normal thymus.

In general, the proportion of cells containing the dark, membrane-bound secretion granules under 300 nm is higher in the polycystic organ than in the normal thymus epithelial component. This finding may be interpreted as a result of the lack of thymic lymphocyte regulatory

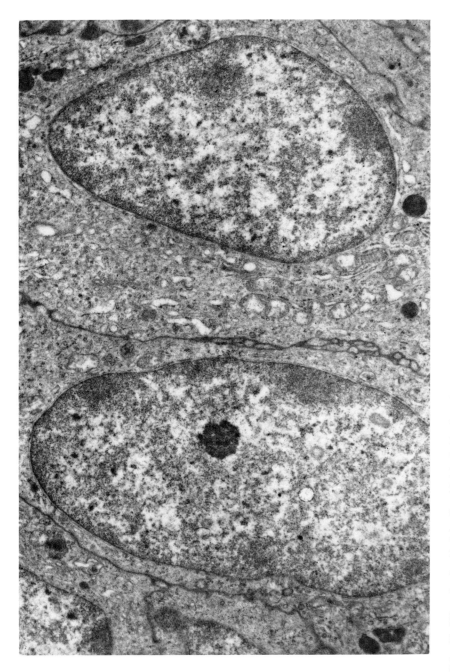

FIGURE 9. Undifferentiated epithelial cells with labyrinthine interdigitations and cystic formations reminiscent of medullary epithelial cells of a normal thymus. Dysgenetic thymus of a BALB/c *nu/nu* male aged 2 months. (Transmission electron microscope; magnification $\times$ 21,000.)

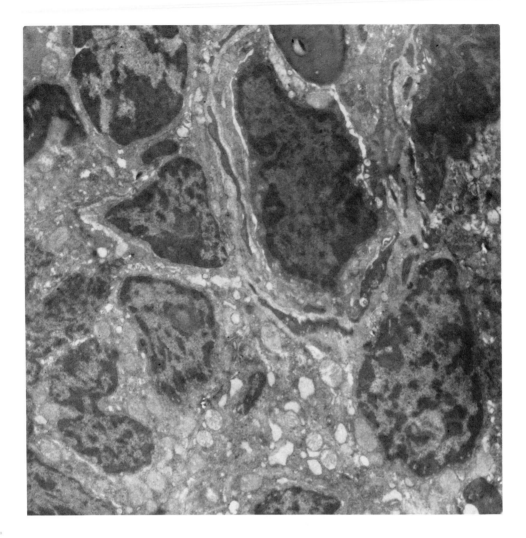

FIGURE 10.   Lymphoid cells surrounded by processes of dark epithelial cells and in the vicinity of undifferentiated epithelial cell clusters in the lining of a small duct of the nude mouse dysgenetic thymus. BALB/c *nu/nu* male, aged 2 months. (Transmission electron microscope; magnification × 13,500.)

influence. Thymus epitheliala cells alone produce in culture more of the specific thymic factors than when cultured with thymic lymphocytes. These may regulate the inductive action of epithelium-derived hormones by some sort of negative feedback.[102] Consequently, it is unlikely that the thymic epithelia in the polycystic organ would be ultrastructurally close to normal thymic epithelial cells, even if they had been identical in their ontogeny, in the epithelial anlage.

The last type of epthelial cell found in the cyst lining, usually among the cylindrical epithelia, is the mucous cell containing large, tightly packed clear vacuoles in the apical portion. These cells correspond to mucous medullary epithelial cells occasionally assembled into acini, in the normal mouse thymus,[103] and in the lining of intrathymic cysts in aging mice[42] (Figure 12).

These mucous cells are the dominant type in the acinar components. They are usually located at the caudal pole of the polycystic organ, on the blind ending of single ducts.[43] Mucous cells in the acini are in tightly packed five-to-ten cell groups, in different stages of

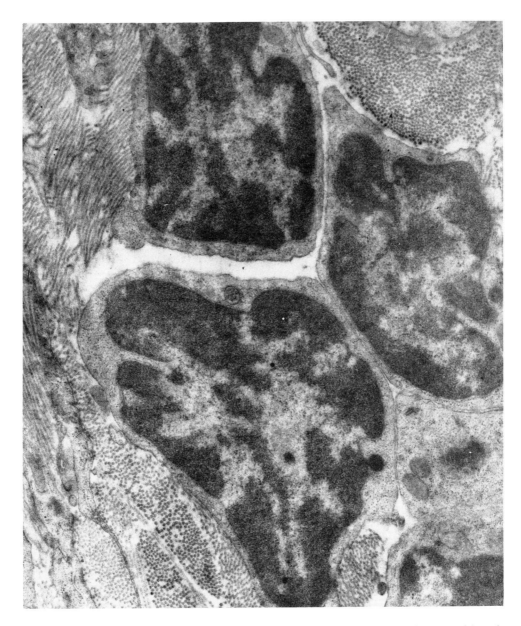

FIGURE 11. A layer of lymphocytes with typical thymic nuclear notching in a connective tissue area of the nude mouse dysgenetic thymus. Tightly clustered lymphocytes are in direct contact with collagen fibers. BALB/c *nu/nu* male, aged 3 months. (Transmission electron microscope; magnification × 20,000.)

the vacuole development, and surrounded by processes of undifferentiated epithelial cells. The base of the mucous cells is filled by a conspicuous array of rough endoplasmic reticulum and attached by desmosomes to the undifferentiated epithelia.[91] The capillary bed of the acini is richer than that of the cyst and duct system[44] and fenestrated capillaries are present,[94] as in the normal thymus. All epithelial cell clusters in the acini are surrounded by a basal membrane. Conspicuous bundles of microfilaments are found associated as a rule with the flat undifferentiated cells[91] and reminiscent of the tonofibrils of medullary epithelial cells in the normal thymus, and of epidermal cells.

Both the cystic portion and the acinar portion of the polycystic organ is surrounded by

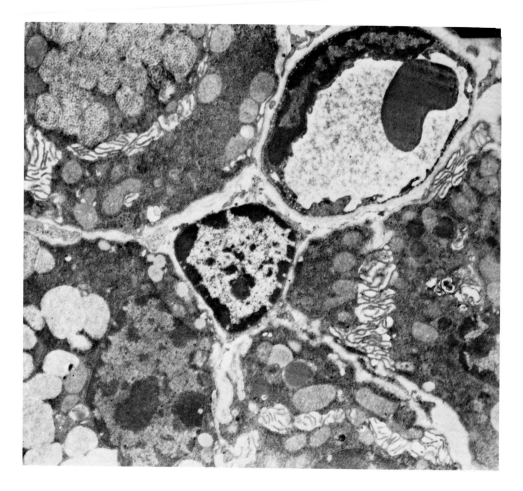

FIGURE 12.   Mucous cells in an epithelial acinus of the dysgenetic thymus of a BALB/c nude female treated with six doses of cyclosporin A. Abundant interdigitations of the mucous cells, variable densities of the product in different cells. A lymphocyte is present in the vicinity of a capillary. (Transmission electron microscope; magnification × 7500.)

very loose connective tissue with fibroblasts and histiocytes, mast cells, lymphoid cells, and many blood vessels.[44,91] No epithelial sheaths surrounding vessels and capillaries can be found; such sheaths form the incomplete blood-thymus barrier in the normal thymus. On the other hand, fenestrated capillaries characteristic of endocrine glands, present in normal thymuses, were also described in the cystic portion.[91]

The lymphatic drainage of the polycystic organ remains to be established; lymph vessels are present in a normal mammalian thymus and drain into the cervical duct (at least in the guinea pig[104]). Afferent lymphatics were never thought of in theories of thymic genesis and dysgenesis, but may still provide some keys.

Myelinated and unmyelinated nerves from the vagus and sympathetic innervation are described in normal thymuses, including murine,[105,106] and sympathetic branches and para-sympathetic nerves are present also in the polycystic organ.[107,108]

In a detailed study of the autonomic nervous system in the normal and dysgenetic thymus of ''B10'' and BALB/c mice, acetylcholinesterase activity was detected for the characterization of cholinergic fibers and glyoxylic acid fluorescence for the characterization of catecholaminergic innervation.[108] Normal thymus of presumably +/+ mice, 6 to 8 weeks old, was innervated by acetylcholinesterase-positive fibers of the vagus, recurrent laryngeal, and phrenic nerves. Intrinsic acetylcholine sterase-positive innervation was evident at the cortico-medullary border and in the subcapsular area. Catecholaminergic innervation was derived from the stellate and other small ganglia of the thoracic sympathetic chain and could be traced within the thymus "along the trabeculae", with perivascular plexuses localized again at the cortico-medullary border and in interlobular septa. Free catecholaminergic fibers could be found both in the cortex and the medulla; they were usually proximal to the cortical autofluorescent cells.[108]

The dysgenetic thymus of young adult nude mice (6 to 8 weeks of age) of both sexes had only scarce catecholaminergic or cholinergic fibers. The majority of the fibers was associated with the acinar component of the organ.[108] The authors suggest that the failure of the nude thymus to receive appropriate innervation by the vagus in early organogenesis might contribute to the dysgenetic process. It may also affect the migrations and interactions of lymphocytes in the epithelial anlage. In a normal thymus, there is a conspicuously dense innervation at the crucial sites of intrathymic events, in the area of large and immature lymphoid cells in the outer cortical zone and at the cortico-medullary border and along the vessels.[108]

This is a new aspect of the nude mouse thymic dysgenesis which may be easily accommodated with other anomalies in the nude mouse nervous systems (Chapter 10, Section III). Again, embryological studies are needed and innervation of the polycystic organ during its conversion to a partly lymphatic tissue (Section VI) must be studied before one could derive a picture of what came first and what is secondary in the dysgenetic process.

Interestingly, there was comparable innervation in mediastinal lymph nodes of the euthymic and nude mice in the Bulloch and Pomerantz observation.[108] Acetylcholinesterase-positive fibers were confined to the subcapsular (marginal) sinus and the vessels of the deeper cortex; catecholaminergic perivascular plexuses were found mainly in the hilar area, with a few free fibers in the subcapsular zone and in the deeper cortex.[108] However, mediastinal lymph nodes were more numerous in nude mice, "large clusters of small lymph nodes" were present in the mediastinal cavity of the nude mice in this experiment,[108] this may have been caused by the microbiological status of the given animals. We did not find this phenomenon in our material (Section VI). In addition, Bulloch and Pomerantz describe multiple accumulations of lymphoid cells in the area; the mean number of these accumulations was 27 in the nudes and 14.6 in the euthymic mice. These accumulations went unnoticed in nonneurological studies. The accumulations , as well as the lymph nodes, were in discrete contact with parasympathetic and sympathetic nerves and ganglia, particularly in *nu/nu* mice.[108]

Bulloch and Pomerantz explain the increased content of lymphoid tissues in the mediastinal area of the nude mouse as a compensatory measure for the lack of thymus (see also Section VI). In fact, in human fetuses the earliest primordia of lymphatic tissues can be seen in perineuronal spaces, first mesenchymal slits are formed in the region of future jugular vein and vagus, fuse into a primary sac, later the primary sacs join together and form a common jugoaxillar sac opening into the jugular vein and situated in close apposition to the nerves.[109] Finally, at 3 months in the human fetus, lymphatic sacs are penetrated by mesenchyme and become restructured into lymphatic vessels and node primordia.[109] This process may well be delayed and prolonged by a general mesenchymal defect and may proceed at different times in the area of the dysgenetic thymus as well as in other loose connective tissue areas affected by chronic inflammations and immunological stimuli.[110] A strong argument for the important morphogenetic and regulatory action of innervation for lymphoid tissues and the nude mouse dysgenetic thymus in particular is provided by Singh's experiment[107] discussed in Section VI.

The cyst and duct systems together with the epithelial acini are embedded in large layers of brown fat, undifferentiated adipose tissue and occasional lobules of white adipose tissue.[43]

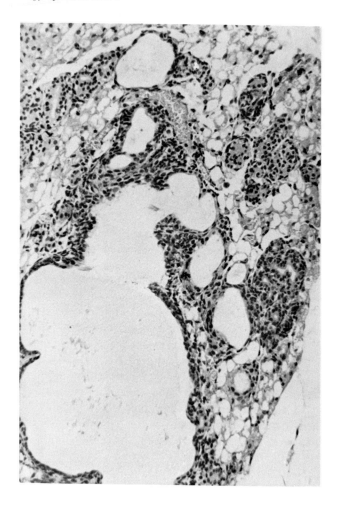

FIGURE 13. Dysgenetic thymus of a 3-week-old CBA/J *nu/nu* male. A large cyst lined by flattened epithelia, ducts with ciliated cylindrical epithelia (right center), Epithelia acini (top right), brown adipose tissue (top left). Sagittal section. (Hem.-eos.; magnification × 120.)

Compared to the normal thymus, the undifferentiated and brown adipose tissue may become strikingly abundant in the vicinity of the dysgenetic thymus (Figures 13 and 14) and appears to be related to nonshivering thermogenesis (Chapter 10, Section II).

With the exception of the few fibroblasts in the loose connective tissue, outside the basal lamina of the epithelial cell formations, no mesenchymal-mesodermal cells can be found in the polycystic organ.[43,44,91,95] This is the one clear-cut qualitative difference from the cytology of the normal thymic stroma. The second is the Ia defect.

MHC-defined antigens are expressed on both the epithelial and mesenchymal thymic cells; however, as mentioned in the previous section, in ontogeny the entry of mesenchymal cells expressing class II (Ia) antigens may be preconditioned by Thy 1-expressing cells which are missing in the dysgenetic thymus embryonic development, as is the bulk of mesenchymal invasion. No Ia[+] cells have been found in 14 to 16 gestation days *nu/nu* thymic rudiments either *in situ* or in short-term culture. Their "mesenchymal" component separated by microdissection before culture did not express any MHC-defined antigens at all, whereas the epithelial component expressed the H-2K (class I) markers.[32] Under the same conditions euthymic embryos (CBA, C57Bl) expressed both class I and II antigens on the thymic

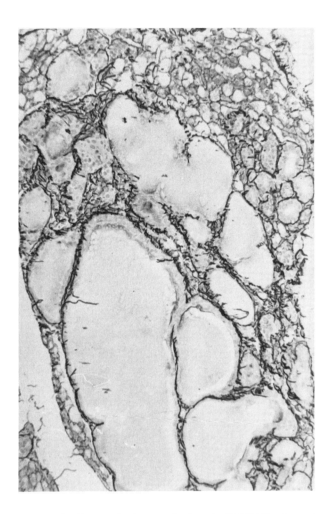

FIGURE 14. Dysgenetic thymus of a 3-week-old CBA/J *nu/nu* male. Silver impregnation disclosing the reticulum lining the cyst and ducts, not penetrating into the epithelial acini (cranial to the large cyst), supporting the undifferentiated and brown fat tissue (top right). Sagittal section, (Gömöry, hem. post stain; magnification × 120.)

epithelia and class I antigens only on the "mesenchymal" cells.[32] Postnatally, there is obviously no major influx of the mesenchymal, blood-borne interdigitating cell and macrophage precursors into the unstimulated polycystic organ and thus the Ia defect becomes permanent or, more exactly, persists in the young adult nudes.

Another analysis of the Ia defect on the nude mouse thymic epithelial cells was performed on the developing thymuses and confirmed the previous finding and assumptions for the given material, i.e., young nude and control mice. Monoclonal antibodies were applied recognizing Ia antigens, GQ gangliosides of neuroendocrine cells, and a determinant associated with the tonofilaments of simple epithelia.[111] It was found in B 10 Br, CBA, and BALB/c mouse fetuses that the neuroendocrine cells form a distict stromal population in the normal thymus and that both these neuroendocrine cells and epithelial Ia antigens appear early in ontogeny (gestation day 15 to 16) and with a similar pattern in vivo and in thymus lobes developing in organ cultures.[111] In the normal thymus, some epithelia expressed both the common epithelial antigens and Ia. In nude mouse thymic rudiments isolated at gestation day 15 to 16, both these antigens were absent and cells positive for the neuroendocrine cell marker were scattered or in clusters in the acinar portions and also in the cyst lining. This is taken as an indication that these cells "are unlikely to share the same developmental origin as the Ia⁺ epithelial population";[111] they may produce some thymic hormones[11] (Section II), but their presence in the nude mouse dysgenetic thymus shows "that alone they are not sufficient for the support of T-cell maturation".[111] Kingston and co-workers[111] suggest that these cells may be of endodermal origin persisting in the dysgenetic thymus[10] which is not fully compatible with other hypotheses on the origin of thymus factor-producing cells (Section II).

The absence of the marker of "simple epithelia tonofilaments" in the dysgenetic thymus is an intriguing problem, since this antigen was found, in the same experiment, to develop on nude mouse salivary gland epithelia;[111] consequently, there is no generalized defect in the nude mouse in the expression of this antigen, the expression fails only in the thymus. The failure may or may not be linked with the absence of Ia antigens which seem to be the key mishap in the dysgenetic thymus.[32,111,112]

Adult nude mice were found (in experiments with cell transfer from F 1 nude mice to lethally irradiated parental mice) to lack any class II (I region) antigen restriction, while the restriction for class I (K/D region) determinants was present.[112] The cytotoxic cells with self-specificity for K/D region determinants could have developed either on the periphery[79,113] or on the epithelial component in the dysgenetic thymus. The same effect could be induced in normal mice treated by a monoclonal anti-Ia antibody in the neonatal period;[73] as in nude mice,[114] also in this model a selective depletion of helper T cells of the L3T4⁺ phenotype was found, whereas the Lyt 2⁺ cytotoxic cell precursor development was undisturbed.[73] The anti-Ia treatment affected presumably the antigen-presenting thymic mesenchymal cells which are missing or almost missing in the dystgenetic thymus. Lo and Sprent[37] endorsed experimentally the supposition that T-cell restriction occurs first by the contact with thymic epithelia and deletion of high affinity for self H 2 determinants later and on interdigitating cells and macrophages;[37] it may be expected that the first step would be less deeply affected in the dysgenetic thymus than the second.

It must be underlined that the polycystic organ is an obviously active epithelial structure with a secretory function, the nature of which is unknown. In the author's view, it is much more likely that the secretion represents rather a residual or minor thymic function than a new and unparalleled function: cyst and duct systems are a component of normal thymi (Section III).

The only indication of one of the possible effects of the secreted material from the dysgenetic thymus comes from experiments with outbred nude mice and our BALB/c *nu/nu* mice which were compared to *nu/+* and *+/+* littermates, all aged 3 to 4 months.[115] Tissue cultures of normal or dysgenetic thymi yielded conditioned media which significantly stimulated the growth of BALB/c bone marrow cell colonies in agar, obviously from macrophage-granulocyte precursors (CFU-GM).[116]

The yield of the secretory product of dysgenetic thymi was per weight or volume higher than the yield from normal lymphoid thymi.[115] As the macrophage colony stimulating factor has been shown to be secreted by cloned human thymic subcapsular cortical epithelial cells,[82a] the activity disclosed by these experiments in the dysgenetic thymus may be taken as an indirect indication of the presence of this key type of the thymic epithelial cell (Section II) in the organ.

It is, in our view, most likely that other effects of the secretory products of dysgenetic thymus epithelia will emerge.

To summarize, the dysgenesis of the nude mutant proceeds through subnormal contact of the endodermal cells with the ectoderm in early ontogeny (day 11 1/2 to the lack of mesenchymal invasion and vascularization of the rudiment which shows little growth, but includes the ectodermal vesicula cervicalis and the duct system derived from the dorsal diverticle of the third pharyngeal pouch as do normal thymi. The morphological and functional state of the epithelial cells in the dysgenetic thymus deviates further from the normal development with altered innervation and by inadequate or negligible traffic of prelymphoid and other mesenchymal/mesodermal cells; thus the acinar arrangement of epithelial (endodermal) cells develops the duct and cyst systems which overgrow and dominate in normal thymi only during involution.

The essential question remains whether this type of dysgenesis allows, under appropriate stimulation, some normal thymic functions to develop in the "polycystic organ", which undergoes no changes comparable with normal thymic involution in aged euthymic mice.

VI. THE LYMPHATIC RUDIMENT AND LYMPHOID INFILTRATIONS IN THE POLYCYSTIC ORGAN

In agreement with the embryonic development from the vesicula cervicalis and the dorsal diverticle, the polycystic organ is situated in the cranial margin of the normal thymic area; this follows from a morphometric analysis of the thymuses of CBA/J and BALB/c mice, with crossing points of the phrenic nerve and internal thoracic vessels taken as topographically invariant points.[117-119] In close proximity to the thymic area there are four, occasionally three, lymph nodes (termed mediastinal or parathymic)[117] They originate from a single lymphatic mass found in 1- to 3-day-old nude mice on either side of the thymic area at the vasa thoracica interna.[117]

Interestingly, in euthymic mice both the left and right lymph nodes are situated laterally to the internal thoracic vessels (85% of cases). In the nudes, the polycystic organ allows a medial shift of both ventromedial nodes which lie on the vessels of 45% of nudes and medially from them in 55%[117] Sometimes, enlarged ventromedial lymph nodes, usually the left node, mimic to some extent the thymic histological architecture. They have an indiscernible subcapsular sinus, cortical, and medullary arrangement of the dense lymphatic and loose reticular tissue.[44] At other instances these nodes are formed by a multilobulated mass of reticular tissue bordered by densely packed lymphocyte layers. These elongated lobuli, or cords, are lined either by strands of loose connective tissue or by widely dilated sinuses; the sinuses may be packed by "histiocytes"[119] (Figure 15).

The occurrence of epithelial cells in these peculiar lymph nodes is not excluded.[44,119,120] This requires corroboration from embryological evidence of a split in the epithelial (endodermal) thymic anlage in the nude mouse.

These lymph nodes receive the lymph from the peritoneal cavity[121] and are the site of the earliest ("local") and quite intensive antibody formation (plaque-forming cell occurrence) following i.p. immunization in the mouse.[122] The distinct nature of peritoneal cell population in normal and in nude mice[123,124] may account in part, together with their high immunological activity, for the specific architecture and cellular content in the nude mouse mediastinal lymph nodes.

There are, apparently, small lymphatic channels connecting the parathymic lymph nodes with the cortical portion of the normal thymus;[125] they may be denoted as afferent lymphatics of the thymus. What happens to these lymphatics traversing the capsule of a normal thymus, in thymic dysgenesis, is unknown, but the lymph circulation and transfer of foreign material[125] from these nodes is obviously altered. This may represent another mechanism of the deviant development of parathymic nodes in the nude mouse.

The anatomical shift of the ventromedial mediastinal node towards the polycystic organ and the eventual atypical architecture of the node is most likely the explanation of the findings of a "normal thymus" or "minute thymus" in 2 out of 60 nude mice in one outbred nude mouse colony[126] and of our "purely lymphatic lobules" located latero-caudally to the polycystic organ and containing Thy-1-positive lymphocytes.[44,120] "Thymus-like lymph nodes" found in 5 out of 74 Swiss nude mice infected with *Trichinella* or *Schizostoma* were reported.[127]

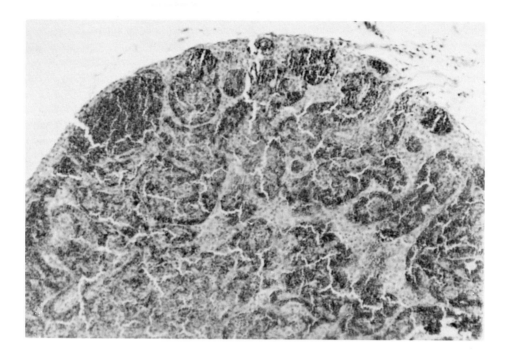

FIGURE 15.   Left cranial mediastinal lymph node of a B10.LP *nu/nu* female, aged 5 weeks, treated with nine doses of levamisole (25 mg/kg s.c.). Sinuses packed with histiocytes penetrate the whole node from cortex to medulla (top right), the paracortex is divided into cords of reticulum cell (interdigitating cells) with layers of cuffs of lymphocytes at the periphery. (Hem.-eos.; magnification × 150.)

No shift in the position of enlarged mediastinal lymph nodes can, however, explain the occurrence of lymphoid cell infiltrates or dense lymphatic nodules within the polycystic organ itself. We have found such lymphatic tranformation in untreated nude mouse polycystic organs, as a rule in one of the epithelial-mucous acini,[119] with lymphocytes present ''inside'' the basal lamina, i.e., among the undifferentiated epithelial cells and ''tonofilament''-rich epithelial cells. The occurrence of the lymphoid infiltration increases with age and can be induced by such treatments as short-term (3 days) administration of levamisole which may rapidly affect the differentiation of maturing thymocyte precursors in the organ itself,[128-131] or transfer of thymocytes or thymic fragments which result in the lymphoid transformation of the organ after months; (Figure 16) an implanted allogeneic thymus is repopulated by most cells after only 2 weeks in the nude mouse.[132]

Both the levamisole administration and thymic lymphocyte transfer resulted in three visible changes in the dysgenetic thymus:

1.   There is increased vascularization and subsequent growth of the epithelial-mucous acini, which become dominated by the tonofilament-rich and dark epithelial cells with frequent keratin-like structures; such proliferation of the solid epithelial acini occurs in polycystic organs transplanted orthotopically (cranially from the normal thymus) into nu/+ littermates in BALB/c mice; after 1 month such a transplant is formed by a solid epithelial mass with a few remaining cysts.[133]

2.   There is an accumulation of lymphocytes among keratinized and dark epithelial cells near the basal lamina of the cyst-lining epithelium, around capillaries in the epithelial acini and in the connective tissue.

3.   There is a formation of giant epithelial cells connected by complex interdigitations, mainly in the growing epithelial acini; these cells display signs of intensive proteo-

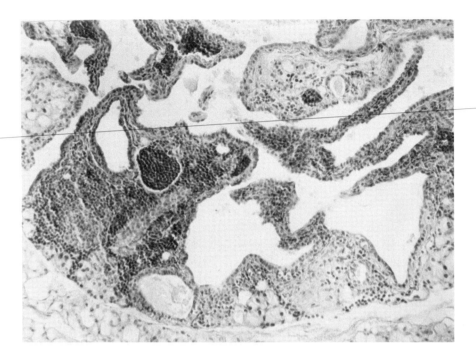

A

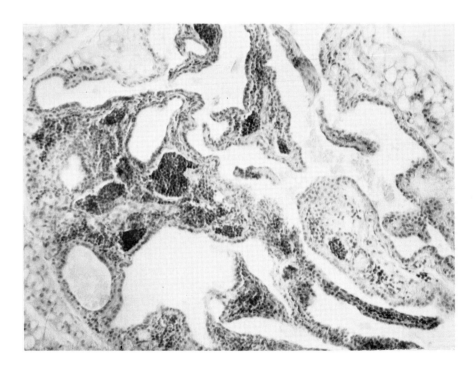

B

FIGURE 16. Three transversal sections (about 10 μ apart) from a dysgenetic thymus of a BALB/c *nu/nu* female, aged 18 months, 16 months after transfer of 4, 8 × 107 cortisone-resistant thymic lymphocytes from a +/+ littermate. Diffuse lymphoid infiltration in the acinar and pericystic areas, dense lymphatic nodules adjacent to the cyst lining. The thymus is surrounded by white adipose tissue only. (Hem.-eos.; magnification × 190.)

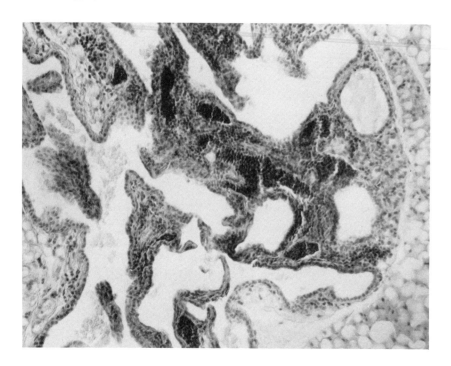

FIGURE 16C

synthesis, abundant stacks of granular endoplasmic reticulum, and contain large accumulations of polymorphous granules of variable density approximately 500 nm in diameter.

In ultrastructural appearance, an increased proportion of the epithelial cells in the transforming polycystic organ resembles the "undifferentiated cells", the "dark cells", and cells of the "subcapsular-perivascular type" adjacent to the basal lamina and possibly contributing to its formation[134] in the normal thymus.

Thy-1.2-positive lymphoid cells could be isolated from the transforming polycystic organ[129] or disclosed *in situ* by immunofluorescence. Thy-1.2-positive lymphoid cells occur, 1 and 2 months after thymocyte transfer, in the vicinity of vessels and in small clusters in the centers of epithelial acini or at the periphery of the thick cyst or duct-lining epithelial layers (Figure 17). Simultaneously, Thy-1.2-positive epithelial cells can be found in the transforming polycystic organ (Thy-1.2-positive epithelial cells have been described so far only in normal thymus of rodents and man[18]).

It seems that both the undifferentiated epithelial cells of the polycystic organ, and lymphocyte precursors in the organ or elsewhere, were affected by the action of levamisole which is likened to that of thymic hormones,[131] or by the transfer of syngeneic thymic lymphocytes which may traffic through the organ, interact with the epithelial cells, and eventually settle in the changed microenvironment. If levamisole really acts as an inducer of "hormone-like products . . . , even in athymic mice",[135] its direct influence on the thymic rudiment would be obvious.

It was noted by Hong et al.[136] that thymic hormones shed by implanted thymic fragments induce a considerable enlargement of the epithelial structures, possibly "vestigial thymic epithelial structures" of the nude mouse polycystic organ. The same is true for the orthotopically transplanted polycystic organ in *nu/+* recipients, as mentioned above.

Also, the precursors of thymic mesenchymal interdigitating cells[80,137] may be assumed to

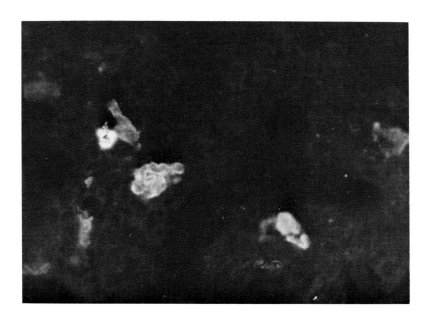

FIGURE 17. Thy-1.2-positive cells in small clusters in the dysgenetic thymus of a BALB/c nude female aged 2 months. Monoclonal anti-Thy 1.2. (SWAM-FITC; magnification × 320.)

infiltrate the connective tissue compartments of the polycystic organ undergoing the partial lymphatic transformation.

Strong support for the assumption that the polycystic organ contains thymus-specific epithelial cells capable of supporting prethymic lymphoid cells to mature into the inductive thymic microenvironment comes from the striking observation of Singh;[107] he found that "thymic rudiments" of nude mouse fetuses implanted into the anterior eye chamber of "syngeneic" nu/+ BALB/c mice are during the 3 weeks of observation repopulated by prethymic lymphoid cells and do support differentiation of murine T cells (Thy 1 positive and binding peanut agglutinins) if cultured in the eye on which side cervical sympathetic ganglia and part of the sympathetic chain have been removed. On the sham-operated side, the anterior eye chamber implant was smaller and contained few lymphoid cells. It was also shown in this study that the polycystic organ of nude fetuses receives sympathetic nerve fibers around gestation day 17 and these fibers increase in density at later stages.[107] Singh suggests that the diminished lymphocyte differentiation on the sham-operated side was due to some inhibitory effect of sympathetic nerves and their transmitters on lymphoid cells bearing beta adrenoreceptors.[138] This is consistent with observations of lymphatic organs in normal mice where the ablation of the sympathetic innervation produced changes in the Thy 1.2 expression (increase in the spleen of adult axotomized mice) and a relative decrease of Lyt-2-positive cells (suppressor/cytotoxic) in neonatally sympathectomized mice.[138] Also, noradrenalin, primarily an alpha adrenergic agent, decreases in normal mouse lymphatic organs during an immune response and is present in considerably larger quantities in nude mouse spleen, compared to the spleen or euthymic mice.[139]

This points to a more universal effect of catecholamines and sympathetic innervation during ontogeny of the nude mouse; the noradrenalin elevation in the nude mouse may also be connected with thermoregulatory problems, but a simple thymic implantation is reported to diminish the noradrenalin level in the spleen of nu/nu mice at 3 weeks of age.[139]

Lymphocytes coming from the transforming polycystic organ are functional T cells. This was found in embryonic (13th day) organs which, when grown in vitro for 1 week, show the same degree of lymphocytopoiesis as thymuses from $+/+$ or $nu/+$ littermates and produce the same graft-vs.-host reaction determined as an increase of labeled amino acid incorporation in semiallogeneic spleen explants.[140] Evidence has also been presented that the numbers of functional T cells increasing in nu/nu mice with age are indeed induced in the dysgenetic thymus.[141] Some low activity in generation helper T cells which can be increased by interleukin 2 was inferred in other experiments.[142]

It can be speculated that manipulations which increase the T-cell differentiation in nude mice, such as the two thymic stromal fractions described by Teodorczyk-Injeyan and Po-tworowski,[143] do act with the help of the dysgenetic thymus; since the insoluble fraction increases migration of precursor cell into the thymus in normal animals.

In conclusion, the nude mouse dysgenetic thymus does contain some rudimentary potential of the thymic inductive microenvironment; it can support to some degree the formation of dense lymphatic tissue.

VII. THE THYMUS OF THE $nu/+$ HYBRID

The effect of the nu gene in the heterozygous mouse is another of the crucial problems of thymic dysgenesis interpretation in the nude mouse. If some thymic alteration also exists in the phenotypically "normal", haired $nu/+$ mouse, it follows that there is a codominant trait in the nu allele in the respect of thymus development (and stem cell potential, see Chapter 6, Section I). The dysgenetic process may then be a quantitative phenomenon with an underlying mechanism caused by the nu gene, but fully expressed only in the homozygous state. Since the nu mutation concerns one gene rather than a very tightly linked gene cluster,[144] a single enzyme defect is likely in the roots of thymic dysgenesis and the mesenchymal stem cell potential. It remains to be seen whether the same defect may also affect hair growth which seems, so far, to be subject to dominant heredity.

There is to date incontestable evidence that the thymus of the $nu/+$ heterozygote is not identical to the thymus of $+/+$ mice of the same background and of the same litter. Scheiff and Cordier[145] have already demonstrated in 1974 that the relative weight of the thymus between 1 and 16 days of age is markedly higher in $+/+$ than in $nu/+$ NMRI mice. The difference was more pronounced immediately after birth. The earliest difference was established by morphometric estimation of thymic volume in fetuses of the 13th gestational day.

We have compared thymuses of mice of C57Bl/10 ScSn background; 3-month-old females had a significant difference in thymus relative weight and a highly significant difference in thymus cellularity, $nu/+$ thymuses being inferior in these respects to $+/+$.[118] In 1-month-old mice, morphometric evaluation of semithin thymus sections revealed that in $nu/+$ there is a 10% lower number of cortical lymphocytes and a highly significant reduction of lymphocytes in the medulla where the number of epithelial elements is proportionally increased.[118] Medullary lymphocytes are more mobile than cortical ones.[146]

The relative position of the $+/+$, $nu/+$, and dysgenetic thymus is given in Figure 18. Decreased relative thymus weight was noted also in 1- to 4-week-old heterozygotes of the C3H/He background; 102-week-old $nu/+$ mice raised in conventional conditions had the same level of leukocytopenia and lymphocytopenia as nu/nu mice of the same age.[147]

In a detailed study, using genetically perfectly defined mice, Zang et al.[148] and Kojima et al.[149,150] have confirmed the size difference. They could exclude the maintenance conditions comparing SPF and clean conventional mice. In C57Bl/6N, C3H/HeN and BALB/cA mice, the relative thymus weights of 7-day-old mice were significantly higher in $+/+$ compared to nu/+ mice and the most pronounced difference was found in highly backcrossed (over 18 times) NFS/N mice, both in 7- and 14-day-old individuals. The difference was easily visible (Figure 19)[149]. By transplantation of the thymi under the kidney capsule of a recipient of the other genotype, an intrinsic defect in the $nu/+$ thymus itself was confirmed.[149] The

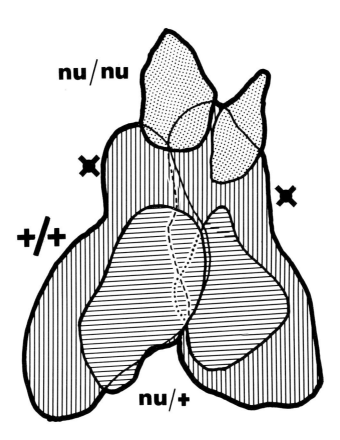

FIGURE 18. Reconstruction of the relative size and position of a *nu/nu* (in caput thymi area), *nu/+* (in corpus thymi area) and *+/+* thymus from morphometric measurements using the crossing point of the phrenic nerve with internal thoracic vessels as reference. Three-month-old CBA/J female mice. The *+/+* thymus was on average 1.6 times heavier than the *nu/+* thymus.

shape of the *nu/+* thymus should also be noted; the right lobe is oval, the left triangular, as indicated in our figure, and the caput thymi is "hypogenetic". In our interpretation, the *nu/+* thymus occupies the corpus thymi area of a normal (*+/+*) thymus.[118] The reduced size (weight) of the *nu/+* thymus was present also in AKR mice, in individuals of the 20th to 22nd backcross. In the AKR-*nu/+* mice, the spontaneous lymphoma had a considerably shorter latent period than in AKR-*+/+* mice.[150]

In conclusion, there is a well-pronounced effect of the *nu* gene on the thymus development of the heterozygous mice. Interestingly, the same is true of the nude rat (A. Kojima, personal communication). In experiments with nude mice, *nu/+* mice cannot be used as "normal" controls and cannot be pooled with *+/+* littermates.

As will be indicated in Chapter 5, Section II, the *nu/+* hybrid is different from *+/+* homozygous mice not only in the white blood counts and thymic size, but also in an antibody-forming capacity.[151,152] A possible cue in the T system of the *nu/+* mice has been suggested in experiments showing a delayed decline of antigen-binding cells, a delayed IgM-IgG switch and a diminished elevation of antigen-induced nonspecific IgG^+ cells during an anti-sheep red blood cell response in BALB/c *nu/+* mice compared to BALB/c *+/+* mice.[153] Some of these functions may be influenced by the leukopenic state of the *nu/+* heterozygote, but the influence of the quantitatively reduced thymic cells and factors supply should have a principal role. A direct evidence is mentioned by Smith and Eaton[154] who observed a

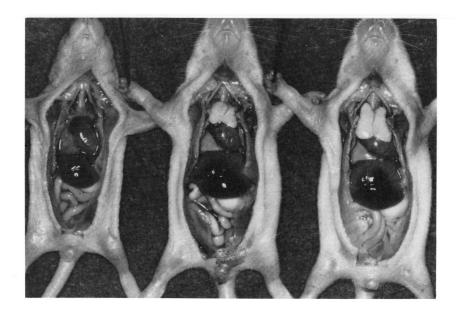

FIGURE 19. Macroscopical appearance of thymuses in 7-day-old NFS/N *nu/nu* male (left), *nu/+* male (center) and +/+ male (right). The +/+ thymus was 1.85 times heavier than the *nu/+* thymus. (From Kojima, A., Saito, M., Hioki, K., Shimanura, K., and Habu, S., *Exp. Cell Biol.*, 52, 107, 1984. With permission.)

strikingly poor response to PHA in some heterozygote individuals with as few as 10% of Thy-1.2-positive cells in the spleen (mice of BALB/c background, 8 to 12 weeks of age). The authors suggest that "some variation in the phenotypic expression of the 'nude' gene may occur" which is what we hinted at in the beginning.

VIII. THYMIC HORMONES

It follows from the ability of the nude mouse dysgenetic thymus to be brought into a state of an inconsistent, spotty thymic microenvironment that some endocrine potential of the epithelium must be preserved in the mutation. There is, however, only one positive report on the detection of thymosin in the acinar epithelial cells 5 in 4 out of 13 dysgenetic thymuses of BALB/c nude mice.[155] Because of the possibility of cross-reactions of the xenoantisera against this crude thymic extract with all kinds of epithelial antigens,[156] definitive proof could be provided using the well-defined and sequenced thymic peptides. Hormone-like, T-cell recruiting and activating products are synthesized after levamisole treatment also in the nude mice.[135]

There is, however, a general belief that the specific thymic hormone activity in the nude mouse blood and peripheral lymphatic organs is absent. This is based mainly on the negative finding on the "facteur thymic sérique" quoted since 1973.[15,157,158]

There is, on the other hand, another component of the crude thymosin fraction 5, namely, thymosin beta 4 which is present in a number of tissues including thymus and brain and is synthesized also in mouse peritoneal macrophages;[159] high levels of this substance are found in the athymic mouse.[159] The authors speculate that thymosin beta 4 may be related to the presence of macrophages in tissues. In respect to these findings, the presence of a "thymic hormone" in spleen, brain, lung, liver, and myocardium[159] and not in the dysgenetic thymus appears very unlikely.

The so-far defined thymic peptidic hormones do exert their effect in the athymic nude mouse and on its cells which serve as one of the main tools for the assays of the hormones.

In vivo, the action of some of the known moieties may proceed also via the thymic rudiment. A synergistic effect of two thymic stromal fractions, one well localized in the thymic perivascular basement membrane, may be needed for the education of T cells in the nude mouse.[143,160] The dysgenetic thymus comprises some basement membrane structures in the cyst and duct systems and lining the epithelial acini which may provide some small-scale effect. The spatial arrangement of a normal thymus is, however, missing.

The target cells of the thymic hormones are obviously the Thy-1-positive precursor cells in the bone marrow and peripheral lymphatic organs of the nude mouse.[132,161] The appearance of Thy 1 is induced by raising the level of intracellular cAMP which is very likely the way of action of thymosins, thymopoietins, and thymic serum factors and also of supernatants of thymic epithelial cell cultures.[162,163]

Also, cells positive for terminal deoxynucleotidyl transferase, the "cellular mutagen", which are depleted in the nude mouse bone marrow, can be induced both in vivo and in vitro by thymosin 5 and specifically by thymosin beta 3.[164,165]

It was suggested for thymopoietin and its synthetic pentapeptide component that it acts not only on the differentiation of T-cell precursors, but also inhibits in vivo the differentiation of some cells of the B lineage. It reduces the numbers of the autologous rosette-forming cells normally present in the spleen of athymic mice.[166]

The T-cell precursors of nude mice could be induced by repeated i.p. injections of bovine or human thymosin 5 or 7 to respond to T-cell mitogens in culture or to home into T-cell areas of lymph nodes.[167,168] Analogous spleen and lymph node cells of nude mice are differentiated by 24 hr culture on normal thymic epithelial cells to T cells responding to concanavalin and in mixed lymphocyte reactions.[169] Also, some increase of the number of antibody-forming cells after a prolonged thymosin treatment[170] or immunization with a hapten-thymosin conjugate[171] was reported, implying the generation of helper T cells.

Suppressor T cells for cytotoxic lymphocytes were generated by a 2-week-long treatment of the nude donors with thymosin 5 (400 μg per s.c. injection);[172] it was reasoned[172] that preferential induction of suppressor cells in nude mouse spleen would prevent the visualization of the hormone effect on accomplished immune reactions such as transplant rejection.[173] In general, there are hints that factors coming from thymic epithelium are more active in inducing helper T cells than substances isolated from entire thymi or from thymocytes,[163,174] albeit some activity could be demonstrated also in spleen and lymph node extracts.[175]

With such a complex compound like thymosin 5-7, the in vivo effect on a thymus (however dysgenetic)-bearing animal obviously creates a very complicated situation,[176] even if all endotoxin effects are really excluded. Among other things, the local processing and the local concentration of different moieties will have some effect. Thymosin 5 was found to stimulate mature thymocytes at high concentrations and induce precursors of helper cells for antibody formation or cells participating in mixed lymphocyte reactions and facilitate the activity of mature specific helper T lymphocytes at low concentrations.[177]

The thymopoietin pentapeptide in 15 i.p. injections of 1 μg for 3 weeks would correct some of the nude mouse spleen cell abnormalities, such as the occurrence of TL$^+$ cells and low diversification of Lyt 123$^+$ cells;[178] these phenotypes are normally confined to the lymphatic thymus; they tend to disappear from the nude mouse spleen after 10 weeks of age without any treatment.[178] There is no indication where they persist, but at that time the lymphocytic content of the dysgenetic thymus increases at least in some individuals. We did not see any consistent effect of thymosin 5 on the status of *nu/nu* and control bone marrow and lymph node cells after 15 daily doses of 100 μg or 3 doses of 1000 μg s.c. per mouse; these treatments caused, however, a decrease in size of both normal and dysgenetic thymus with some loss of the cyst system.[179] Comparing three doses of different preparations of thymosin 5, levamisole (500 μg/mouse s.c.) and thymopoietin pentapeptide

(10 μg/mouse s.c.) given at 3 consecutive days after immunization with sheep red blood cells, we have obtained a 30- to 100-fold increase of the spleen PFC at day 5 of primary antibody response of BALB/c or C57Bl nude mice and lymphatic infiltration and increase of the mucous cell acini in the dysgenetic thymus which was maximal after levamisole, but well pronounced also after the synthetic pentapeptide.

There is little doubt that the nude mouse has the target cells of thymic hormones; it may also be able to produce at least some of the active principles of the known hormones after stimulants (such as levamisole) in the dysgenetic thymus which clearly reacts to the administration of the active hormonal moieties, or elsewhere.

REFERENCES

1. **Rygaard, J.,** *Thymus & Self, Immunobiolgoy of the Mouse Mutant Nude,* F. A. D. L. Copenhagen, 1973.
2. **Miller, J. F. A. P.,** Experimental thymology has come of age, *Thymus,* 1, 3, 1979.
3. **Pahwa, R., Ikehara, S. S., Pahwa, S. G., and Good, R. A.,** Thymic function in man, *Thymus,* 1, 27, 1979.
4. **Zotterman, A.,** Die Schweinethymus als eine Thymus ecto-endodermalis, *Anat. Anz.,* 38, 514, 1911.
5. **Weller, G. L.,** Development of the thyroid, parathyroid and thymus glands, *Carnegie Inst. Contrib. Embryol.,* 24, 93, 1933.
6. **Norris, E. H.,** The morphogenesis and histogenesis of the thymus gland in man: in which the origin of the Hassall's corpuscles of the human thymus is discovered, *Carnegie Inst. Contrib. Embryol.,* 27, 191, 1938.
7. **Crisan, C.,** Die Entwicklung der Thyreo-Parathyreo-Thymischen Systems der weissen Maus, *Z. Anat. Entwicklungsgesch,* 104, 326, 1935.
8. **Hsi, B. L., Yeh, C. J. G., and Faulk, W. P.,** Human thymus contains amnion epithelial antigens, *Immunology,* 49, 289, 1983.
9. **Faulk, W. P. and McIntire, J. A.,** Immunological studies of human trophoblast: markers, subsets and functions, *Immunol. Rev.,* 75, 139, 1983.
10. **Cordier, A. C. and Haumont, S. M.,** Development of thymus, parathyroids, and ultimo-branchial bodies in NMRI and nude mice, *Am. J. Anat.,* 157, 227, 1980.
11. **Haynes, B. F.,** The human thymic microenvironment, *Adv. Immunol.,* 36, 87, 1984.
12. **Mandel, T.,** Differentiation of epithelial cells in the mouse thymus, *Z. Zellforsch. Mikrosk. Anat.,* 106, 408, 1970.
13. **Oláh, I., Röhlich, P., and Törö, I.,** *Ultrastructure of Lymphoid Organs,* Akadémiai Kiadó, Budapest, 1975, 105.
14. **Koninkx, J. F., Schreurs, A. J., Penninks, A. H., and Seinen, W.,** Induction of postthymic T-cell maturation by thymic humoral factor(s) derived from a tumor cell of thymic epithelial origin, *Thymus,* 6, 395, 1984.
15. **Monier, J. C., Dardenne, M., Pléau, J. M., Schmitt, D., Deschaux, P., and Bach, J. F.,** Characterization of facteur thymique sérique (FTS) in the thymus. I. Fixation of anti-FTS antibodies on thymic reticulo-epithelial cells, *Clin. Exp. Immunol.,* 42, 470, 1980.
16. **Ritter, M. A., Sauvage, C. A., and Cotmore, S. F.,** The human thymus microenvironment: in vivo identification of thymic nurse cells and other antigenically distinct subpopulations of epithelial cells, *Immunology,* 44, 439, 1981.
17. **Ritter, M. A. and Morris, R. J.,** Thy-1 antigen: selective association in lymphoid organs with the vascular basement membrane involved in lymphocyte recirculation, *Immunology,* 39, 85, 1980.
18. **Raedler, A., Arndt, R., Raedler, E., Jablonski, D., and Thiele, H. G.,** Evidence for the presence of Thy-1 on cultured thymic epithelial cells of mice and rats, *Eur. J. Immunol.,* 8, 728, 1978.
19. **Raedler, A., Arndt, R., and Thiele, H. G.,** Evidence for the expression of Thy-1 analogous structures in human thymic epithelial cells, *Scand. J. Immunol.,* 10, 69, 1979.
20. **Weissman, I. L.,** Thymus cell maturation, *J. Exp. Med.,* 137, 504, 1973.
21. **Shortman, K. and Jackson, H.,** The differentiation of T-lymphocytes. I. Proliferation kinetics and interrelationships of subpopulations of mouse thymus cells, *Cell. Immunol.,* 12, 230, 1974.
22. **Fathman, C. G., Small, M., Herzenberg, L. A., and Weissman, I. L.,** Thymus cell maturation. II. Differentiation of three mature subclasses in vivo, *Cell. Immunol.,* 15, 109, 1975.
23. **Scollay, R., Butcher, E., and Weissman, I.,** Thymus migration: quantitative studies on the rate of migration of cells from the thymus to the periphery in mice, *Eur. J. Immunol.,* 10, 210, 1980.

24. **Reichert, R. A., Gallatin, W. M., Butcher, E. C., and Weissman, I. L.,** A homing receptor-bearing cortical thymocyte subset: implications for thymus cell migration and the nature of cortisone-resistant thymocytes, *Cell,* 38, 89, 1984.

25. **Andrews, P., Shortman, K., Scollay, R., Potworowski, E. F., Kruisbeek, A. M., Goldstein, G., Trainin, N., and Bach, J.-F.,** Thymic hormones do not induce proliferative ability or cytolytic function in PNA⁺ cortical thymocytes, *Cell. Immunol.,* 91, 455, 1985.

26. **Scollay, R., Barlett, P., and Shortman, K.,** T cell development in the adult murine thymus: changes in the expression of the surface antigens Ly 2, L3T4 and B2A2 during development from early precursor cells to emigrants, *Immunol. Rev.,* 82, 79, 1984.

27. **Wekerle, H., Ketelsen, U. P., and Ernst, M.,** Thymic nurse cells. Lymphoepithelial cell complexes in murine thymuses: morphological and serological characterization, *J. Exp. Med.,* 151, 925, 1980.

28. **van de Wijngaert, F. P., Rademakers, L. H. P. M., Schuurman, H. J., de Weger, R. A., and Kater, L.,** Identification and in situ localization of the "thymic nurse cell" in man, *J. Immunol.,* 130, 2348, 1983.

29. **Andrews, P., Boyd, R. L., and Shortman, K.,** The limited immunocompetence of thymocytes within thymic nurse cells, *Eur. J. Immunol.,* 15, 1043, 1985.

30. **Rouse, R. V., van Ewijk, W., Jones, P. P., and Weissman, I. L.,** Expression of MHC antigens by mouse thymic dendritic cells, *J. Immunol.,* 122, 2508, 1979.

31. **Janossy, G., Thomas, J. A., Bollum, F. J., Granger, S., Pizzolo, G., Brandstock, K. F., Wong, L., McMichael, A., Ganeshaguru, K., and Hoffbrand, A. V.,** The human thymic microenvironment: an immunohistologic study, *J. Immunol.,* 125, 202, 1980.

32. **Jenkinson, E. J., van Ewijk, W., and Owen, J. J. T.,** Major histocompatibility complex antigen expression on the epithelium of the developing thymus in normal and nude mice, *J. Exp. Med.,* 153, 280, 1981.

33. **Van Vliet, E., Melis, M., and Van Ewijk, W.,** Monoclonal antibodies to stromal cell types of the mouse thymus, *Eur. J. Immunol.,* 14, 524, 1984.

34. **Kruisbeek, A. M., Sharrow, S. O., Mathieson, B. J., and Singer, A.,** The H-2 phenotype of the thymus dictates the self-specificity expressed by thymic but not splenic T lymphocyte precursors in thymus-engrafted nude mice, *J. Immunol.,* 127, 2168, 1981.

35. **Kast, W. M., De Waal, L. P., and Melief, C. J. M.,** Thymus dictates major histocompatibility complex (MHC) specificity and immune response gene phenotype of class II MHC-restricted T cells but not of class I MHC-restricted T cells, *J. Exp. Med.,* 160, 1752, 1984.

36. **Schuurman, H. J., Vaessen, L. M. B., Vos, J. G., Hertogh, A., Geertzema, J. G. N., Brandt, C. J. W. M., and Rozing, J.,** Implantation of cultured thymic fragments in congenitally athymic nude rats: ignorance of thymic epithelial haplotype in generation of alloreactivity, *J. Immunol.,* 137, 2440, 1986.

37. **Lo, D. and Sprent, J.,** Identity of cells that imprint H-2-restricted T-cell specificity in the thymus, *Nature,* 319, 672, 1986.

38. **Rimmer, J. J.,** Myoid cells and myasthenia gravis: a phylogenetic overview, *Dev. Comp. Immunol.,* 4, 385, 1980.

39. **Puchtler, H., Meloan, S. N., Branch, B. W., and Gropp, S.,** Myoepithelial cells in human thymus: staining, polarization and fluorescence microscopic studies, *Histochemistry,* 45, 163, 1975.

40. **Wekerle, H., Ketelsen, U. P., Zurn, A. D., and Fulpius, B. W.,** Intrathymic pathogenesis of myasthenia gravis: transient expression of acetylcholine receptors on thymus-derived myogenic cells, *Eur. J. Immunol.,* 8, 579, 1978.

41. **Bargmann, W.,** Der Thymus, in *Handbuch der mikroskopischen Anatomie des Menschen,* Vol. 6 (Part 4), v. Möllendorff, W., Ed., Springer, Berlin, 1943, 1.

42. **Arnesen, K.,** The secretory apparatus in the thymus of mice, *Acta Pathol. Scand.,* 43, 339, 1958.

43. **Groscurth, P., Müntener, M., and Töndury, G.,** Histogenese des Immunsystems der "nude" Maus. II. Postnatale Entwicklung des Thymus: eine lichtmikroskopische Studie, *Beitr. Pathol.,* 154, 125, 1975.

44. **Holub, M., Vaněček, R., and Rossmann, P.,** The polycystic organ in senescent athymic nude mice and in euthymic mice, *Folia Biol. (Prague),* 21, 382, 1975.

45. **Senelar, R., Catayee, G., Escola, R., Escola, M.-J., and Bureau, J.-P.,** Contribution a l' étude des kystes épithéliaux du thymus du rat Wistar et de leur variations sous l'influence des hormones sexuelles et thyroïdiennes, *Pathol. Biol.,* 21, 937, 1973.

46. **Linhartová, A.,** Experimentelle Zystose des Thymus, *Zbl. Allg. Pathol. Pathol. Anat.,* 105, 340, 1964.

47. **Oksanen, A.,** Multilocular fat in thymuses of rats and mice associated with thymus involution: a light- and electron-microscope and histochemical study, *J. Pathol.,* 105, 223, 1971.

48. **Tachibana, F., Imai, Y., and Kojima, M.,** Development and regeneration of the thymus: the epithelial origin of the lymphocytes of the mouse and chick, *J. RES Soc.,* 15, 475, 1974.

49. **Hammar, J. A.,** Zur Histogenese und Involution der Thymusdrübe, *Anat. Anz.,* 27, 23 and 41, 1905.

50. **Maximow, A.,** Untersuchungen über Blut und Bindegewebe. II. Über die Histogenese der Thymus bei Säugetieren, *Arch. Mikroskop. Anat.,* 74, 525, 1909.

51. **Moore, M. A. S. and Owen, J. J. T.,** Experimental studies on the development of the thymus, *J. Exp. Med.,* 126, 715, 1967.

52. **Metcalf, D. and Moore, M. A. S.,** *Haemopoietic Cells,* North-Holland, Amsterdam, 1971, chap. 4.

53. **Mandel, T. and Russel, P. J.,** Differentiation of foetal mouse thymus. Ultrastructure of organ cultures and of subcapsular grafts, *Immunology,* 21, 659, 1971.

54. **Harris, J. E., Ford, C. E., Barnes, D. W. H., and Evans, E. P.,** Cellular trafic of the thymus: experiments with chromosome markers. Evidence from parabiosis for an afferent stream of cells, *Nature,* 201, 886, 1964.

55. **Scollay, R., Smith, J., and Stauffer, V.,** Dynamics of early T cells; prothymocyte migration and proliferation in the adult mouse thymus, *Immunol. Rev.,* 91, 129, 1986.

56. **Van Ewijk, W., Jenkinson, E., and Owen, J.,** Detection of Thy-1, T-200, Lyt-1 and Lyt-2-bearing cells in the developing lymphoid organs of the mouse embryo in vivo and in vitro, *Eur. J. Immunol.,* 12, 262, 1982.

57. **Singh, U. and Owen, J. J. T.,** Studies on the effect of various agents on the maturation of thymus stem cells, *Eur. J. Immunol.,* 5, 286, 1975.

58. **Habu, S., Okumura, K., Diamantstein, T., and Shevach, E. M.,** Expression of interleukin 2 receptor on murine fetal thymocytes, *Eur. J. Immunol.,* 15, 456, 1985.

59. **Lugo, J. P., Krishnan, S. N., Sailor, R. D., Koen, P., Malek, T., and Rothenberg, E.,** Proliferation of thymic stem cells with and without receptors for interleukin 2. Implications for intrathymic antigen recognition, *J. Exp. Med.,* 161, 1048, 1985.

60. **Le Douarin, N.,** Thymus ontogeny studied in interspecific chimeras, in *Development of Host Defenses,* Cooper, M. D. and Dayton, D. H., Eds., Raven Press, New York, 1977, 107.

61. **Pritchard, H. and Micklem, H. S.,** Haemopoietic stem cells and progenitors of functional T-lymphocytes in the bone marrow of "nude" mice, *Clin. Exp. Immunol.,* 14, 597, 1973.

62. **Auerbach, R.,** Morphogenetic interactions in the development of the mouse thymus gland, *Dev. Biol.,* 2, 271, 1960.

63. **Le Douarin, N. M. and Jotereau, F. V.,** Tracing of cells of the avian thymus through embryonic life in interspecific chimeras, *J. Exp. Med.,* 142, 17, 1975.

64. **Bockman, D. E. and Kirby, M. L.,** Dependence of thymus development on derivatives of the neural crest, *Science,* 223, 498, 1984.

65. **Le Lièvre, C. and Le Douarin, N.,** Mesenchymal derivatives of the neural crest: analysis of chimaeric quail and chick embryos, *J. Embryol. Exp. Morphol.,* 34, 124, 1975.

66. **Jenkinson, E. J., Owen, J. J. T., and Aspinall, R.,** Lymphocyte differentiation and major histocompatibility complex antigen expression in the embryonic thymus, *Nature,* 284, 177, 1980.

67. **Duijvestijn, A. M., Sminia, T., Köhler, Y. G., Janse, E. M., and Hoefsmit, E. C. M.,** Ontogeny of the rat thymus micro-environment: development of the interdigitating cell and macrophage populations, *Dev. Comp. Immunol.,* 8, 451, 1984.

68. **Barlett, P. F. and Pyke, K. W.,** Evidence for extrinsic origin of Ia-positive cells in the embryonic murine thymus, in *In Vivo Immunology,* Nieuwenhuis, P., v. d. Broek, A. A., and Hanna, M. G., Jr., Eds., Plenum Press, New York, 1982, 375.

69. **von Gaudecker, B. and Müller-Hermelink, H. K.,** Ontogeny and organization of the stationary non-lymphoid cells in the human thymus, *Cell Tissue Res.,* 209, 287, 1980.

70. **Duijvestijn, A. M. and Kamperdijk, E. W. A.,** Birbeck granules in interdigitating cells of thymus and lymph node, *Cell. Biol. Int. Rep.,* 6, 655, 1982.

71. **Higley, H. R. and O'Morchoe, C. C. C.,** Morphometric analysis of thymic medullary non-lymphoid cell changes during postnatal development, *Dev. Comp. Immunol.,* 8, 711, 1984.

72. **Naparstek, Y., Holoshitz, J., Eisenstein, S., Reshef, T., Rappaport, S., Chemke, J., Ben-Nun, A., and Cohen, I. R.,** Effector T lymphocyte line cells migrate to the thymus and persist there, *Nature,* 300, 262, 1982.

72a. **O'Neil, H. C.,** Isolation of a thymus-homing Lyt-2⁻, L3T4 T-cell line from mouse spleen, *Cell. Immunol.,* 109, 222, 1987.

73. **Kruisbeek, A. M., Mond, J. J., Fowlkes, B. J., Carmen, J. A., Bridges, S., and Longo, D. L.,** Absence of the Lyt-2⁻ L3T4⁺ lineage of T cells in mice treated neonatally with anti-I-A antibody correlates with the absence of intrathymic I-A bearing antigen-presenting cell function, *J. Exp. Med.,* 161, 1029, 1985.

74. **Papiernik, M., Nabarra, B., Savino, W., Pontoux, C., and Barbey, S.,** Thymic reticulum in mice. II. Culture and characterization of nonepithelial phagocytic cells of the thymic reticulum: their role in the syngeneic stimulation of thymic medullary lymphocytes, *Eur. J. Immunol.,* 13, 147, 1983.

75. **Beller, D. I. and Unanue, E. R.,** Thymic macrophages modulate one stage of T cell differentiation in vitro, *J. Immunol.,* 121, 1861, 1978.

76. **Barclay, A. N. and Mayrhofer, G.,** Bone marrow origin of Ia-positive cells in the medulla of rat thymus, *J. Exp. Med.,* 153, 1666, 1981.

77. **Longo, D. L., Kruisbeek, A. M., Davis, M. L., and Matis, L. A.,** Bone marrow-derived thymic antigen-presenting cells determine self-recognition of Ia-restricted T lymphocytes, *Proc. Natl. Acad. Sci. U.S.A.,* 82, 5900, 1985.

78. **Bradley, S. M., Morrissey, P. J., Sharrow, S. O., and Singer, A.,** Tolerance of thymic cytotoxic T lymphocytes to allogeneic H-2 determinants encountered prethymically: evidence for expression of anti-H-2 receptors prior to entry into the thymus, *Proc. Natl. Acad. Sci. U.S.A.,* 79, 2003, 1982.

79. **Reimann, J. and Miller, R. G.,** Differentiation from precursors in athymic nude mouse bone marrow of unusual spontaneously cytolytic cells showing anti-self-H-2 specificity and bearing T cell markers, *J. Exp. Med.,* 158, 1672, 1983.

80. **Hong, R. and Klopp, R.,** Transplantation of cultured thymus fragments. III. Induction of allotolerance, *Thymus,* 4, 91, 1982.

81. **Hays, E. F. and Beardsley, T. R.,** Immunologic effects of human thymic stromal grafts and cell lines, *Clin. Immunol. Immunopathol.,* 33, 381, 1984.

81a. **Lo, D. and Sprent, J.,** Exogenous control of I-a expression in fetal thymus explants, *J. Immunol.,* 137, 1772, 1986.

82. **Bourgeois, N., Bergmans, G., and Buyssens, N.,** The thymus as haematopoietic tissue of non-lymphoid cells, *Virchows Arch. A,* 391, 81, 1981.

82a. **Mizutani, S., Watts, S. M., Robertson, D., Hussein, S., Healy, L. E., Furley, A. J. W., and Greaves, M. F.,** Cloning of hyman thymic subcapsular cortex epithelial cells with T-lymphocyte binding sites and hemopoietic growth factor activity, *Proc. Natl. Acad. Sci. U.S.A.,* 84, 4999, 1987.

83. **Kendall, M. D. and Singh, J.,** The presence of erythroid cells in the thymus gland of man, *J. Anat.,* 130, 183, 1980.

84. **Albert, S., Wolf, P., Pryjma, I., and Vazquez, J.,** Variations in morphology of erythroblasts of normal mouse thymus, *J. RES Soc.,* 2, 158, 1965.

85. **Kendall, M. D.,** The effect of haemorhage on the cell populations of the thymus and bone marrow in wild starlings *(Sturgus vulgaris), Cell Tissue Res.,* 190, 459, 1978.

86. **Pantelouris, E. M.,** Absence of thymus in a mouse mutant, *Nature,* 217, 370, 1968.

87. **Pantelouris, E. M. and Hair, J.,** Thymus dysgenesis in nude (*nu/nu*) mice, *J. Embryol. Exp. Morphol.,* 24, 615, 1970.

88. **Wortis, H. H., Nehlsen, S., and Owen, J. J.,** Abnormal development of the thymus in "nude" mice, *J. Exp. Med.,* 134, 681, 1971.

89. **Groscurth, P., Müntener, M., and Töndury, G.,** The postnatal development of the thymus in the nude mouse. I. Light microscopic observations, in *Proc. 1st Int. Workshop on Nude Mice,* Rygaard, J. and Povlsen, C. O., Eds., G. Fischer, Stuttgart, 1974, 31.

90. **Tamaoki, N. and Esaki, K.,** Electron microscopic observation of the thymus and lymph nodes of the nude mouse, in *Proc. 1st Int. Workshop on Nude Mice,* Rygaard, J. and Povlsen, C.O., Eds., G. Fischer, Stuttgart, 1974, 43.

91. **Cordier, A.,** Ultrastructure of the thymus in "nude" mice, *J. Ultrastruct. Res.,* 47, 26, 1974.

92. **Groscurth, P. and Kistler, G.,** Histogenese des Immunsystems der "nude" Maus. I. Pränatale Entwicklung des Thymus: eine lichtmikroskopische Studie, *Beitr. Pathol.,* 154, 109, 1975.

93. **Owen, J. J. T., Jordan, R. K., and Raff, M. C.,** The development of the thymus in the nude mouse, *Eur. J. Immunol.,* 5, 653, 1975.

94. **Ebbensen, P. and Nielsen, M. H.,** Thymic cysts in oestrogenized BALB/c mice, *Acta Pathol. Microbiol. Scand. Sect A,* 80, 211, 1972.

95. **Groscurth, P. and Kistler, G.,** Histogenese des Immunsystems der "nude" Maus. IV. Ultrastruktur der Thymusanlage 12- und 13-tägigen Embryonen, *Beitr. Pathol.,* 156, 359, 1975.

96. **Habu, S. and Tamaoki, N.,** Thymocyte differentiation from precursor cells in the embryonic thymus of nude and normal mice, in *Proc. 2nd Int. Workshop on Nude Mice,* Nomura, T., Oshawa, N., Tamaoki, N., and Fujiwara, K., Eds., University of Tokyo Press, Tokyo, 1977, 197.

97. **Jordan, R. K.,** Ultrastructure studies on cells containing secretory granules in the early embryonic thymus, in *The Biological Activity of Thymic Hormones,* van Bekkum, D. W., Ed., Kooyker, Rotterdam, 1975, 49.

98. **Cordier, A. C.,** Ultrastructure of the cilia of thymic cysts in "nude" mice, *Anat. Rec.,* 181, 227, 1975.

99. **Fukuda, T., Kistler, G. S., and Groscurth, P.,** The early postnatal development of the thymus in the nude mouse. II. Electron microscopic observations, in *Proc. 1st Int. Workshop on Nude Mice,* Rygaard, J. and Povlsen, C. O., Eds., G. Fischer, Stuttgart, 1974, 37.

100. **Djaczenko, W. and Garaci, E.,** Dark reticular epithelial cells of the thymus as the primary target of heterologous anti-lymphocyte serum in BALB/c mice, *Clin. Immunol. Immunopathol.,* 6, 213, 1976.

101. **Hoffmann-Fezer, G., Rodt, H., and Thierfelder, S.,** Immunohistochemical identification of T- and B-lymphocytes delineated by the unlabeled antibody enzyme method. II. Anatomical distribution of T- and B-cells in lymphoid organs of nude mice, *Beitr. Pathol.,* 161, 17, 1977.

102. **de Souza, M. and Incefy, G.,** The possible contribution of the thymus lymphocyte to thymus humoral function, in *The Biological Activity of Thymic Hormones,* van Bekkum, D. W., Ed., Kooyker, Rotterdam, 1975, 49.

103. **Clark, S. L., Jr.,** Electron microscopy of the thymus in mice of strain 129/J, in *The Thymus in Immunobiology, Structure, Function and Role in Disease,* Good, R. A. and Gabrielsen, A. E., Eds, Harper Row-Hoeber Medical Division, New York, 1964, 85.

104. **Kotani, M., Seiki, K., Yamashita, A., and Horii, I.,** Lymphatic drainage of thymocytes to the circulation in the guinea-pig, *Blood,* 27, 511, 1966.

105. **Williams, J. M. and Felten, D. L.,** Sympathetic innervation of murine thymus and spleen: a comparative histofluorescence study, *Anat. Rec.,* 199, 531, 1981.

106. **Bulloch, K. and Moore, R. Y.,** Innervation of the thymus gland by brain stem and spinal cord in mouse and rat, *Am. J. Anat.,* 162, 157, 1981.

107. **Singh, U.,** Lymphopoiesis in the nude fetal thymus following sympathectomy, *Cell. Immunol.,* 93, 222, 1985.

108. **Bulloch, K. and Pomerantz, W.,** Autonomic nervous system innervation of thymic-related lymphoid tissue in wildtype and nude mice, *J. Comp. Neurol.,* 228(1), 57, 1984.

109. **Kočová, J. and Slípka, J.,** To the morphogenesis of the lymphatic system, in *Lymphology, Proc. 6th Int. Congr.,* Málek, P., Bartoš, V., Weissleder, H., and Witte, M. H., Eds., G. Thieme, Stuttgart and Avicenum, Prague, 1978, 14.

110. **Holub, M.,** Immunological and histological changes in immunization with aid of a lipoid adjuvant, *Folia Biol.* (Prague), 3, 297, 1957.

111. **Kingston, R., Jenkinson, E. J., and Owen, J. J. T.,** Characterization of stromal cell populations in the developing thymus of normal and nude mice, *Eur. J. Immunol.,* 14, 1052, 1984.

112. **Kruisbeek, A. M., Davis, M. L., Matis, L. A., and Longo, D. L.,** Self-recognition specificity expressed by T cells from nude mice. Absence of detectable Ia-restricted T cells in nude mice that do exhibit self-K/D-restricted T cell responses, *J. Exp. Med.,* 160, 839, 1984.

113. **Besedovsky, H. O., del Rey, A., and Sorkin, E.,** Role of prethymic cells in acquisition of self-tolerance, *J. Exp. Med.,* 150, 1351, 1979.

114. **MacDonald, H. R., Blanc, C., Lees, R. K., and Sordat, B.,** Abnormal distribution of T cell subsets in athymic mice, *J. Immunol.,* 136, 4337, 1986.

115. **Jirásková, Z. and Nečas, E.,** Hemopoietic colony-stimulating factors in conditioned media from cultures of the normal and dysgenetic mouse thymus, *Folia Biol. (Prague),* 1989, in press.

116. **Metcalf, D.,** *The Hemopoietic Colony Stimulating Factors,* Elsevier, Amsterdam, 1984, 315.

117. **Rychter, Z., Holub, M., and Vaněčk, R.,** Topical and quantitative analysis of the thymus region in the nude mouse, *Folia Biol. (Prague),* 24, 414, 1978.

118. **Barták, A., Bokorová, M., Rychter, Z., and Holub, M.,** The thymus of the *nu/+* hybrid, *Folia Biol. (Prague),* 24, 419, 1978.

119. **Holub, M., Rossmann, P., Rychter, Z., and Vaněček, A.,** The dysplastic thymus of the mouse mutant nude, in *21st Colloq. Scientificum Facultatis Medicae University Carolinae* and *19th Congr. Morphologicus Symp.,* Klika, E., Ed., Charles University, Prague, 1978, 305.

120. **Holub, M., Rossmann, P., Tlaskalová, and Vidmarová, H.,** Thymus rudiment of the athymic nude mouse, *Nature,* 256, 491, 1975.

121. **Yoffey, J. M. and Courtice, F. C.,** *Lymphatics, Lymph and the Lymphomyeloid Complex,* Academic Press, London, 1970, 295.

122. **Hill, S. W.,** Distribution of plaque-forming cells in the mouse for a protein antigen. Evidence for highly active parathymic lymph nodes following intraperitoneal injection of hen lysozyme, *Immunology,* 30, 895, 1976.

123. **Jarošková, L., Trebichavský, I., Tučková, L., Jankásková, D., and Holub, M.,** The omental immune apparatus of athymic nude mice, *Folia Biol. (Prague),* 24, 432, 1978.

124. **Ishikawa, H. and Saito, K.,** Congenitally athymic nude *(nu/nu)* mice have Thy-1-bearing immunocompetent helper T cells in their peritoneal cavity, *J. Exp. Med.,* 151, 965, 1980.

125. **Eggli, P., Schaffner, T., Gerber, H. A., Hess, M. W., and Cottier, H.,** Accessibility of thymic cortical lymphocytes to particles translocated from the peritoneal cavity to parathymic lymph nodes, *Thymus,* 8, 129, 1986.

126. **Pantelouris, E. M.,** Nude mice with normal thymus, *Nature,* 254, 140, 1975.

127. **Hsu, C. K., Whitney, R. A., and Hansen, C. T.,** Thymus-like lymph node in nude mice, *Nature,* 257, 681, 1975.

128. **Holub, M., Rychter, Z., and Machoninová, A.,** Induction of lymphatic tissue in the nude mouse dysgenetic thymus, in *Proc. 3rd Int. Workshop on Nude Mice,* Reed, N. D., Ed., G. Fischer, New York, 1982, 197.

129. **Amery, W. K.,** The mechanism of action of levamisole: immune restoration through enhanced cell maturation, *J. RES Soc.,* 24, 187, 1978.

130. **Otterness, I. G., Lachman, L. B., and Bliven, M. L.,** Effect of levamisole on the proliferation of thymic lymphocyte subpopulations, *Immunopharmacology,* 3, 61, 1981.
131. **Renoux, G. and Renoux, M.,** Thymus-like activities of sulphur derivatives on T-cell differentiation, *J. Exp. Med.,* 145, 466, 1977.
132. **Loor, F. and Kindred, B.,** Differentiation of T-cell precursors in nude mice demonstrated by immuno-fluorescence of T-cell membrane markers, *J. Exp. Med.,* 138, 1044, 1973.
133. **Holub, M., Rossmann, P., and Mándi, B.,** The dysgenetic thymic complex of the nude mouse, *Folia Biol. (Prague),* 24, 416, 1978.
134. **van de Wijngaert, F. P., Kendall, M. D., Schuurman, H.-J., Rademakers, L. H. P. M., and Kater, L.,** Heterogene of epithelial cells in the human thymus. An ultrastructural study, *Cell Tissue Res.,* 237, 227, 1984.
135. **Renoux, G. and Renoux, M.,** Immunostimulation par le levamisole: cibles et mechanismes, *Nouv. Presse Med.,* 7, 197, 1978.
136. **Hong, R., Schulte-Wissermann, H., Jarret-Toth, E., Horowitz, S. D., and Manning, D. D.,** Transplantation of cultured thymic fragments. II. Results in nude mice, *J. Exp. Med.,* 149, 398, 1979.
137. **Schuurman, H. J., Vos, J. G., Broekhuizen, R., Brandt, C. J. W. M., and Kater, L.,** In vivo biological effect of allogeneic cultured thymic epithelium on thymus-dependent immunity in athymic nude rats, *Scand. J. Immunol.,* 21, 21, 1985.
138. **Miles, K., Chemicka-Schorr, E., Atweh, S., Otten, G., and Arnason, B. G. W.,** Sympathetic ablation alters lymphocytes membrane properties, *J. Immunol.,* 135, 797s, 1985.
139. **Besedowski, H. O., del Rey, A., and Sorkin, E.,** Immune-neuroendocrine interactions, *J. Immunol.,* 135, 750s, 1985.
140. **Chakravarty, A., Kubai, L., Sidky, Y., and Auerbach, R.,** Ontogeny of thymus cell function, *Ann. N.Y. Acad. Sci.,* 249, 34, 1975.
141. **Ikehara, S., Yasumizu, R., Nakamura, T., Sekita, K., Muso, E., Ohtsuki, H., Ogura, M., Toki, J., Inoue, N., Suguira, K., Iwai, H., Shintaku, M., Ihara, N., Hamashima, Y., and Good, R. A.,** Role of the thymus and the stem cells in the differentiation of T cells, in *Immune-Deficient Animals in Biomedical Research, Proc. 5th IWIDA,* Rygaard, J. et al., Eds., S. Karger, Basel, 1987, 69.
142. **Stötter, H., Rüde, E., and Wagner, H.,** T cell factor (interleukin 2) allows in vivo induction of T helper cells against heterologous erythrocytes in athymic (*nu/nu*) mice, *Eur. J. Immunol.,* 10, 719, 1980.
143. **Teodorczyk-Injeyan, J. and Potworowski, E. F.,** Synergism between two thymic stromal fractions in the development of T-helper function in nude mice, *Immunol. Lett.,* 2, 29, 1980.
144. **Hansen, C. T.,** The nude gene and its effects, in *The Nude Mouse in Experimental and Clinical Research,* Fogh, J. and Giovanella, B. C., Eds., Academic Press, New York, 1978, 1.
145. **Scheiff, J. M. and Cordier, A.,** Étude quantitative du thymus de la souris heterozygote pour le gene nu, *Bull. Assoc. Anat.,* 58, 163, 1974.
146. **Sainte-Marie, G. and Leblond, C. P.,** Origin and fate of cells in the medulla of rat thymus, *Proc. Soc. Exp. Biol. Med.,* 98, 909, 1958.
147. **Yunker, V. M., Gruntenko, E. V., and Moroskova, T. S.,** Leucocyte blood composition in mice C3H/He *nu/nu,* C3H/He *nu/+* and C3H/He, *Folia Biol. (Prague),* 24, 437, 1978.
148. **Zhang, M., Kojima, A., Hata, M., Nishizuka, Y., and Suchi, T.,** Developmental abnormality of the thymus in NFS/N-*nu/+* mice (transl.), *Igaku No Ayumi,* 127, 189, 1983.
149. **Kojima, A., Saito, M., Hioki, K., Shimanura, K., and Habu, S.,** NFS/N-*nu/+* mice can macroscopically be distinguished from NFS/N-*+/+* littermates by their thymic size and shape, *Exp. Cell Biol.,* 52, 107, 1984.
150. **Shisa, H., Kojima, A., and Hiai, H.,** Accelerating effect of nude gene heterozygosity on spontaneous AKR thymic lymphomagenesis, *Jpn. J. Cancer Res.,* 77, 568, 1986.
151. **Holub, M., Hajdu, I., Jarošková, L., and Trebichavský, I.,** Lymphatic tissues and antibody-forming cells of athymic nude mice, *Z. Immunitactsforsch.,* 146, 322, 1974.
152. **Tlaskalová-Hogenová, H. and Holub, M.,** The effect of fed xenogeneic red blood cells on the immune response of euthymic and athymic mice, in *Immune-Deficient Animals in Biomedical Research, Proc. 5th IWIDA,* Rygaard, J. et al., Eds, S. Karger, Basel, 1987, 101.
153. **Fehniger, T. E., Martínez-Maza, O., Kanovith-Klein, S., and Ashman, R. F.,** Analysis of antigen-binding cell surface Ig profiles and Ig-secreting cells in mice carrying the nu allele: immune regulation abnormality in heterozygous nu/+ mice, *J. Immunol.,* 128, 568, 1982.
154. **Smith, L. B. and Eaton, G. J.,** Suppressor cells in spleens from ''nude'' mice: their effect on the mitogenic response of B lymphocytes, *J. Immunol.,* 117, 319, 1976.
155. **Mándi, B., Holub, M., Rossmann, P., Csaba, B., Glant, T., and Ölveti, E.,** Detection of thymosin 5 in calf and mouse thymus and in nude mouse dysgenetic thymus, *Folia Biol. (Prague),* 25, 49, 1979.
156. **van den Tweel, J. G., Taylor, C. R., McClure, J., and Goldstein, A. L.,** Detection of thymosin in thymic epithelial cells by an immunoperoxidase method, in *Function and Structure of the Immune System,* Müller-Ruchholz, W. and Müller-Hermelink, H. K., Eds., Plenum Press, New York, 1979, 511.

157. **Bach, J.-F., Dardenne, M., and Bach, M.-A.,** Detection of a circulating thymic hormone using T-rosette forming cells, in *Proc. 7th Leucocyte Culture Conf.,* Daquillard, F., Ed., Academic Press, New York, 1973, 271.

158. **Cohen, S., Berrih, S., Dardenne, M., and Bach, J.-F.,** Feedback regulation of the secretion of a thymic hormone (thymulin) by human thymic epithelial cells in culture, *Thymus,* 8, 109, 1986.

159. **Xu, G. J., Hannappel, E., Morgan, J., Hemstead, J., and Horecker, B. L.,** Synthesis of thymosin beta 4 by peritoneal macrophages and adherent spleen cells, *Proc. Natl. Acad. Sci. U.S.A.,* 79, 4006, 1982.

160. **Potworowski, E. F.,** The thymic microenvironment; localization of a biologically active insoluble fraction, *Clin. Exp. Immunol.,* 30, 305, 1977.

161. **Roelants, G. E., Mayor, K. S., Hägg, L. B., and Loor, F.,** Immature T lineage lymphocytes in athymic mice: presence of TL, lifespan and homeostatic regulation, *Eur. J. Immunol.,* 6, 75, 1976.

162. **Bach, M. A., Fournier, C., and Bach, J. F.,** Regulation of theta-antigen expression by agents altering cyclic AMP level and by thymic factor, *Ann. N.Y. Acad. Sci.,* 249, 316, 1975.

163. **Kruisbeek, A. M., Astaldi, G. C. B., Blankwater, M.-J., Zijlstra, J. J., Levert, L. A., and Astaldi, A.,** The in vitro effect of a thymic epithelial culture supernatant on mixed lymphocyte reactivity and intracellular cAMP levels of thymocytes and on antibody production to SRBC by *nu/nu* spleen cells, *Cell. Immunol.,* 35, 134, 1978.

164. **Pazmino, N. H., Ihle, J. N., McEwan, R. N., and Goldstein, A. L.,** Control of differentiation of thymocyte precursors in the bone marrow by thymic hormones, *Cancer Treat, Rep.,* 62, 1749, 1978.

165. **Pazmino, N. H., Ihle, J. N., and Goldstein, A. L.,** Induction in vivo and in vitro of terminal deoxynucleotidyl transferase by thymosin in bone marrow cells from athymic mice, *J. Exp. Med.,* 147, 708, 1978.

166. **Goldstein, G., Scheid, M. P., Boyse, E. A., Schlesinger, D. H., and Van Wauwe, J.,** A synthetic pentapeptide with biological activity characteristic of the thymic hormone thymopoietin, *Science,* 204, 1309, 1979.

167. **Thurman, G. B., Silver, B. B., Hooper, J. A., Giovanella, B. C., and Goldstein, A. L.,** In vitro mitogenic responses of spleen cells and ultrastructural studies of lymph nodes from nude mice following thymosin administration in vivo, in *Proc. 1st Int. Workshop on Nude Mice,* Rygaard, J. and Povlsen, C. O., Eds., G., Fischer, Stuttgart, 1975, 105.

168. **Thurman, G. B., Ahmed, A., Strong, D. M., Gershwin, M. E., Steinberg, A. D., and Goldstein, A. L.,** Thymosin-induced increase in mitogenic responsiveness of lymphocytes of C57B1/6J, NZB/W and nude mice, *Transplant. Proc.,* 7, 299, 1975.

169. **Satton, V. L., Waksal, S. D., and Herzenberg, L. A.,** Identification and separation of pre T-cells from *nu/nu* mice: differentiation by preculture with thymic reticuloepithelial cells, *Cell. Immunol.,* 24, 173, 1976.

170. **Ikehara, S., Hamashima, Y., and Masuda, T.,** Immunological restoration of both thymectomized and athymic nude mice by a thymic factor, *Nature,* 258, 335, 1975.

171. **Ahmed, A., Smith, A. H., Sell, K. W., Gershwin, M. E., Steinberg, A. D., Thurman, G. B., and Goldstein, A. L.,** Thymic-dependent anti-hapten response in congenitally athymic (nude) mice immunized with DNP-thymosin, *Immunology,* 33, 757, 1977.

172. **Marshall, G. D., Thurman, G. B., Rossio, J. L., and Goldstein, A. L.,** In vivo generation of suppressor T cells by thymosin in congenitally athymic nude mice, *J. Immunol.,* 126, 741, 1981.

173. **Pierpaoli, W. and Besedovsky, H. O.,** Failure of "thymus factor" to restore transplantation immunity in athymic mice, *Br. J. Exp. Pathol.,* 56, 180, 1975.

174. **van Bekkum, D. W., Betel, I., Blankwater, M. J., Kruisbeek, A. M., and Swart, A. C.,** Biologic activities of various thymus preparations, *Transplant. Proc.,* 9, 1197, 1977.

175. **Blankwater, M. J., Levert, L. A., Swart, A. C. W., and van Bekkum, D. W.,** Effect of various thymic and nonthymic factors on in vitro antibody formation by spleen cells from nude mice, *Cell. Immunol.,* 35, 242, 1978.

176. **Ahmed, A., Smith, A. H., Wong, D. M., Thurman, G. B., Goldstein, A. L., and Sell, K. W.,** In vitro induction of Lyt surface markers on precursor cells incubated with thymosin polypeptides, *Cancer Treat. Rep.,* 62, 1739, 1978.

177. **Armerding, D. and Katz, D. H.,** Activation of T and B lymphocytes in vitro. IV. Regulatory influence on specific T cell functions by a thymus extract factor, *J. Immunol.,* 114, 1248, 1975.

178. **Ranges, G. E., Goldstein, G., Boyse, E. A., and Schield, M. P.,** T cell development in normal and thymopentin-treated nude mice, *J. Exp. Med.,* 156, 1057, 1982.

179. **Machoninová, A., Rychter, Z., Holub, M., Korčáková, L., and Mándi, B.,** Influence of thymosin and levamisole on dysgenetic thymus of the nude mouse, *Folia Biol. (Prague),* 24, 424, 1978.

Chapter 4

T CELLS

I. T-CELL DIFFERENTIATION AND FUNCTION

Since the earliest days of the discovery of "athymia", or, more exactly, thymic dysgenesis in the nude mouse, it has been known that the animal is not entirely devoid of the T-lineage cells. Raff's studies have revealed small but significant numbers of Thy-1-positive cells in nude mouse spleens and lymph nodes;[1,2] 3 to 20% of Thy-1-positive cells were demonstrated by a variety of techniques and their immaturity confirmed by the finding of TL expression which is normally confined to the thymus.[3-5] In a pioneer study with fluorescence-activated cell sorting, Cantor et al.[6] found two populations of Thy-1.2-positive cells: "bright T cells" (with high Thy 1 expression), preferentially homing to the spleen and present in normal mice (BALB/c) in constant numbers from birth to 30 weeks of age; and "dull T cells", homing more to lymph nodes, increasing in numbers with age, not affected by adult thymectomy and rapidly recirculating. In nude mice, the dull T cells are much less reduced than the bright T cells which amount here to about 20% of the dull T cells.[6]

There are many more *nu/nu* spleen and lymph node cells, which are positive for the brain-derived antigen.[7] The xenoantiserum defining this antigen possibly reacts with more epitopes on the same antigenic molecule[7] and is found in 16 to 32% of nude spleen cells and 26 to 35% of nude lymph node cells (BALB/c and C57Bl backgrounds). The positive cells are comparatively large and could be induced — as pre-T cells — to respond to concanavalin A and in the mixed lymphocyte reaction after preculture on normal thymic stromal cells.[7]

The presence of these T-lineage cells was a stirring fact, since it was assumed that (1) Thy-1-positive cells of the T lineage should be thymus-dependent and (2) the nude mouse has no thymus and thymus-dependent function whatsoever. Both suppositions were a little exaggerated. It was well known before that cells able to mount upon transfer T-cell reactions such as graft vs. host appear in mice prior to the thymic anlage, on the 9th to 10th day of intrauterine life, in the liver and placenta.[8] It was obvious that these precursor cells may persist during athymic development. It was already stated during the first workshop on nude mice that there is "little serious doubt that T-cell progenitors exist in adult nude mice";[9] they have a low density of the Thy 1 antigen, slow electrophoretic mobility, do not recirculate through the thoracic duct, are TL[+], and have a life-span of 1 to 2 days.[5] Their presence in peripheral lymphatic organs is under homeostatic regulation by a normal thymus since they appear after thymectomy in normal mice and disappear after thymus implantation in athymic mice.[5]

The Thy 1 surface antigen was redefined as "one of the set of Ig-related structures that mediate cell recognition in morphogenesis".[10-12] Observations on transgenic mice show that Thy-1 glycoprotein plays an important role in the activation, differentiation and proliferation of many different cell and tissue types.[13] It may be said that thymus development is Thy 1 expression-dependent rather than that Thy-1-positive cells must be thymus-induced. The thymus epithelial stroma seems to need few fully competent T-cell progenitors to be primed for its normal development[14] and it has been suggested for human thymic dysgenesis that it may be caused by the failure of T-cell progenitors to populate the epithelial anlage:[15] the same may be true for the earliest development of the nude thymus.[9] This, of course, implies that Thy 1 expression in pre-T cells and elsewhere[11,12] in nude mouse tissues would be insufficient in the early "prethymic" ontogeny.

There is no consensus whether Thy 1 expression in nude mouse lymphocytes can be influenced during intrauterine life. Loor[16,17] has found similar numbers of Thy-1-positive lymphocytes in nudes born to homozygous and heterozygous mothers, other reports[18,19] indicate slightly higher numbers in nudes born to euthymic mothers. This would most likely suggest a humoral influence of the maternal thymus on the development of Thy-1-positive cells. Such an influence could also be traced in the anti-sheep red blood cells antibody response.[20]

Viral hepatitis was found to induce up to 40% Thy-1-positive and TL positive cells in the spleens of adult nude mice, also of the "supernude" type (from homozygous matings).[21] The same could be achieved by a series of injections of the hormone thymopoietin or ubiquitin.[21] Obviously, the pool of lymphocytes which can be induced to express higher densities of Thy 1, TL, and possibly also markers of more mature T cells not only increases with age,[17] but can be triggered into differentiation by extreme conditions. No data are available on viral or hormonal manipulation of nude embryos or fetuses.

The nude mouse spleen and bone marrow contain cells which are capable of being transformed by Moloney murine leukemia virus into lymphoma cells and to develop enzymatic markers (terminal deoxynucleotidyl transferase or 20 alpha-hydroxysteroid dehydrogenase) typical for the analogous cells in euthymic mice (Chapter 9 Section I).

Also, lymphocytes already bearing the Thy 1, Lyt 1, and Lyt 2 markers increase in numbers with the age of the nude mice[22-24] and their differentiation may be due to the pressure of "environmental antigens".[28] These "strongly Thy 1 positive" lymphocytes[25] amount in the spleen of nude mice (BALB/c and C57Bl background) older than 6 months to about 10%, in the lymph nodes to about 20%.[24] The percentage of these cells in the spleen and lymph nodes of the respective control (*nu/+*) mice was about three times higher. In aged mice with a combined immunodefect, N:NIH(s)II *nu/nu*, the percentage of Thy 1[+] cells was elevated about threefold and almost identical with that of control mice.[24] These cells localized in thymus-dependent areas of the spleen, lymph nodes, and Peyer's patches in nude mice over 3 to 4 months of age;[26] in mice older than 7 months Thy 1[+] cells were clustered in the spleen periarteriolar areas; Lyt 2[+] were less numerous, but in the same areas as Thy 1[+] cells.[26] Thus, in the phenotypical characteristics of peripheral T cells, this type of nude mice develops very closely to its euthymic counterpart.

Since there is incontestable evidence that the T cells or T-like cells in nude mice do not come from their euthymic mothers,[17,27] their identity with T cells from thymus-bearing animals has to be shown. Formally, these T cells may be prethymic cells maturing in an abnormal way.

Cytotoxic T lymphocytes of nude mice have been invariably shown to be Thy 1[+] in the precursor stage and Thy 1[+] Lyt 2[+] in the effector stage, as are analogous cells of euthymic mice.[23,24,27] The expression of Lyt 1 and Lyt 2 antigens relative to the proportion of Thy 1[+] lymphocytes is again similar in nude and control mice.[22] Also, the T-cell help for B-cell responses of nude mice is provided by Thy-1-positive cells[28,29] and IL-2-producing cells inducible in the nudes are Thy 1[+] Lyt 2[−] as in controls.[30] Suppressor cells, possibly lymphocytes, demonstrable by the effect of the response to a B-cell mitogen in vitro have been described in the spleen of young BALB/c nude mice and were Thy 1[+].[31]

It can be stated that "functional nude T cells are phenotypically indistinguishable from normal T cells"[23] with a few reservations.

It has been conclusively shown by flow cytometric analysis of forward light scatter that nude Thy 1[+] and Lyt 2[+] lymphocytes are larger than their control counterparts.[7,22,24,26] The larger lymphocytes were found in N:NIH(s) II mice aged 7 months especially in the lymph nodes.[26] Otherwise, they had the ultrastructural features of mature lymphocytes,[26] possibly only with more abundant ribosomal fields. This is reminiscent of the situation in other hematopoietic cell series (myeloid, erythroid) where less mature, usually larger, stages may acquire fully differentiated characteristics and functions; this may be associated with the omission of one or more mitoses in the proliferating precursor compartments and provoked by a high turnover of the functional stages. In the nude mouse blood granulocytes (bands) are also of a larger size than the respective leukocytes in euthymic littermates, though there is no difference in nuclear maturation.[32]

The abnormal maturation of phenotypically characterized *nu/nu* T cells is revealed also by the occurrence of the TL marker in the spleen[5] and its association with Thy 1 and Lyt 123 in all splenic T cells at 2 months of age in BALB/c nude mice.[33] Also, the expression of the Qa 1 marker on splenic cells is different in nude and *nu/+* mice.[33] Again, only in older mice (after 10 weeks of age) the diversification of Lyt 123 precursors into Lyt 1 and Lyt 2 subsets occurs spontaneously and TL positivity decreases; this process can be attained also by treatment with a thymic hormone (thymopentin, the synthetic pentapetide fragment of thymopoietin).[33]

Also, the advantage presented by the peritoneal cavity microenvironment (possibly due to the presence of activated macrophages) to the development or sojourn of Thy 1^+ helper T cells of young (2 months old) BALB/c nude mice points to a peculiar trait of this otherwise normal and immunocompetent population.[29]

Helper T lymphocytes also express the L3T4 antigen which is — unlike Lyt 1 — mutually exclusive with Lyt 2 in peripheral lymphocytes.[34] It was revealed by flow microfluorometry that the proportion of L3T4-positive cells is reduced much more than the proportion of Lyt 2^+ (or Thy 1^+) cells in aged nude C57Bl or BALB/c mice: the L3T4:Lyt 2 ratio was 1.4 in nu/+ C57Bl mice and 0.4 in *nu/nu* C57Bl mice aged over 6 months.[35] Again, possible precursor cells with the ontogenetically early phenotype Thy 1^+ Lyt 2^- L3T4^{-34} were found in elevated numbers in nude mouse lymph nodes and spleen suspensions, but the phenotype Lyt 2^+ L3T4$^+$ which makes up 80 to 85% of normal thymocytes[36,37] was missing.[35] It is likely that the L3T4 differentiation marker is almost exclusively dependent on the thymic Ia-positive stroma[38] and can only be induced in a minimal degree by other microenvironments. A high individual variation of the expression of L3T4 was found among nude C57Bl mice.[35] Also in the nude athymic rat a deeper defect in cells with the phenotype and function of helper T cells than in cytotoxic T cells was established, using 16- to 18-month-old animals.[39]

The occurrence of nude mouse T-lineage cells defined in functional assays seems to follow the pattern of delayed and stimulus-dependent appearance. In C57Bl mice aged 5 to 8 months, the cytolytic activity of splenic cells stimulated in a mixed lymphocyte culture was (on a per cell basis) about 25 times lower in nu/nu mice than in euthymic mice after 5 days of culture and 2 to 5 times lower after 7 days.[40] The frequency of cytolytic T lymphocyte precursors in old C57Bl nude mice was again by two to three orders lower than in euthymic controls.[41] The frequency of IL-2-producing cells increased with age and in N:NIH(s)II mice the increment was as high as three orders of magnitude between nudes aged 1.5 month and 4 to 5 months. In control *nu/+* mice the frequency was stable and even in aged mice by one order higher than in nudes.[30,42] Endogenous production of IL 2 and immune interferon in aged (9 months) but not young (2 months) CBA *nu/nu* mice spleen cells has been described; the production was similar to that of *nu/+* controls and appeared to be closely linked to the generation of cytotoxic T cells.[43]

The first report on in vitro generation of cytotoxic T lymphocytes from nude mouse spleen cell suspensions (in the presence of exogenous IL 2) already noted that these cells were able to respond to alloantigens (H-2 disparate cells).[44] In an isolated report, nude mouse T-cells helpers specific for the bacterial antigen flagellin were pointed out.[45] This means that the key role of T cells, i.e., alloantigen and conventional antigen recognition, exists among nude mouse T cells.

Mapping studies indicated that nude cytotoxic T cells recognized H-2 K and H-2 D region-encoded antigens[27] and even a mutated H-2 K^b gene product.[27] Also, a response to xenogeneic (rat) stimulator cells could be induced.[46] The responses of nude mouse T cells to conventional antigens were confirmed on TNP-modified syngeneic cells and the H-2 restriction (recog-

Table 1
PROPERTIES OF NUDE MOUSE T CELLS

Thy 1 expression	Weak: numbers of positive cells increase with age; strong: few positive cells, small increase with age
Lyt 123 expression; TL expression	Positive cells present in peripheral lymphatic tissues
Lyt 1+-L3T4+ helper cells	Low numbers, delayed appearance
Lyt 2+ suppressor cells, cytotoxic cell precursors	Low numbers, delayed appearance
Anatomic distribution	Normal
Cell size	Cells larger than their counterparts from normal mice
IL 2 production and receptors	Low, delayed appearance
Functional T cells	Low proportion among cells of the respective phenotype
Specificity repertoire	Oligoclonal; individual variations in dominant clones; driven by natural pathogens
Precursor supply	Reduced; possible lack of Thy 1 expression in prethymic ontogeny

nition of conventional antigens only in the context with self determinants) proven by most experiments.[23,46-48] This extends the salient qualification of nude T cells to the recognition of H-2 antigens in general and makes them into something which would be in a euthymic animal labeled as the post-thymic cell. However, class II (Ia)-restricted T cells were undetectable by the techniques used so far in nude mice exhibiting self-KD-restricted responses.[49] This is obviously witnessed by the very low level of L3T4-positive helper cells mentioned above.[35] Also, in the nude mouse the marked specificity of the responses of T-cell subsets holds true; L3T4+ cells respond only to class II antigens, Lyt 2+ cells only to class I antigens.[50]

There is evidence that cytotoxic T-cell precursors, concanavalin A-responsive cells, and IL 2 production can be detected also in young supernudes (born and nursed by nude mothers) of NIH, BALB/c, and C57Bl/6J strains; the numbers of these functional T cells were smaller in supernudes than in conventional nudes, but they were "clearly present".[19] Consequently, in the *nu/nu* "athymic" model, full functional maturation can be achieved in different T-cell subsets without any intervention of a normal lymphatic thymus. The T-cell defect in the nude mice is deep, but basically quantitative. At least two studies implicate the possibility of some role of the dysgenetic thymus in differentiation of the few *nu/nu* "postthymic" cells.[19,28] The delayed development of T cells is coincident with an increase of the dysgenetic thymus and its different components.[51]

It cannot be ruled out that some of the mature T-cell functions such as IL 2 production may be due to NK cells[52] which are present in nude mice of all strains tested in increasing numbers after 4 weeks of age; their proportion culminates between 5 to 8 weeks of age and decreases thereafter. Their decrease is slower in nude mice than in euthymic controls.[53]

The peculiarities of the T lymphocytes developing in nude mouse tissues are surveyed in Table 1. The inevitable conclusion is that in addition to some Thy-1-positive progenitor population which is evidently prethymic and to immature T lymphocytes, a minimal population of typical and competent T lymphocytes does hesitatingly develop in the nude mouse.

II. THE SPECIFICITY PATTERN OF T CELLS

Even if we take into account the age dependence of T-cell marker expression, there is some discrepancy between the occurrence of different defined T-cell subsets and the demonstrable immune reactivity of nude mice. In our view the high incidence of T cells in aged nude mice is, as a rule, associated with a decline of phagocytosis[54] and sometimes perhaps with incipient exhaustion of precursor cell compartments.[55] Therefore, it does not necessarily lead to a marked increase of reactivity in all or most individuals. Also, as will be mentioned in Chapter 10, Section II, nude mice dependent on social thermoregulation (i.e., not individually caged) may be affected by thermoregulatory stresses in variable degrees.

In addition, there may be an abnormal specificity repertoire and an abnormal distribution of T-cell clones in nude mice.[23] The lack of processing by a normal thymus may result in a low cross-reactivity of alloreactive cytotoxic T cells and in the presence of H-2-restricted T cells for a reduced range of conventional antigens.[23] The high degree of variability in the specificity pattern of IL-2-producing cells and L3T4-positive T-helper cells among individual nude mice[35,56] and the high degree of variability of the specificity pattern of cytotoxic cell precursors among individual nude mice[46] appears to be consistent with the hypothesis that there is no qualitative difference in this respect between nude and euthymic mice. However, the slow and less effective differentiation of *nu/nu* T cells tends to result in an oligoclonal repertoire.[23,56] Also, the occasional "dramatic cross-reactivity patterns" of IL-2-producing cells in individual nude mice suggest the oligoclonal type of response,[56] the dominance of different T-cell clones in individual animals.

There is the logical possibility that few maturing T cells may fill the peripheral compartments by clonal expansion even without antigenic stimulation.[23] Alternatively, the pressure of a limited range of natural pathogens which the nude mouse cannot effectively cope with[57] provokes in aged, possibly pathogen-selected, nude mice the limited specificity repertoire of T-cell clones which reflect this driving force;[23] the occurrence of T cells primed for flagellin in CBA/J nude mice reported in one of the earliest contributions to the nude mice T-cell story[45] points in this direction.

In general, there is a low frequency of functional effectors among nude mouse T cell subsets phenotypically qualified for single functions. A "significant proportion of nude T cells may be fundamentally nonresponsive to antigens or mitogens",[56] the low frequency of responding cells appeared to be an "intrinsic property" of these cells.[58] In a high cloning efficiency system only 10% of mature T cells could be stimulated by a combination of concanavalin A and soluble factors.[59] Almost no T-cell receptor genes rearrangement and transcription were found in concanavalin A-activated *nu/nu* Thy-1[+] cells.[60] However, these studies "did not confirm the presence of other T-cell-specific messages in the RNA preparations used";[61] only 2- 3-month-old mice with a low T-cell occurrence[22] were used.

Using also 20-week-old BALB/c nude mice and the cloned genes of the alpha and beta chains of the T-cell receptor, low levels of the alpha and beta gene transcripts were found, with a prominent truncated message of the beta gene.[62] Interestingly, in this study an increased level of expression of full length gamma-chain messages were obtained; these nude T-receptor gamma gene products were functional and were suggested to be a specific trait of T-cell recognition of the "athymic" mouse.[62]

In 4- to 5-month-old N:NIH(s)II mice, meritorious in this field, MacDonald et al.[61] have established full-length transcripts for the alpha and beta genes, at a level two- to threefold lower in *nu/nu* than in *nu/+* mice. Monoclonal antibodies against a protein product of a beta chain variable region revealed a striking heterogeneity in the proportion of nude T cells expressing this protein. The expression was frequently associated only with the L3T4[+] or only with the Lyt 2[+] subset of T cells and it was found (by Southern blotting) that the pattern of beta-chain rearrangements is restricted in nude T cells compared to normal T cells.[61] It was concluded again that the restricted functional repertoire in individual nude mice may result from an oligoclonal expansion of T cells that have "randomly rearranged and expressed" the beta chain of the T-cell receptor.[61]

Essentially the same results were obtained in BALB/c nudes aged 20 months, full length alpha- and beta-chain messages were found in concentrated splenic T cells and sequence analysis of cDNA revealed completely rearranged V./D/-J-C gene segments which encode potentially functional proteins.[63] The T-cell receptor repertoire resulting from the slow gene rearrangements was suggested to be limited.[63]

Interestingly, studying cells with NK activity, Habu and co-workers have found the rearrangement of beta-chain gene of the T receptor in both nude mouse NK populations (one Thy 1[+] GA1[+], the second Thy 1[-] GA1[+]).[64]

Also, the IL 2 receptor and transferrin receptor expression which is of prime importance for T-cell proliferation, especially in the early stages of their development, has received some attention in nude mice studies. From experiments using exogenous IL 2 for the generation of T-cell-dependent functions in nude mouse cells it must be inferred that they express IL 2 receptors even before demonstrable endogenous IL 2 production.[44,27,28,65] On the other hand, Habu did not find IL-2 receptor-positive cells in nude mice spleens and uses this direct observation as evidence for the intrathymic expression of IL 2 receptor molecules.[66] Demonstrable IL 2 production in aged mice may, however, enhance the receptor expression.[28]

On the other hand, an IL-2-independent T-cell precursor compartment was thought upon as the site for T-cell diversification.[67,68] In the nude mouse, such an extrathymic T-cell subset would explain the somewhat surprising possibility to induce T-cell-mediated or -dependent functions including IgG responses, concanavalin A, and PHA responsiveness even in young individuals by i.p. injection of xenogeneic (human), heavily in vitro irradiated T lymphocytes in a narrow cell dose range.[69] Leukemic lymphoblasts which were completely unable to produce IL 2 in vitro were effective, leukemic cells producing IL 2 (Jurkat line) were without effect.[69] A model was suggested implying two extrathymic and thymus relatively independent T-cell pools; in the first, IL-2-independent, diversification, and clonal expansion would be induced by postthymic cells and the resulting T cells would populate the second, IL-2-dependent pool of cells competent to respond to antigens and mitogens. The first pool of T cells fails to expand in the nude mice because of the lack of postthymic inducer T cells. The second pool is consequently small and can be exhausted by artificial IL 2 treatment. In old nude mice both T-cell pools would slowly grow, "directed by nonspecific signals", until sufficient pool sizes and repertoires of T cells eventually develop.[69]

All work on nude mouse T cells, their receptor expression, and function may be complicated by the high levels of nude mouse NK cells and more generally of large granular lymphocytes comprising also the natural suppressor cells. Some of the suppressor activity found in young nude mice spleen[70] may be attributed to these cells, present at sites of "considerable hematopoiesis"[71] which is eminent in the *nu/nu* spleen.

The normal thymus, as shown by postirradiation repopulation experiments, does not contain a self-sustaining stem cell pool and must be continually supplied with exogenous precursors,[72] some of which may have a weak Thy 1 positivity[73] as the bulk of young nude mouse T-like cells. This continual supply of prethymic cells regulated at nude mouse hemopoietic sites by a low stem cell potential (Chapter 6, Section I) and possibly by an increased occurrence of large granular lymphocytes provides reduced numbers of T-cell clones which manage to mature into phenotypically and even functionally normal T cells; this may occur under the influence of factors of the dysgenetic thymus[74] and at extrathymic sites such as spleen with its thymocyte maturational factor or skin with its epidermal epithelial factors and Thy 1[+] or Ia[+] dendritic cells (Chapter 9, Section I). There is, however, growing evidence that the recognition of the self-H-2 determinants is already present in the prethymic cells both in the normal and athymic mouse.[75-77] Under the pressure of natural pathogens in adult and aging nude mice the extrathymic recruitment and restriction of the T cells may also be enhanced.

Analogous age-related development of mature T-cell phenotypes (associated with increased mitogen reactivity, but not with an in vivo immune response to a protein antigen) was observed in SPF nude rats.[39,78]

Since sex-related changes in mitogen and mixed lymphocyte reactivity have been described in some BALB/c mouse substrains (females being superior to males in some T-cell-mediated functions from 3 months to 1 year of age),[79] the development of T cells in nude mice should be analyzed also in this relation.

In sum, the athymic nude mouse stands as an excellent example for the general notion formulated by Stutman, that "postthymic T cells can express a thymus-independent state and can show extensive self-renewal, expansion, and functional activity in the absence of the thymus"[79] We would only add . . . in the absence of the normal lymphatic thymus. Stutman concludes: "While the degree of thymus-dependency of postthymic expansion needs some study, it is apparent that 'true' extrathymic T-cell differentiation in the absence of a thymus from putative 'prethymic' cells is a highly inefficient procedure for the generation of functional T cells".[80] To assure the biological success of the organism, this almost thymus-independent system must be supplemented by compensatory measures in other cellular defenses.

III. NATURAL KILLER AND CYTOTOXIC CELLS

Kindred[57] rates the natural killer (NK) cells as the "not depressed immune mechanisms" of the nude mouse and we have invoked the NK cells several times as a possible factor in both the defense systems and hematopoiesis regulations. NK cells belong, together with natural cytotoxic (NC) and natural suppressor (NS) cells, to the morphologically assessed large granular lymphocyte (LGL) family which appears to be a typical component of the nude mouse blood and spleen lymphoid population. In our SPF BALB/c females aged 4 to 7 weeks there were 18.3% of LGL of all lymphocytes, compared to 2.5% in +/+ controls; in BALB/c males of this age group 13.5% LGL in *nu/nu* against 2.7% in +/+ (means from 10 mice, tail vein blood). The numbers were slightly higher in the 8 to 12 week age groups and a little lower in B10LP mice of the respective genotype and age. This corresponds to the levels of NK activity in the original observations of Herberman[53] and Kiessling.[81] BALB/c and C57Bl mice belong to "moderate NK activity" strains.[82,84] It has been directly shown in BALB/c mice that LGL follow the NK activity in *nu/nu* vs. +/+ mice.[85] In C3H and BALB/c mice, LGL also followed the NK activity in organ distribution (peripheral blood, spleen, gut, lung, to a lesser extent bone marrow, and lymph nodes) and in age dependence.[85]

NK cells, in general, are more frequent in the spleens of nude mice older than 3 weeks. Cytotoxic activity appears at 4 to 5 weeks and reaches peak levels between 5 and 8 weeks of age in mice of all genotypes, the highest activity being attained in CBA and C3H mice and nudes being always superior to euthymic mice.[53,81-83] The decline of activity thereafter is steeper in euthymic mice, where no detectable activity is found in most animals over 12 weeks of age. In the nudes, the decline is much more gradual.[82]

The high frequency of NK cells was logically associated with the resistance of not-too-old nudes to spontaneous tumors[82,86-88] and to the oncogenic effects of methylcholantrene, urethane,[89] pristane, estrogen, transplacental oncogene 1-ethyl-1-nitrosurea and viruses (polyoma, Moloney sarcoma, Friend leukemia),[88] the resistance which might have been surprising in view of the immune surveillance theory[90] but, in fact, represents only an "alternative pathway of immunological responses against antigenic tumors".[88] This pathway was suggested by Herberman's hypothesis to be based on NK activity.[82] In Stutman's words, "there is no clear correlation between the remarkable immune deficit of the nude mouse and any form of peculiar risk for tumor development, either spontaneously or after exposure to a variety of oncogenic agents".[88] This is the effect of some "primitive immune surveillance"[91] shown to be based, in some situations, mainly on NK cells,[82,84,91,92] in others rather on macrophages and minor agents provoked by the specific properties of the tumor line in question.[93-96] In any case, NK cells helped in the hectic history of nude mouse oncological application to ruin the career of the mouse as a predictive test system in clinical oncology, of course, in combination with the tremendous heterogeneity of the human tumors cultivated in this model.[97]

The clear strain-dependence of the proportion of NK activity in nude mice[82,94,96] excludes the possibility that increased differentiation of NK cells, (LGL in general) is an obligatory compensation of the "athymic" state or a correlate to another compensatory factor. They may not simply be the pre-T cells which have missed the thymic inductive microenvironment. In parabiosed nude mice of the CBA background carrying the *xid* gene and a ten times higher NK activity in the spleen than their partners (Swiss outbred background), the level of NK activity was "at the lowest common denominator".[96] That means that the "low NK" partner has replaced some defect in the *xid-nu* mouse and in this way the need for, or mechanism of a high NK activity. The thymic dysgenesis was not the only cause. The association with a B-cell subpopulation is suggested also by the observation that the relative resistance to polyoma oncogenesis of 3-month-old nudes could be transferred to unprotected, sensitive newborn nudes by spleen cells sensitive both to anti-Thy 1.2 and anti-Ig treatment, i.e., the resistance of the respective (CBA/H background) *nu/nu* mice was due also to a late differentiation of some B-cell lineage.[98]

In the case of lymphoma development in the nudes, it is intriguing that the induction by skin painting with methylcholantrene appears not to correlate with the basal NK activity nor with interferon augmentation of NK activity;[94] on the other hand, an anti-μ-chain antibody induces lymphomas in *nu/nu* mice, in spite of high NK activity not affected or even induced by the anti-μ treatment.[99] This points to some B-cell peculiarity and questions the role of NK cells. It must be noted that natural cytotoxic cells[71] may act synergistically with NK in handling small numbers of tumor cells; their cytotoxic capacity does not require the presence of the conventional tumor-associated transplantation antigen,[94,100] their levels are not well documented in nude mice, and not well demarcated from the natural suppressor cells.[71]

Stutman[94] concludes that natural cell-mediated cytotoxicity develops its antitumor potential as "a by-product of its true function which was to act as a defense mechanism against bacterial, viral and parasitic invaders". We are here back at the beginnings of the great surveillance debate where the argument has been that "the rejection of allografts is a tiresome by-product of the existence of a body-wide monitoring system, of which the primary purpose is to identify and cause the rejection of malignant variants to normal tissue cells".[101]

The survival of both euthymic and athymic C57Bl/6 mice infected with herpes simplex virus type 1 was dramatically shortened after the NK activity had been almost eliminated by antibodies to asialo GM1 (a surface glycolipid ganglio-*N*-tetraosylceramide, typical of murine NK) and NK cells were suggested as one of the main barriers against herpetic infections.[102] Permanently virus-infected tumors were rejected by nude mice, but nude mouse NK cells failed to show cytotoxicity for the same lines when uninfected.[84,103] The experimental xenogeneic tumor cell lines infected with RNA viruses (mumps, measles, vesicular stomatitis, influenza, rabies) triggered a high cytotoxic activity in vitro in *nu/nu* (BALB/c) mice spleen cells; the activity was due to NK cells of two populations characterized by the presence of the asialo GM1 and Lyt 5 surface marker and differing in the presence of Thy 1.2.[84] The same populations sorted out by flow cytometry were lineaged with respect to the rearrangement of the T-receptor beta chain genes and showed a reduction of the germ line band of DNA, in other words, belong to the T-cell lineage[64] which is in accord with the demonstration T-cell receptors in rat and human LGL[104] and with the in vitro propagation by interleukin 2 of at least two NK clones derived from nude mice and reactive either against lymphoid tumor cells or lymphoid and solid tumor cells.[105]

The NK populations were obviously responsible for interferon production upon cocultivation of the virus-infected cell line with nude mouse spleen cells.[84] In vivo, only heavy irradiation or pretreatment with anti-mouse interferon (type I) could break the NK barrier of the nudes and induce invasiveness and metastases even of the virus-infected tumor cell lines.[84]

Interferon is very likely a regulator of NK activity and its production in nude mice seems not to be much different from normal in many situations. Nude mouse spleen cells pretreated with pure interferon had a markedly enhanced NK activity[78] and when cocultured with virus-infected cell lines released interferon into the medium.[106] Induction of interferon in vivo, in nude mice infected with herpes simplex virus, appeared to be normal,[107,108] induction with Newcastle disease virus was described as low in the nudes,[109] or at least delayed.[110] Even the production of interferon in the cultures of nude lymphoid cells stimulated with PHA (but not concanavalin A) was normal, in spite of the fact that the cells did not proliferate.[111,112]

Taken together, the antiviral defense based on mononuclear phagocytes (Chapter 6) and NK-interferon systems and lacking the bulk of cytotoxic T cells which recognize and kill virus-infected cells of the self H-2[113] seems to be sufficient for virulent, not specific, pathogens, but less effective with natural pathogens.[57]

Also, spontaneous neoplasms, lymphomas, which were described in some long-living nude mice (7 to 34 months) and affect as much as one half of the nude homozygotes, compared to 7% of the heterozygotes of the NIH/s strain, could suggest an inadequate barrier or countermeasure against a protracted irritation of lymphoid cells by RNA viruses carried both by NIH/s and BALB/c strains.[114] However, lymphoma incidence is by no means a general phenomenon in other nude mice strains or breeding colonies (Chapter 9, Section II).

It is likely that NK cells are connected with antimicrobial protection in general as a local effector with a major role in the first line defense,[115] in close relation with the phagocytic defense. In the case of *Toxoplasma* infection, it has been shown that the protozoon modulates the NK activity in the spleen and peritoneum and that the augmentation of NK activity is macrophage dependent.[116] Also, the localization and homing of specifically labeled LGL in athymic animals in close association with interdigitating cells, intestinal epithelia, in bronchus-associated lymphatic tissue, along capillaries in the liver, kidney, and bone marrow, and especially large numbers of LGL in lesions caused by bacteria and viruses (suppurative pneumonia, ulcers, enteritis, sialoadenitis)[117] correspond to a local antimicrobial defense role. LGL are usually in close contact with microbe-containing cells; we have observed such a situation in athymic nude mice infected with *Mycobacteria*. LGL identified ultrastructurally were localized in substantial numbers in the hyperplastic interdigitating cell network in the lymph node paracortex, and many LGL were closely apposed to *Mycobacteria*-loaded macrophages.[118]

There is also some evidence that infections contribute to the nude mouse resistance to skin tumor induction and prevention of wasting is essential for establishing the susceptibility of the nudes to chemical skin carcinogenesis.[119]

The nude mouse has decisively contributed to the definition of NK cells and appears to be a model of "paraimmunological" defense[94] based on natural cytotoxicity, interferon, and chronic activation of phagocytic systems.

The broader regulatory implications of the enhanced NK-NS activity on hematopoietic processes whichg may be affected by a humoral colony-inhibiting factor from these cells[120] and even on antibody response which may be limited by NK-based elimination of antigen-exposed accessory cells[121] is an open problem of the nude mouse immunology as is the presence of something like natural cytotoxic cells in the yolk sac of a 10-day mouse embryo.[122]

REFERENCES

1. **Raff, M. C. and Wortis, H. H.,** Thymus dependence of Θ-bearing cells in the peripheral tissues of mice, *Immunology,* 18, 931, 1970.
2. **Raff, M. C.,** Θ-bearing lymphocytes in nude mice, *Nature,* 246, 350, 1973.
3. **Lamelin, J. P., Lisowska-Bernstein, B., Matter, A., Ryser, J. E., and Vassali, P.,** Mouse thymus-independent and thymus-derived lymphoid cells. I. Immunofluorescent and functional studies, *J. Exp. Med.,* 136, 984, 1972.
4. **Loor, F. and Roelants, G. E.,** High frequency of T lineage lymphocytes in nude mouse spleen, *Nature,* 251, 229, 1974.
5. **Roelants, G. E., Mayor, K. S., Hägg, L. B., and Loor, F.,** Immature T lineage lymphocytes in athymic mice. Presence of TL, lifespan and homeostatic regulation, *Eur. J. Immunol.,* 6, 75, 1976.
6. **Cantor, H., Simpson, E., Sato, V. L., Fathman, C. G., and Herzenberg, L. A.,** Characterization of subpopulations of T lymphocytes. I. Separation and functional studies of peripheral T-cells binding different amounts of fluorescent anti-Thy 1.2 (theta) antibody using a fluorescence-activated cell sorter (FACS), *Cell. Immunol.,* 15, 180, 1975.
7. **Sato, V. L., Waksal, S. D., and Herzenberg, L. A.,** Identification and separation of pre T-cells from *nu/nu* mice: differentiation by preculture with thymic reticuloepithelial cells, *Cell. Immunol.,* 24, 173, 1976.
8. **Tyan, M. L.,** Studies on the ontogeny of the mouse immune system. I. Cell-bound immunity, *J. Immunol.,* 100, 535, 1968.
9. **Pritchard, H. and Micklem, H. S.,** The nude (*nu/nu*) mouse as a model of thymus and T-lymphocyte deficiency, in *Proc. 1st Int. Workshop on Nude Mice,* Rygaard, J. and Povlsen, C. O., Eds., G. Fischer, Stuttgart, 1974, 127.
10. **Cohen, F. E., Novotný, J., Sternberg, M. J. E., Campbell, G., and Williams, A. F.,** Analysis of structural similarities between brain Thy-1 antigen and immunoglobulin domains, *Biochem. J.,* 195, 31, 1981.
11. **Williams, A. F. and Gagnon, J.,** Neuronal cell Thy-1 glycoprotein: homology with immunoglobulin, *Science,* 216, 696, 1982.
12. **Bukovský, A., Presl, J., and Holub, M.,** The ovarian follicle as a model for the cell-mediated control of tissue growth, *Cell Tissue Res.,* 236, 717, 1984.
13. **Kollias, G., Evans, D. J., Ritter, M., Beech, J., Morris, R., and Grosveld, F.,** Ectopic expression of Thy-1 in the kidneys of transgenic mice induces functional and proliferative abnormalities, *Cell,* 51, 21, 1987.
14. **Ford, C. E., Micklem, H. S., Evans, E. P., Gray, J. G., and Ogden, D. A.,** The inflow of bone marrow cells to the thymus: studies with part-body irradiated mice injected with chromosome-marked bone-marrow and subjected to antigenic stimulation, *Ann. N.Y. Acad. Sci.,* 129, 283, 1966.
15. **Rosen, F. S.,** Defects in immunological development in man, in Ciba Foundation Symp. Ontogeny of Acquired Immunity, Associated Science, Amsterdam, 1972, 213.
16. **Loor, F., Hägg, L. B., Mayor, K. S., and Roelants, G. E.,** θ-positive cells in nude mice born from homozygous nu/nu mothers, *Nature,* 255, 657, 1975.
17. **Loor, F., Amstutz, H., Hägg, L.-B., Mayor, K. S., and Roelants, G. E.,** T lineage lymphocytes in nude mice born from homozygous nu/nu parents, *Eur. J. Immunol.,* 6, 663, 1976.
18. **Kramer, M. H. and Gershwin, M. E.,** Immune competency of nude mice bred from homozygous and heterozygous mothers, *Transplantation,* 22, 539, 1976.
19. **Ikehara, S., Pahwa, R. N., Fernandes, G., Hansen, C. T., and Good, R. A.,** Functional T cells in athymic nude mice, *Proc. Natl. Acad. Sci. U.S.A.,* 81, 886, 1984.
20. **Hale, M. L., Hanna, E. E., and Hansen, C. T.,** Nude mice from homozygous parents show smaller PFC response to sheep erythrocytes than nude mice from heterozygous mothers, *Nature,* 260, 44, 1976.
21. **Scheid, M. P., Goldstein, G., and Boyse, E. A.,** Differentiation of T cells in nude mice, *Science,* 190, 1211, 1975.
22. **MacDonald, H. R., Lees, R. K., Sordat, B., Zaech, J., Maryanski, J., and Bron, C.,** Age-associated increase in expression of the T cell surface markers Thy-1, Lyt-1 and Lyt-2 in congenitally athymic *nu/nu* mice: analysis by flow microfluorometry, *J. Immunol.,* 126, 865, 1981.
23. **Hünig, T.,** T-cell function and specificity in athymic mice, *Immunol. Today,* 4, 84, 1983.
24. **MacDonald, H. R.,** Phenotypic and functional characteristics of T-like cells in nude mice, *Exp. Cell Biol.,* 52, 2, 1984.
25. **Kindred, B.,** T cell functions in nude mice: lack of secondary antibody response in vitro, *Exp. Cell Biol.,* 52, 17, 1984.
26. **Bamat, J., Sordat, B., Lees, R. K., Zaech, P., Ceredig, R., and MacDonald, H. R.,** Development and localization of 'T-like' cells in the nude mouse, *Exp. Cell Biol.,* 52, 25, 1984.

27. **Hünig, T. and Bevan, M. J.**, Specificity of cytotoxic T cells from athymic mice, *J. Exp. Med.*, 152, 688, 1980.
28. **Stötter, H., Rüde, E., and Wagner, H.**, T cell factor (interleukin 2) allows in vivo induction of T helper cells against heterologous erythrocytes in athymic (*nu/nu*) mice, *Eur. J. Immunol.*, 10, 719, 1980.
29. **Ishikawa, H. and Saito, K.**, Congenitally athymic nude (*nu/nu*) mice have Thy-1-bearing immunocompetent helper T cells in their peritoneal cavity, *J. Exp. Med.*, 151, 965, 1980.
30. **MacDonald, H. R., Lees, R. M., Glasebrook, A. L., and Sordat, B.**, Interleukin 2 production by lymphoid cells from congenitally athymic (*nu/nu*) mice, *J. Immunol.*, 129, 521, 1982.
31. **Smith, J. B. and Eaton, G. J.**, Suppressor cells in spleens from "nude" mice: their effect on the mitogenic response of B lymphocytes, *J. Immunol.*, 117, 319, 1976.
32. **Holub, M., Fornůsek, L., Větvička, V., and Chalupná, J.**, Enhanced phagocytic activity of blood leukocytes in athymic nude mice, *J. Leukocyte Biol.*, 35, 605, 1984.
33. **Ranges, G. E., Goldstein, G., Boyse, E. A., and Scheid, M. P.**, T cell development in normal and thymopoietin-treated nude mice, *J. Exp. Med.*, 156, 1057, 1982.
34. **Ceredig, R., Dialynas, D. P., Fitch, F. W., and MacDonald, H. R.**, Precursors of T cell growth factor producing cells in the thymus ontogeny, frequency and quantitative recovery in a subpopulation of phenotypically mature thymocytes defined by monoclonal antibody GK-1.5, *J. Exp. Med.*, 158, 1654, 1983.
35. **MacDonald, H. R., Blanc, C., Lees, R. K., and Sordat, B.**, Abnormal distribution of T cell subsets in athymic mice, *J. Immunol.*, 136, 4337, 1986.
36. **Scollay, R.**, Intrathymic events in the differentiation of T lymphocytes: a continuing enigma, *Immunol. Today*, 4, 282, 1983.
37. **Mathieson, B. J. and Fowlkes, B. J.**, Cell surface antigen expression on thymocytes: development and phenotypic differentiation of intrathymic subsets, *Immunol. Rev.*, 82, 141, 1984.
38. **Kast, W. M., de Waal, L. P., and Melief, C. J. M.**, Thymus dictates major histocompatibility complex (MHC) specificity and immune response gene phenotype of class II MHC-restricted T cells but not of class I MHC-restricted T cells, *J. Exp. Med.*, 160, 1752, 1984.
39. **Vaessen, L. M. B., Schuurman, H.-J., Tielen, F. J., Hertogh, J. M. A., Broekhuizen, R., Vos, J. G., and Rozing, J.**, Phenotype and functional capacity of T-like cells in spleen of young and adult athymic (nude) rats, *Transpl. Proc.*, 19, 3127, 1987.
40. **Maryanski, J. L., MacDonald, H. R., Lees, R. K., Sordat, B., and Cerottini, J.-C.**, Alloreactive cytolytic T lymphocyte precursor cells in aged C57B1/6 *nu/nu* mice: frequency and cell surface phenotype, *Exp. Cell Biol.*, 52, 21, 1984.
41. **Maryanski, J. L., MacDonald, II. R., Sordat, B., and Cerottini, J. C.**, Cytolytic T lymphocyte precursor cells in congenitally athymic C57B1/6 *nu/nu* mice: quantitation, enrichment and specificity, *J. Immunol.*, 126, 871, 1981.
42. **Lees, R. K., MacDonald, H. R., Glasebrook, A. L., and Sordat, B.**, Interleukin-2 production by lymphoid cells from nude mice. A comparison of bulk culture and limiting dilution analysis, *Exp. Cell Biol.*, 52, 12, 1984.
43. **Klein, J. R. and Bevan, M. J.**, Secretion of immune interferon and generation of cytotoxic T cell activity in nude mice are dependent on interleukin 2: age-associated endogenous production of interleukin 2 in nude mice, *J. Immunol.*, 130, 1780, 1983.
44. **Gillis, S., Union, N. A., Baker, P. E., and Smith, K. A.**, The in vitro generation and sustained culture of nude mouse cytolytic T-lymphocytes, *J. Exp. Med.*, 149, 1460, 1979.
45. **Kirov, S. M.**, An anti-theta sensitive hapten-carrier response in nude mice, *Eur. J. Immunol.*, 4, 739, 1974.
46. **Hünig, T. and Bevan, M. J.**, Ability of nude mice to generate alloreactive, xenoreactive and H-2-restricted cytotoxic T-lymphocyte responses, *Exp. Cell Biol.*, 52, 7, 1984.
47. **Ando, I. and Hurme, M.**, Self-MHC-restricted cytotoxic T-cell responses without thymic influences, *Nature*, 289, 494, 1981.
48. **Wagner, H., Hardt, C., Bartlett, R., Pfizenmaier, K., Röllinghoff, M., and Heeg, K.**, T-lymphocyte progenitors from thymus deficient (*nu/nu*) mice differentiate in vitro in H-2 restricted hapten-specific cytotoxic effector cells, *Behring Inst. Mitt.*, 67, 105, 1980.
49. **Kruisbeek, A. M., Davis, M. L., Matis, L. A., and Longo, D. L.**, Self recognition specificity expressed by T cells from nude mice. Absence of detectable Ia-restricted T cells in nude mice that do exhibit self-KD-restricted T cell responses, *J. Exp. Med.*, 160, 839, 1984.
50. **Sprent, J., Schaefer, M., Lo, D., and Korngold, R.**, Functions of purified L3T4⁺ and Lyt 2⁺ cells in vitro and in vivo, *Immunol. Rev.*, 91, 195, 1986.
51. **Holub, M., Vaněček, R., and Rossman, P.**, The polycystic organ in senescent athymic nude mice and in euthymic mice, *Folia Biol. (Prague)*, 21, 382, 1975.
52. **Kasahara, T., Djeu, J. Y., Dougherty, S. F., and Oppenheim, J. J.**, Capacity of human large granular lymphocytes (LGL) to produce multiple lymphokines: interleukin 2, interferon, and colony stimulating factor, *J. Immunol.*, 131, 2379, 1983.

53. **Herberman, R. B., Nunn, M. E., and Lavrin, D. H.,** Natural cytotoxic reactivity of mouse lymphoid cells against syngeneic and allogeneic tumors. I. Distribution of reactivity and specificity, *Int. J. Cancer,* 16, 216, 1975.

54. **Holub, M., Větvička, V., Fornůsek, L., and Paluska, E.,** Phagocytic cells of athymic nude mice in fetal life, in *Immune-Deficient Animals in Biomedical Research, Proc. 5th IWIDA,* Rygaard, J. et al., Eds., S. Karger, Basel, 1987, 59.

55. **Holub, M., Hajdu, I., Jarošková, L., and Trebichavský, I.,** Lymphatic tissues and antibody-forming cells of athymic nude mice, *Z. Immunitactsforsch.* 146, 322, 1974.

56. **MacDonald, H. R. and Lees, R. K.,** Frequency and specificity of precursors of interleukin 2-producing cells in nude mice, *J. Immunol.,* 132, 605, 1984.

57. **Kindred, B.,** Deficient and sufficient immune systems in the nude mice, in *Immunologic Defects in Laboratory Animals,* Vol. 1, Gershwin, M. E. and Merchant, B., Eds., Plenum Press, New York, 1981, 215.

58. **MacDonald, R., Blanc, C., Lees, R. K., and Sordat, B.,** Development of T-dependent immune function in nude mice, in *Immune-Deficient Animals in Biomedical Research, Proc. 5th IWIDA,* Rygaard, J. et al., Eds, S. Karger, Basel, 1987, 51.

59. **Chen, W. F., Scollay, R., Shortman, K., Skinner, M., and Marbrook, J.,** T-cell development in the absence of a thymus: the number, the phenotype, and the functional capacity of T lymphocytes in nude mice, *Am. J. Anat.,* 170, 339, 1984.

60. **Owen, M. J., Jenkinson, E. J., Williams, G. T., Kingston, R., and Owen, J. J. T.,** An investigation of T cell receptor gene rearrangement and expression in organ cultures of normal embryonic thymus and Thy-1$^+$ cells of nude mice, *Eur. J. Immunol.,* 16, 875, 1986.

61. **MacDonald, H. R., Lees, R. K., Bron, C., Sordat, B., and Miescher, G.,** T cell antigen receptor expression in athymic (*nu/nu*) mice. Evidence for an oligoclonal β chain repertoire, *J. Exp. Med.,* 166, 195, 1987.

62. **Yoshikai, Y., Reis, M. D., and Mak, T. W.,** Athymic mice express a high level of functional γ-chain but greatly reduced levels of α- and β-chain T cell receptor messages, *Nature,* 324, 482, 1986.

63. **Kishihara, K., Yoshikai, Y., Matsuzaki, G., Mak, T. W., and Nomoto, K.,** Functional α and β T cell chain receptor messages can be detected in old but not in young athymic mice, *Eur. J. Immunol.,* 17, 477, 1987.

64. **Habu, S., Shimamura, K., Tamaoki, N., Kumagai, Y., and Okumura, K.,** Two natural killer cell populations which belong to the T lineage in nude mice, *Eur. J. Immunol.,* 16, 1453, 1986.

65. **Wagner, H., Hardt, C., Heeg, K., Röllinghoff, M., and Pfitzenmaier, K.,** T-cell-derived helper factor allows in vivo induction of cytotoxic T cells in *nu/nu* mice, *Nature,* 284, 278, 1980.

66. **Habu, S.,** IL 2 receptor expression on differentiating lymphocytes in the murine thymocyte, *Immunol. Rev.,* 92, 67, 1986.

67. **Ching, L. M. and Miller, R. G.,** Generation of cytotoxic T lymphocyte precursor cells in T cell colonies grown in vitro, *Nature,* 289, 802, 1981.

68. **Ching, L. M. and Miller, R. G.,** Development of cytotoxic t lymphocyte precursor cells in T cell colonies grown in vitro, *J. Immunol.,* 129, 2345, 1982.

69. **Dosch, H.-M., White, D., and Grant, C.,** Reconstitution of nude mouse T cell function in vivo: IL 2-independent effect of human T cells, *J. Immunol.,* 134, 336, 1985.

70. **Miller, R. G. and Derry, H.,** A cell propulation in *nu/nu* spleen can prevent generation of cytotoxic lymphocytes by normal spleen cells against self antigens of the *nu/nu* spleen, *J. Immunol.,* 122, 1502, 1979.

71. **Maier, T., Holda, J. H., and Claman, H. N.,** Natural suppressor (NS) cells. Members of the LGL regulatory family, *Immunol. Today,* 7, 312, 1986.

72. **Scollay, R., Smith, J., and Stauffer, V.,** Dynamics of early T cells: prothymocyte migration and proliferation in the adult mouse thymus, *Immunol. Rev.,* 91, 129, 1986.

73. **Basch, R. S. and Berman, J. W.,** Thy-1 determinants are present on many murine hematopoietic cells other than T cells, *Eur. J. Immunol.,* 12, 359, 1982.

74. **Ikehara, S., Yasumizu, R., Nakamura, T., Sekita, K., Muso, E., Ohtsuki, H., Ogura, M., Toki, J., Inoue, N., Sugiura, K., Iwai, H., Shintaku, M., Ihara, N., Hamashima, Y., and Good, R. A.,** Role of the thymus and the stem cells in the differentiation of T cells, in *Immune-Deficient Animals in Biomedical Research, Proc. 5th IWIDA,* Rygaard, J. et al., Eds., S. Karger, Basel, 1987, 69.

75. **Besedovsky, H. O., del Rey, A., and Sorkin, E.,** Role of prethymic cells inacquisition of self-tolerance, *J. Exp. Med.,* 150, 1351, 1979.

76. **Morrissey, P. J., Kruisbeek, A. M., Sharrow, S. O., and Singer, A.,** Tolerance of thymic cytotoxic T lymphocytes to allogeneic H-2 determinants encountered prethymically: evidence for expression of anti-H-2 receptors prior to entry into the thymus, *Proc. Natl. Acad. Sci. U.S.A.,* 79, 2003, 1982.

77. **Reimann, J. and Miller, R. G.,** Differentiation from precursors in athymic nude mouse bone marrow of unusual spontaneously cytolytic cells showing anti-self-H-2 specificity and bearing T cell markers, *J. Exp. Med.,* 158, 1672, 1983.

78. **Vaessen, L. M. B., Broekhuizen, R., Rozing, J., Vos, J. G., and Schuurman, H.-J.,** T-cell development during ageing in congenitally athymic (nude) rats, *Scand. J. Immunol.,* 24, 223, 1986.

79. **Belisle, E. H. and Strausser, H. R.,** Sex-related immunocompetence of Balb/c mice. II. Study of immunologic responsiveness of young, adult and aged mice, *Dev. Comp. Immunol.,* 5, 661, 1981.

80. **Stutman, O.,** Postthymic T-cell development, *Immunol. Rev.,* 91, 159, 1986.

81. **Kiessling, R., Klein, E., and Wigzell, H.,** "Natural" killer cells in the mouse. I. Cytotoxic cells with specificity for mouse Moloney leukemia cells. Specificity and distribution according to genotype, *Eur. J. Immunol.,* 5, 112, 1975.

82. **Herberman, R. B.,** Natural cell-mediated cytotoxicity in nude mice, in *The Nude Mouse in Experimental and Clinical Research,* Fogh, J. and Giovanella, B. C., Eds., Academic Press, New York, 1978, 135.

83. **Tamaoki, N., Habu, S., Okumura, K., Kasai, M., Akatsuka, A., Sato, T., Shimamura, K., and Saito, M.,** Characterization and strain difference of natural killer cells in nude mice, in *Proc. 3rd Int. Workshop on Nude Mice,* Reed, N. D., Ed., G. Fischer, New York, 1982, 413.

84. **Reid, L. M., Minato, N., Jones, C., Bloom, B., and Holland, J.,** Rejection of virus persistently infected tumor cells and its implications for regulation of tumor growth and metastasis in athymic nude mice, in *Proc. 3rd Int. Workshop on Nude Mice,* Reed, N. D., Ed., G. Fischer, New York, 1982, 505.

85. **Luini, W., Borasci, D., Alberti, S., Aleotti, A., and Tagliabue, A.,** Morphological characterization of a cell population responsible for natural killer activity, *Immunology,* 43, 663, 1981.

86. **Rygaard, J.,** *Thymus & Self, Immunobiology of the Mouse Mutant Nude,* F. A. D. L., Copenhagen, 1973, 163.

87. **Gershwin, M. E., Merchant, B., Gelfand, M. C., Vickers, J., Steinberg, A. D., and Hansen, C. T.,** The natural history and immunopathology of outbred athymic (nude) mice, *Clin. Immunol. Immunopathol.,* 4, 324, 1975.

88. **Stutman, O.,** Spontaneous, viral, and chemically induced tumors in the nude mouse, in *The Nude Mouse in Experimental and Clinical Research,* Fogh, J. and Giovanella, B. C., Eds., Academic Press, New York, 1978, 411.

89. **Stutman, O.,** Tumor development in immunologically deficient nude mice after exposure to chemical carcinogenesis, in *Proc. 1st Int. Workshop on Nude Mice,* Rygaard, J. and Povlsen, C. E., Eds., G. Fischer, Stuttgart, 1974, 257.

90. **Burnet, F. M.,** Immunological surveillance in neoplasia, *Transplant. Rev.,* 7, 3, 1971.

91. **Habu, S., Shimamura, K., Akamatsu, K., Okomura, K., and Tamaoki, N.,** Protective role of natural killer cells in tumor growth and viral infection in mice, *Exp. Cell Biol.,* 52, 40, 1984.

92. **Gorelik, E. and Herberman, R. B.,** Radioisotope assay for evaluation of in vivo natural cell-mediated resistance of mice to local transplantation of tumor cells, *Int. J. Cancer,* 27, 709, 1981.

93. **Simon, R. S., Klein, A. S., Kim, U., Freedman, V. H., and Shin, S.,** Thymus-independent host resistance against the growth and metastases of allogeneic and xenogeneic tumors in nude mice, in *Proc. 3rd Int. Workshop on Nude Mice,* Reed, N. D., Ed., G. Fischer, New York, 1982, 379.

94. **Stutman, O.,** Natural antitumor resistance in immuno-deficient mice, *Exp. Cell Biol.,* 52, 30, 1984.

95. **Jacubovich, R., Cabrillat, H., and Dore, J. F.,** Natural resistance to xenografts of human malignant melanoma cell lines in nude mice, *Exp. Cell Biol.,* 52, 48, 1984.

96. **Giovanella, B. C., Hunter, J. T., Gary, D. W., Stehlin, J. S., and Ledbetter, J.,** Nude mice of different strains in parabiosis for prolonged periods of time, *Exp. Cell Biol.,* 52, 114, 1984.

97. **Spang-Thomsen, M., Brünner, N., Engelholm, S. A., and Vindeløv, L. L.,** Therapy studies in nude mice, in *Immune-Deficient Animals in Biomedical Research, Proc. 5th IWIDA,* Rygaard, J. et al., Eds., S. Karger, Basel, 1987, 316.

98. **Stutman, O.,** Tumor development after polyoma infection in athymic nude mice, *J. Immunol.,* 114, 1213, 1975.

99. **Brodt, P. and Gordon, J.,** Antitumor-immunity in B-lymphocyte-deprived mice. II. In vitro studies, *Cell. Immunol.,* 65, 20, 1981.

100. **Stutman, O., Lattime, E. C., and Figarella, E. F.,** Natural cytotoxic cells against solid tumors in mice. A comparison with natural killer cells, *Fed. Proc. Fed. Am. Soc. Exp. Biol.,* 40, 2699, 1981.

101. **Medawar, P. B. and Medawar, J. S.,** *Aristotle to Zoos,* Harvard University Press, Cambridge, Mass., 1983, 156.

102. **Welsh, R. M.,** Mouse natural killer cells: induction, specificity and function, *J. Immunol.,* 121, 1631, 1978.

103. **Minato, N., Bloom, B., Jones, C., Holland, J., and Reid, L.,** Mechanism of rejection of virus persistently infected tumor cells by athymic nude mice, *J. Exp. Med.,* 149, 1117, 1979.

104. **Young, H. A., Ortaldo, J. R., Herberman, R. B., and Reynolds, C. W.,** Analysis of T cell receptors in highly purified rat and human large granular lymphocytes (LGL): lack of functional 1.3kb β-chain mRNA, *J. Immunol.,* 136, 2701, 1986.

105. **Kedar, E., Ikejiri, B. L., Sredni, B., Bonavida, B., and Herberman, R. B.,** Propagation of mouse cytotoxic clones with characteristics of natural killer (NK) cells, *Cell. Immunol.,* 69, 305, 1982.

106. **Minato, N., Reid, L., Cantor, H., Lengyel, P., and Bloom, B.,** Mode of regulation of natural killer cell activity by interferon, *J. Exp. Med.,* 152, 124, 1980.

107. **Zawatsky, R., Hilfenhaus, J., and Kirchner, H.,** Resistance of nude mice to Herpes simplex virus and correlation with in vitro production of interferon, *Cell. Immunol.,* 47, 424, 1979.

108. **Kirchner, H., Keyssner, K., Zawatsky, R., and Hilfenhaus, J.,** Interferon production in mouse spleen cells. II. Studies of the producer cell of Herpes simplex virus-induced interferon, *Immunobiology,* 157, 401, 1980.

109. **Yokota, Y., Kishida, T., Esaki, K., and Kawamata, J.,** Lower production of circulating interferon in congenitally athymic (nude) mice induced by intravenous administration of Newcastle disease virus, *Biken J.,* 18, 275, 1975.

110. **Pantelouris, E. M. and Pringle, C. R.,** Interferon production in athymic nude mice, *J. Gen. Virol.,* 32, 149, 1976.

111. **Wietzerbin, J., Sefanos, S., Falcoff, R., Lucero, M., Calinot, L., and Falcoff, E.,** Immune interferon induced by phytohemagglutinin in nude mouse spleen cells, *Infect. Immun.,* 21, 966, 1978.

112. **Kirchner, H., Fenkl, H., Zawatsky, R., Engler, H., and Becker, H.,** Interferon production in mouse spleen cells. I. Dissociation between interferon production induced by phytohemagglutinin and concanavalin A in spleen cell cultures of nude mice, *Eur. J. Immunol.,* 10, 224, 1980.

113. **Zingernagel, R. M., Althage, A., Waterfield, E., Kindred, B., Welsh, R. M., Callahan, G., and Pincetl, P.,** Restriction specificities, alloreactivity and allotolerance expressed by T cell from nude mice reconstituted with H-2 compatible or incompatible thymus grafts, *J. Exp. Med.,* 151, 376, 1980.

114. **Parker, J. W., Joyce, J., and Pattengale, P.,** Spontaneous neoplasms in aged athymic (nude) mice, in *Proc. 3rd Int. Workshop on Nude Mice,* Reed, N. D., Ed., G. Fischer, New York, 1982, 347.

115. **Herberman, R. B. and Ortaldo, J. R.,** Natural killer cells: their role in defenses against disease, *Science,* 214, 24, 1981.

116. **Hauser, W. E., Sharma, S. D., and Remington, J. S.,** Natural killer cells induced by acute and chronic Toxoplasma infection, *Cell. Immunol.,* 69, 330, 1982.

117. **Ward, J. M., Argilan, F., and Reynolds, C. W.,** Immunoperoxidase localization of large granular lymphocytes in normal tissues and lesions of athymic nude rats, *J. Immunol.,* 131, 132, 1983.

118. **Kubín, M., Holub, M., Mohelská, H., and Schlegerová, D.,** Experimental infection with *Mycobacterium kansasii* in athymic nude mice, *Exp. Pathol.,* 25, 233, 1984.

119. **Holland, J. M. and Perkins, E. H.,** Resistance of germ-free athymic nude mice to two-stage skin cancerogenesis, in *Proc. 3rd Int. Workshop on Nude Mice,* Reed, N. D., Ed., G. Fischer, New York, 1982, 423.

120. **Degliantoni, G., Perussia, B., Mangoni, L., and Trinchieri, G.,** Inhibition of bone marrow colony formation by human natural killer cells and by natural killer cell-derived colony-inhibiting activity, *J. Exp. Med.,* 161, 1152, 1985.

121. **Abruzzo, L. V. and Rowley, D. A.,** Homeostasis of the antibody response: immunoregulation by NK cells, *Science,* 222, 581, 1983.

122. **Dahl, C. A.,** Natural cytotoxicity in the mouse embryo: characterization of yolk sac-associated natural cytotoxic cells and their activity, *Eur. J. Immunol.,* 13, 747, 1983.

Chapter 5

B CELLS AND IMMUNOGLOBULINS

I. INTRODUCTION

The nude mouse is by no means a B mouse, even if the surprisingly high proportion of non-B cells occurs only in the spleen, and the blood and lymph appear to carry almost pure B cells.[1-3] The essential question pertaining to B-cell populations is whether they are just B cells left alone, or more or less altered clones of cells affected by genetic or epigenetic factors of the nude mouse lymphatic tissues and/or hormonal and metabolic peculiarities. The deep depression of responses to thymus-dependent antigens, of some immunoglobulin isotypes, of memory and tolerance induction[4] was explainable by the lack of T-cell regulation as a dominant trait of nude mouse B cells and thus, most interpretations were centered on athymic state and not at more basic, prethymic defects which would be reflected also by B cells.

II. B-CELL TURNOVER AND DIFFERENTIATION

In lymphatic tissues and in circulation, the nude mouse B cells seem to be numerically about equal to B cells of euthymic mice, just stripped of the bulk of the T-cell population. Sprent has shown in the thoracic duct lymph surprisingly corresponding numbers of B cells (Fc receptor- or sIg-bearing cells) in CBA $+/+$, nu/nu, and "littermates of nu/nu".[3,5] In lymphatic tissues B-cell areas are packed with lymphocytes, T-cell areas are reticular and populated only by scarce lymphocytes.[6] One important difference in the B-cell areas resides in the fact established very early in the era of basic nude mouse studies, namely that the nude mouse lymphocytes residing in the cortex of lymph nodes, the B area, have a longer life-span and are more sessile than paracortical, T area-resident, lymphocytes;[7,8] in euthymic mice long-lived T lymphocytes dominate the paracortex and newly formed cells, mostly B, concentrate in the cortex.[9] Most of the data come from experiments with young (4- to 6-week-old) NMRI or CBA nude mice; there is no information whether the atypical homing and/or turnover of lymph node B cells would occur also in older nudes. Here, the B lymphocytes are confronted and regulated by progressively increasing numbers of T cells of different subsets (Chapter 4).

During prolonged thoracic duct drainage in the nude mice, the number of newly formed cells, coming mostly through the paracortical areas of the lymph nodes, decreases as these cells are obviously drained away[10] and replaced by sessile long-lived B cells from the cortical nodules. This is again in opposition to the kinetics of thoracic duct cells in normal mice.[8] The normal overall input of B cells into the thoracic duct lymph declines only slowly, from 1.2×10^7 cells per 12 hr at day 1 of cannulation to 5×10^6 cells per 12 hr at day 10, showing an adequate supply of precursors. Prolonged administration of 3H thymidine showed that nude mouse thoracic duct cells have a much shorter life-span than the T and B thoracic duct lymphocytes of euthymic CBA mice. The majority of B cells from nude lymphatic organs display a similar life-span of 5 to 7 weeks.[7,8] However, there is about 15% of rapidly proliferating cells in the spleen[8] and small lymphocytes with a life-span of a few days exist in the bone marrow; these cells may either die there or emigrate.[7]

In the adult bone marrow there are far more B lymphocytes produced than are needed to maintain the B-cell pool on the periphery. Virgin B cells are short-lived, unless they are recruited in peripheral tissues following antigen activation or following depletion of the peripheral B-cell pool.[11] Under normal conditions, the bone marrow of young adult mice produces about 50×10^6 B lymphocytes per day and the nude mouse bone marrow seems to be equivalent to the bone marrow of euthymic mice in this respect, with variations due to age and exogenous antigen pressure.[12] Stem cells enumerated in transplantation assays (Chapter 6, Section I) and defective in the nudes are obviously irrelevant to the B-cell lineage representing mostly precursors committed to erythroid and myeloid lineages.[13] Alternatively, if the putative lymphoid stem cell and B progenitors mirror the nude mesenchymal defect, they may be upregulated by exogenous or internal factors such as interleukin 1, which has been shown to enhance the functional maturation of normal surface Ig-positive B-cell precursors[14] as well as the in vitro response of nude spleen cells to sheep red blood cells.[15]

The economy and internal regulation of lymphoid cell lineages, of the B-cell lineage(s) in the first place, appears to be quite different from those of the myeloid cell families: the lymphoid lineages establish a system memory, among other things by the return of mature stages to the central organ or central inducing microenvironment, the bone marrow in the case of B cells. Reentering mature-memory B cells render the cellular interactions and kinetics in the bone marrow too complicated for simple turnover and life-span assays.

As mentioned, a majority of B-lineage cells in the bone marrow are newly formed from precursor pools. They are continuously disseminated during terminal maturation and rapidly renewed. They acquire low densities of surface IgM already in the hemopoietic tissue and mature already within bone marrow sinusoids.[16] The bone marrow virgin B cells repopulate and maintain the pools of rapidly renewed virgin B cells in the lymphatic tissues. There these cells die after a short time unless they receive an appropriate signal.

It has been proposed[11] that the first phase of activation requires T-cell help and is initiated by antigen presented on interdigitating cells in the lymph node paracortex, in the splenic periarteriolar area, and other "T cell sites". The interdigitating cell networks are well developed in the nude mouse lymphatic organs (Chapter 8), but the process seems to be confined to short periods following antigen localization and does not proceed in later phases of responses to thymus-dependent antigens.[11] In the nude mouse tissue, this process may become important only during infections connected with the trapping of microbes in the interdigitating cell mesh.[17] By this process, the incoming virgin B cells are converted into memory B cells and antibody-secreting plasma cells which are markedly short-lived, with an average life-span of 3 days.[11] The rapid plasma cell turnover would then be associated with the active selection of B cells from the germ line repertoire. During the recruitment of virgin B cells, the immunoglobulin gene rearrangement occurs as a sequential process involving, first, by the time the bone marrow B precursor cells express the B-lineage antigens, the heavy chains; the light chain rearrangement occurs later, during the period of postmitotic maturation.[18] Already in these rapidly renewed virgin B cell pools in the lymphatic tissue, novel clonotypes may be created, anticipating further antigenic challenges.[16]

The second phase of B-cell activation is centered in the lymph node cortical follicles, splenic follicles, and other "B cell" sites, and is driven by an antigen exposed as immune complexes on the dendritic follicular cells during prolonged immune responses. Somatic mutations in rearranged immunoglobulin V-region genes may occur mainly here.[11] Memory B cells and long-lived virgin B cells are able to migrate into the follicular stroma and give rise to the germinal center formation. It is conjectured that somatic mutations in the DNA of V-region sequences occur especially in the centroblastic, rapidly proliferating stage of B cells;[11] centroblasts lose their surface immunoglobulins[19] which have been instrumental during the first phase of activation and can, consequently, expose the mutated gene product. This may also be the process of affinity maturation of the response. The cells not selected may die in the process within the germinal centers. Plasma cells generated in this phase have an average life-span of over 20 days and memory B cells, activated or not in this phase, may recirculate from the follicular locations.[11]

It is this second phase of B-cell activation which is severely limited in the nude mice and can be partly recovered only by thymus cells installed months before the B-cell activation by antigen.[20] Interleukin 2 failed to provoke the secondary response to SRBC in vivo[21] and no secondary response could be obtained after transfer of the spleen cells into another nude or an irradiated recipient or put in tissue culture;[22,21] only another primary (IgM) response resulted.

Activation by antigens which have multiple repeating determinants and are only slowly metabolized ("thymus-independent antigens") may occur by another cellular interaction, e.g., with the dendritic cells in the perifollicular, marginal zone in the spleen.

The recruitment of nude mouse B cells is not defective in the responses to thymus-independent antigens;[23,24] however, antilymphocyte sera which are supposed to neutralize the T suppressors of the response but not the T "amplifiers" do not enhance the B-cell response in nude 2- to 3-month-old mice, but provoke an enormous increase in euthymic controls.[23,24] Instead of postulating some ALS-resistant T-cell enhancement of the response, an explanation may be looked for in some B-cell limiting factor in the nude mouse.

Antigen-activated long-living B cells enter the B-cell recirculation pool on the periphery or, usually during a secondary response, recirculate back into the bone marrow and mature there to antibody-secreting plasma cells.[25] The number and repertoire of these bone marrow immunoglobulin-containing and secreting cells increases with age and contributes to the pool of free antibody (immunoglobulin) molecules which exceeds by several orders the number of B-cell receptors.[25] Also, a small part of the recirculating B-memory cells from the periphery reenters the bone marrow and forms a minority population of long-lived B lymphocytes.[16]

The reentry of recirculating B cells into the bone marrow is not seriously hampered in nude mice.[26] However, the recruitment of these cells, their idiotypic and antibody repertoire may be different from those of euthymic mice because one of the selective mechanisms, the T-cell help, is defective,[25] especially in the young nudes. This applies of course to all randomly activated B cells in all lymphatic organs.

Homing, activation phases, and eventual interactions with T cells of nude B cells seem to be affected by an additional disorder of stromal cells in the lymphatic organs which prevent normal migration of lymphocytes (presumably T cells) from euthymic mice.[24]

A decisive answer to the intrinsic B-lineage defect in the nude mouse which further complicates the above-mentioned disorders of inducing interactions has been provided by the studies of lipopolysaccharide (LPS) stimulation and of the mice carrying a combined defect of sex-linked immunodeficiency (xid) and nude. LPS acts as a polyclonal activator of nude mouse cells in vitro, but it is incapable of inducing responsiveness to sheep red blood cells (SRBC) or a protein antigen in vivo; it was concluded that nu/nu mice might be deficient in a B-cell population responsive to both the antigen and the polyclonal B-cell activator.[28]

The xid and nude mutations appear to provoke complementary defects in antibody formation.[29] Mice of the CBA/N background bred to express both mutations were found to lack mature B lymphocytes, there was a virtual absence of surface μ, κ, or λ₁ chains, no spleen cell responses to thymus-independent antigen and to LPS, less than 10% of a normal serum immunoglobulin level and no lymph node cortical follicles. It was concluded that there must be an intrinsic defect in one B-cell lineage due to the nude mutation, or a defect in the tissue normally inducing this lineage.[26] The intrinsic defect was suggested also by the differing electrophoretic mobility of nude and normal B cells[30] and by the observation of an abnormal binding of nude B cells to macrophages.[29]

The defective B-cell lineage was finally defined by Palacios and Leu.[31] A monoclonal antibody was developed, specific for mouse immature B cells sensitive for interleukin 3 (IL 3 supporting the growth and long-term cultures of the sensitive cells is produced by T cells). Using again the combined defect in xid-nude mice, the authors were able to show that the xid mutation renders the environment for B-cell precursors inefficient and nude mutation

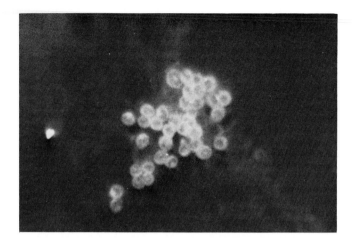

FIGURE 1.   Cluster of large lymphoid cells positive for Lyt 1 and sIgM, situated on the omentum of B10.LP *nu/nu* female, aged 6 weeks, injected with LPS i.p. 30 min before sacrifice. (Rat anti-μ-chain polyclonal antibody — SwARa-TRITC, mouse anti-Lyt-1 monoclonal antibody + biotin — avidin + FITC; magnification × 400.)

affects the capacity of precursors of IL-3-insensitive (IL 3 receptor-missing) B cells to differentiate.[31] IL-3-sensitive B-cell precursors are normal in *nu/nu* mice and IL 3 may be produced there by some bone marrow and spleen cells which are Thy 1[+] and negative for more mature T-cell markers.[31] The results are compatible with the assumption of two B-cell lineages, both having "B stem cells",[31] one sensitive for IL 3, one missing the receptors. The IL 3 R[+] lineage would split into precursors of cells bearing surface IgM and maturing B-cell markers and into precursors of Lyt 1[+] sIgM[+] B cells which do not recirculate back into the bone marrow, but give rise to a self-supplementing subset in the peritoneal cavity which produces autoantibodies[32,33] and is not missing in nude mice (Figure 1).

The nude mutant misses the maturing cells of the IL 3 R[-] lineage which use an unknown growth factor and may be responsible for the intrinsic peculiarities described in the nude mouse B-cell system. In this way, the problem again points back to the mesenchymal defect affecting the bone marrow stem cell potential and recruitment.

III. ANTIBODY FORMATION

It can be expected — as mentioned in the previous section — that the specificity repertoire of nude mouse B cells may be different from that of euthymic mice, due to changed selective mechanisms. The repertoire diversity is determined to a high degree by inheritance,[34,35] however, the control of the phenotypic expression is multigenic[36] and the microenvironments of the precursor cells affect the process considerably.[37,38]

By characterization of influenza virus hemagglutinin-specific antibodies in reactivity pattern analysis it was found that in 2- to 3-month-old BALB/c and BALB/c nude mice the repertoires are about equal, extremely diverse, and only the expansion of single clones was reduced in the *nu/nu* model.[39] This was not observed with some other antigens, e.g., the frequency of B cells responsive to sheep erythrocytes was normal in the microculture system of Lefkowitz.[40] In the same system, the frequencies of precursors for anti-NIP or anti-DNP haptens were even greater[41,42] and increasing with age. In the neonatal nude spleen, the anti-NIP precursors were by one order less numerous but increased about 17 times upon 72-hr culture.[43]

In the commonly studied response to SRBC, the nude mouse is agreed to be inferior to euthymic controls especially in indirect (IgG) plaque-forming cells (PFC).[44-49] Cells with high antigen-binding capacity are present in the nude mouse spleen, albeit in smaller numbers (BALB/c strain).[50a]

In the enumeration of plaque-forming cells of the spleen, the nude mouse may give lower counts, if the PFC are expressed per all nucleated cells and the erythroblasts which look in suspensions very much like small lymphocytes are not subtracted. Erythropoiesis is much higher in the spleen red pulp of nude mice than in the spleen of euthymic $+/+$ mice up to the 5th month of age.[50] Discrepancies in PFC counts in the nudes should be confirmed by serum antibody titers. In general, high individual variability among nude mice obviously reflects the nature of their T-cell systems (Chapter 4, Section II) and variations of some physiological parameters (Chapter 10).

Some disagreement of the results among single laboratories, especially from the early days of nude mouse housing, may be due also to the epidemiologic status in conventional colonies defined too liberally, and to the age of experimental animals. Infections, as opposed to experimentally applied bacterial adjuvants, tend to have an enhancing action on the humoral responses to xenogeneic erythrocytes; in the case of pinworms (*Aspicularis, Syphacia*), a marked correlation of hemagglutinating antibodies with the infection was described.[51]

Additional confusion may be caused by the reference-control euthymic animal and its response. There is no doubt that the *nu/+* heterozygote is markedly different in its antigen-binding cells, surface IgG-expressing cells, and antibody forming cells from $+/+$ mice.[50,52]

In the primary response, the numbers of plaque-forming cells (IgM) were comparable to the responses of the haired littermates in an unspecified colony and at the age of 5 to 6 weeks; the main difference was the early decline after day 4 of response in the nudes, whereas the peak in the controls was attained at day 6 both in PFC and serum hemolysins.[44]

A systematic study of the effect of antigen dose on the anti-SRBC response of nude mice and nonspecified haired littermates[46] has shown that the nude mice mount higher primary responses (day 5) at high SRBC doses (10^9 to 10^{10}), but they never match the euthymic controls.[46]

A comparison of nude mice of three different backgrounds has shown that they follow the reactivity (anti-SRBC IgM PFC primary response day 5) of the normal mice of the respective strain and display a ratio of 1.6% of the control (euthymic) IgM PFC number in C3H, 6.1% in BALB/c and 13.5% in C57Bl/6 which was the best responder in these experiments.[1] We have found some differences between BALB/c nudes and C57Bl/10 ScSn nudes in terms of IgM PFC and enhancement of the responses by levamisole,[53] which may correspond to the genetic differences of the background strains.[54]

The secondary response to SRBC looked very much like the primary in IgM PFC, the IgG secondary response hardly climbed above the background.[44] In one outbred nude mouse colony of very good viability and survival time — N:NIH(s) background — no increase of the PFC response, measured at day 4 of the primary IgM PFC production, with the age of the nudes, was described, not even in 1-year-old mice.[49]

Also, no basic differences were established in the anti-SRBC responses in nude mice raised under germ-free, specific pathogen-free (SPF) and conventional conditions[55] which is rather striking in view of a very likely dependence of the nude mouse T-cell maturation on their epidemiological status (Chapter 4, Section I). In any case, the reservation must be made that "conventional" has a very broad sense and should not include colonies heavily infested and limited by parasites and dying of mouse hepatitis virus during the first months of life, as was the case in the earliest days of nude mouse experimentation.

In a careful analysis of the anti-SRBC response in BALB/c mice, females, aged 10 to 14 weeks and housed in SPF conditions, it was found that antigen-binding cells (ABC) increased 11-fold in $+/+$ mice, 24-fold in *nu/+* at day 5, and only about twice after 25 days in *nu/*

nu. Among the antigen-binding B cells, there was an increase of sIgG cells to about 65% in *nu/+* and *+/+* mice and only to 38% (from 18% at day 0) in *nu/nu*. On day 12 there was a decline of sIgG cells in *+/+* and *nu/nu* mice, but not in *nu/+*. Minor changes occurred in sIgM expression of ABC in mice of all genotypes. Surface IgD expression on ABC declined between day 0 and 5 only in *nu/+* mice and not in *nu/nu* (36 and 27%) or *+/+* (37 and 37%).[52]

IgM-secreting cells (PFC in the protein A-SRBC plaque assay) had the highest level in *nu/nu* before and after SRBC immunization and no significant increase of the total IgM-secreting cells was seen in any group.[52] On the contrary, total IgG-secreting cells expanded 100-fold between day 0 and 5 in *+/+* mice reaching a double of the level of the *nu/+*, whereas in the *nu/nu* there was a very slow twofold increase from day 0 to day 25.[52] Specific anti-SRBC PFC of the IgM isotype reached a maximum at day 5 (no earlier days were investigated); the increase in *+/+* was more than 100-fold; *nu/+* had 1.5 times more PFC than *+/+*, and *nu/nu* had one tenth of those of *+/+*. All counts declined on days 12 and 25. Specific anti-SRBC PFC of the IgG isotypes increased by more than three orders in *+/+* and *nu/+* mice from day 0 to day 5, however, *nu/+* reached only two thirds of the *+/+* level and declined more slowly in the later days. In the *nu/nu* group, only individual animals had some IgG PFC at day 5 with some increase to day 12.[52] It is evident that the nudes slightly increase the antigen-binding cells and the expression of surface IgG on antigen-binding cells during the primary response. The response of secretory cells is confined almost entirely to the IgM isotype but, in addition to the high level of total IgM-secreting cells, there is a proportion of nonspecific IgG-secreting cells increasing very slowly during the response. The lack of expansion of the activated B-cell clones is compatible with the view that B cells of the primary response stop just short of cell division.[56] or, alternatively, that the intrinsic nude B-cell defect of the non-IL-3-reactive population becomes visible. In favor of the second possibility speaks the fact that we could restore the secondary response and IgG PFC by transfer of bone marrow cells from a *nu/+* littermate (CBA/J) immediately after birth (immunization at 2 months).[50]

The *nu* gene-bearing euthymic mice (*nu/+*) — compared to *+/+* — have a delayed switch from IgM to IgG production, persisting higher numbers of antigen-binding cells expressing surface IgG, but a lower number of specific IgG-secreting cells on day 5 of the primary response. Fehninger and co-authors conclude that *nu/+* mice may be deficient in a T-suppressor population as documented also by cell transfer experiments; in addition, the *nu/+* heterozygote may be lacking some isotype-specific T helper cells[57] involved in the development of SRBC-induced nonspecific PFC.[52]

Abnormalities in the splenic microenvironment were not ruled out in the heterozygous mouse,[52] but there are no data which would suggest some changes comparable with the *nu/nu* B-cell microenvironment (Chapter 8, Section I). Differences between *nu/+* and *+/+* were found also in the responses to thyroglobulin, both in terms of histopathologic changes and antibody production.[57a]

An interesting difference in antibody formation was observed also among all three genotypes of our BALB/c and C57 Bl ScSn and LP mice after immunization with BSA (bovine serum albumin) or with a PEG_{29}-BSA polymer.[58] After three i.p. injections of 100 μg of alum-precipitated BSA in 2-week intervals and 7 days after the last injection, antibodies were measured by an ELISA test, using BSA or PEG_{29}-BSA as the antigen. The titers against BSA were 1:32,000 in BALB/c *nu/+* mice and 1:64,000 in BALB/c *+/+*, 1:64,000 in B10.LP *nu/+*, and 1:2000 in B10.LP *+/+* (groups of seven mice). Nude homozygotes of both backgrounds had only 1:32 to 1:64 titers. The titers of antibodies after BSA immunization, but with PEG_{29}-BSA as antigen in the ELISA test, were lower in all *nu/+* and *+/+* animals, on the same marginal level in the nudes. When, however, the less immunogenic PEG_{29}-BSA polymer was used for immunization according to the same schedule, there was a striking reduction of the *nu/+* response. In mice of the BALB/c background, the response of +/+ mice was 1:16,000 (measured against BSA or against PEG_{29}-BSA), *nu/+* mice had titers of 1:256 and 1:32, respectively. In the C27Bl strains the responses of +/+ were 1:1000 against both antigens, the responses of *nu/+* were 1:32 against PEG_{29}-BSA and 1:16 against BSA, *nu/nu* mice of both backgrounds had titers of 1:64 (PEG_{29}-BSA) and 1:8 (BSA).[58]

Since the PEG-BSA polymer has a different distribution and persists longer in the organism, the involvement of the phagocytic systems in the reaction may be different and may be implicated in the differences between the BALB/c and C57Bl mice.[59] Phagocytic systems of *nu/+* heterozygotes do, however, not differ from +/+ mice (Chapter 7) and consequently could not explain the impressive difference in antibody formation against the less immunogenic PEG_{29}-BSA. The response to different epitopes on the BSA molecule exposed or hidden in the PEG polymer may be one of the cues, in addition to some T-cell deficit of the *nu/+* mice; these are very likely connected with the quantitative (if not qualitative) alteration of the *nu/+* thymus as described in Chapter 3, Section V). Not all euthymic mice are equally euthymic. The *nu/+* littermate "cannot be used as a normal control for any *nu/nu* immune function unless it is also compared to +/+ animals of the same strains".[52]

The nude mouse lack of IgG response against SRBC,[47,52] lack of memory cells, and secondary response induction[44] is associated with the lack of plasma cell differentiation in the primary response or after booster stimulation, on day 5 or 10. Compared to 22% of plasma cells in +/+ mice (CBA/J) we have found 2 to 5% of plasma cells in the centers of the hemolytic plaques of *nu/nu* mice, the majority of PFC in *nu/nu* were lymphocytes.[50,60] The proportion of plasma cells could be brought to normal by the transfer of different kinds of peritoneal exudate cells from littermates at the time of immunization.[50,61] This type of supplementation of the CBA/J nude mice led also to an improvement of the primary response to SRBC and suggested an additional defect in antigen processing present in the nudes and to some extent also in the heterozygous mice with low blood leukocyte counts.[50,60,61] Transfer of bone marrow cells from a *nu/+* donor to newborn nudes resulted in an increase of plasma cell differentiation in both the primary and secondary responses; among the IgG PFC the plasma cell proportion was 45%.

Kindred and Weiler[62] obtained in a partially backcrossed stock of BALB/c nude mice an analogous improvement of the hemagglutinin response with spleen, lymph node, and peritoneal cells; they have shown that the antibodies are mostly produced by the nude host. Transfer of bone marrow cells and fetal liver, spleen, and thymus cells were unsuccessful with the exception of one bone marrow transfer.[62] The central defect in the B lineages can presumably be corrected to a higher degree only during the perinatal period.

The lack of plasma cell differentiation in nonsupplemented nude mice was also observed in the response against horseradish peroxidase administered intraperitoneally; in the omentum, the antibody-containing cells were detected by horseradish peroxidase labeling. The proportion of plasma cells in the omental pseudofollicles was 5 to 7% on day 6 and 3 to 6% on day 7 of the response, the majority of antibody-containing cells being ribosome-rich lymphocytes.[60] Types of antibody-secreting cells of the nude mouse are given in Figure 2. It is obvious that the rate of synthesis, glycosylation, intracellular transport, secretion, and storage of the IgM or IgG antibody in these ultrastructural types of cells must be very diverse.[63] Some of the nude mouse antibody-secreting (-releasing) cells were never found in euthymic animals (Figure 2C). No mitoses were recorded among the PFC of nude mice in accordance with the assumptions mentioned above.

A lower proportion of plasma cells among PFC was noted also in the leukopenic littermates, the bulk of which might have been of the *nu/+* genotype.[50] In these CBA/J mice the primary response to SRBC was on day 5 considerably lower than that of the CBA/J +/+.[50] In mice of the BALB/c background we noted a dependence of the response of the *nu/+* heterozygote

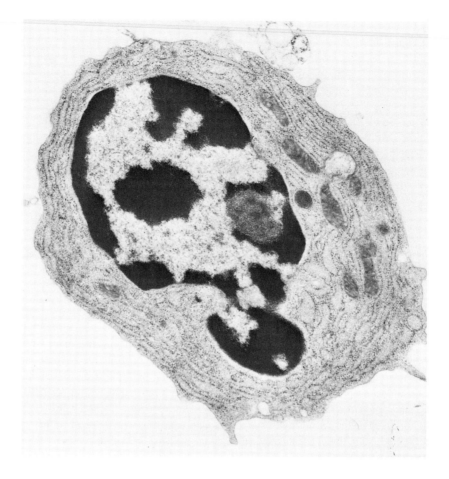

A

FIGURE 2.   Plaque-forming cells from CBA/J *nu/nu* mouse spleen, day 5 of primary response against sheep erythrocytes. Transmission electron microscopy (A) plasma cell; magnification × 18,000, (B) small lymphocyte; magnification × 20,000, (C) cell of a mixed morphology, with a number of mononuclear traits (residual bodies, dense bodies, projections), magnification × 16,000. (Dr. I. Hajdu.)

on the amount of SRBC injected, the response to 10^8 being higher than that to 10^7. The latter dose gave at day 5 of the primary response less IgM PFC in *nu/+* than in *+/+*.[64] In general, some essential difference in the regulation of the primary response between *+/+* and *nu/+* mice clearly shown by Fehninger and collaborators[52] in different sublines of BALB/c is present also in mice of other strains. No clear-cut results are available with other antigens. All work done has been centered on the "athymic" responses.

With bacteriophages, the "SRBC type" of response was obtained in the case of fd phage where the secondary is the same as primary; T4 phage gave no secondary response at all.[65,66] Interestingly, phage ϕx elicited a low secondary response[66] including, possibly, IgG.

The antibacterial response *(Brucella abortus)* consisted in *nu/nu* of IgM antibodies and was considerably prolonged over the control (BALB/c) response.[67] *Bordetella pertussis* had only a limited adjuvant effect on the primary response to SRBC and the background PFC, a slight increase of IgG PFC occurred in the primary response but no secondary response could be incuded in NMRI nude mice of uncertain health status.[68] Gnotobiotic *nu/nu* mice recovering from Campylobacter infection were found to produce specific antibodies of the

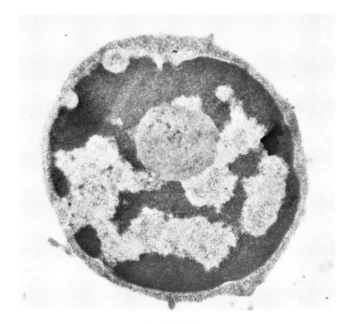

FIGURE 2B

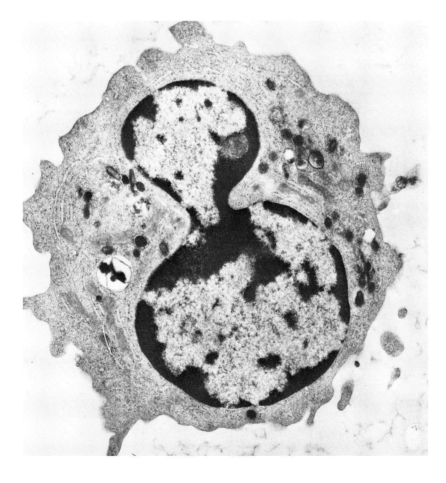

FIGURE 2C

IgG class.[70a] An IgG response could be produced in BALB/c nudes also by mucosal stimulation with *Mycoplasma pulmonis*.[71a]

No response was obtained in the *nu/nu* mice with Maia squinado hemocyanin (MSH), dinitrophenol-human globulin and DNP-polymerized flagellin.[67] No adjuvant effect of *Bordetella* was seen for the immunogenicity of MSH.[69] However, impressive high levels of background (spontaneous) PFC to a score of large synthetic haptens coupled to lysine residues on indicator SRBC were found in nudes in an outbred colony with a long survival time.[49] The highest numbers of PFC were recorded for tripeptide-enlarged representatives of dansyl, trinitrophenyl, and dinitrophenyl groups.[49]

To make the story even more complicated, N:NIH nude mice gave, under SPF conditions, a higher in vitro PFC response to TNP on rabbit erythrocytes when born to *nu/+* mothers than "supernudes" born to *nu/nu* mothers.[70] The response of supernude splenocytes could be supplemented by the splenocytes of "normal" nudes and it has been shown that the reason may be a higher T-precursor population in the spleens of the 5 to 8 week-old nudes.[70]

Also, the response to thymus-independent antigens in the nudes is not simply higher; generally, *nu/nu* and their cells in vitro respond as well as, or better than, euthymic mice.[23,50,71,72-80] Thymus-independent carriers like Ficoll coupled with a hapten (DNP) can induce a nude mice a "strong IgM and modest IgG memory" which is carrier specific. The IgM memory was not found in euthymic controls of the N:NIH background. IgG production in nude mice immunized by thymus-independent antigens has been repeatedly observed.[75,79] and a secondary response was also obtained with LPS,[74] but not with DNP-AE-dextran.[79] An intriguing observation on the mechanism of action of a thymus-independent antigen which elicits, in normal mice, responses in one class of Ig only, mostly IgM, comes from an experiment of Schuler and co-workers.[81] It was found by means of isoelectric focusing, hemagglutination, and immuno-diffusion techniques that perfectly backcrossed BALB/c nudes (8 to 14 weeks of age) produce after one i.p. injection of $\alpha(1\rightarrow3)$ dextran not only IgM, but also IgG antibodies of all IgG subclasses and so do almost all germ-free $+/+$ mice; however, conventionally raised euthymic BALB/c mice exhibit only a weak IgG response. Reconstitution of the *nu/nu* mice by splenic T cells from conventionally raised $+/+$ mice reduced the capacity of the *nu/nu* recipients to produce IgG anti-Dex antibodies.[81] T-cell-mediated suppression, neonatally induced in euthymic mice by the first contact with bacterial antigens, is postulated[81] and the "failure of *nu/nu* to suppress their IgG response" ascribed, e.g., to their inability to produce autologous anti-idiotypic antibodies.[81] This leaves open the question of why the *nu/nu* response to some other thymus-independent antigen is so defective in IgG and what would happen to the anti-Dex response in nudes which have developed more Lyt 2$^+$ cells (Chapter 4).

The nude mouse IgG antibodies displayed predominantly λ chains in the primary anti-Dex response[81] as noted in a different situation also by Wortis et al.[29]

A limited B-cell amplification mechanism in the nudes is suggested by the findings that they are more sensitive than euthymic mice to anti-heavy chain sera in neonatal life: treatment with anti-μ serum resulted in a complete loss of IgM and IgG with no recovery 2 months later, treatment with anti-α gave suppression of IgA, and anti-$\gamma_1\gamma_2$ caused subtotal suppression of IgG$_1$ and IgG$_2$.[82] This suggests that *nu/nu* mice in general may have a comparatively high proportion of B cells in a not fully differentiated state with multiple Ig isotypes expressed on the surface, as shown directly by Bankhurst and Warner.[83]

The literature on antibody formation could have yielded more insight into the mechanisms were it less extensive and more intensive, centered on standard mice and comparable techniques. The specificity repertoire and the IgM responses of the nude mice seem to be close to normal, only the expansion of clones and of antigen-binding cells may be limited and slowed down, leading to very depressed numbers of IgG antibody-producing plasma cells.

Table 1
PROPERTIES OF NUDE MOUSE B CELLS

sIg expression	Multiple sIg isotypes on a high proportion of B cells; low increase of sIgG on antigen-binding cells
Specificity repertoire	Normal or subnormal; expansion of clones markedly reduced
Ig secretion	High proportion of homogenous IgG_1, IgG generally reduced, IgA deeply defective; variation in individual mouse colonies and in individual mice
Antibody formation	IgM responses to thymus-dependent antigens low, IgG and secondary responses mostly absent; with thymus-independent antigens, IgM responses normal or supranormal, IgG responses may occur in all isotypes
Cytology	Low plasma cell differentiation in most reactions; antibody produced mostly by lymphocytic types
Precursor supply	Normal?
Bone marrow output and reentry	Normal, variations with age and different antigenic pressures
Anatomic distribution	Normal; in follicles (spleen, lymph nodes) a high proportion of sessile, long-living cells
Activation in lymphatic tissues	Nondefective with some thymus-independent antigens and polyclonal activators; with thymus-dependent antigens, defects in intercellular interaction visible especially in follicles — no germinal center formation
Subpopulations	Possible defect of Il-3-receptor-negative lineage

A lack of T regulation and a possible intrinsic defect in a B-cell subpopulation can be overcome with some thymus-independent antigens giving also IgG production of all subclasses and IgG memory. Defective T suppression of the IgG responses plays some role and this trait makes also the responses of $nu/+$ heterozygotes different from normal.

A tentative survey of some nude mouse B-cell properties is given in Table 1.

IV. TOLERANCE

Under the assumption that an antigen load leads in the absence of adequate T-cell help to specific unresponsiveness, nude mice have been injected with thymus-dependent antigens, notably sheep red blood cells (SRBC) or xenogenic α globulins. Later, with the same antigen and reconstituting T cells, specific unresponsiveness resulted.[28,84-87] A rather complicated immunological situation of the reconstituted nudes made it difficult to conclude on the recovery of responsivness in vivo, but the specific unresponsiveness could be transferred into irradiated hosts[84,86,87] and the unresponsive B cells could be induced by a variety of treatments before transfer to an active state.[86] Transfer into culture resulted in poor responsiveness.[85,88] and this was unaffected by the addition of allogeneic cells,[85] unlike the responses dependent on suppressor T cells. Increase of the number of responsive B cells upon 3 days of culture of bone marrow cells was inhibited by the presence of antigen in culture which was taken as evidence for clonal abortion.[89] Also, in vitro tolerance could be induced to different antigens.[42,90,91] The most likely interpretation was a tolerant state induced in the immature, unprotected, or deficient nude mouse B cells, e.g., inhibition of sIgG B cells in the absence of T cells.[84]

Avoiding the need of T-cell reconstitution of the nude mice for the visualization of the tolerant state, we used different schemes of levamisole administration after or during tolerization of nude mice of the BALB/c or C57B1/10 ScSn background (SPF, aged 5 to 7 weeks).[53] Levamisole is known to improve the anti-SRBC response of nude mice.[92] Pretreatment of nude mice by 10^8 or 10^9 SRBC i.p. 14 and 7 weeks before challenge with 10^8

Table 2
**INFLUENCE OF PRETREATMENT OF
BALB/c *nu/nu* RECIPIENTS WITH TWO
DOSES OF 10⁹ SRBC i.p. AT DAY 14 AND 7
ON PFC FORMATION AFTER TRANSFER
OF 10⁷ SPLEEN CELLS FROM A +/+
DONOR WITH 10⁸ SRBC i.v. (MEANS ±
SEM OF PFC)10⁶ SPLEEN CELLS, DAY 5**

nu/nu recipient (saline injected) (n)	*nu/nu* recipient (SRBC pretreated) (n)
Nonimmunized donor	
(IgM)[a] 518,95 ± 180.16 (6)	6.89 ± 4.48[b] (6)
Donor immunized 30 days previously (10⁸ SRBC)	
(IgM) 202.20 ± 54.55 (9)	52.34 ± 14.44[b] (13)
(IgG) 363.39 ± 104.9 (9)	446.59 ± 159.2 (13)

[a]   IgG PFC negligible.
[b]   Significant difference; $p < 0.05$.

SRBC resulted in suppression of the levamisole-augmented IgM PFC response. Pretreatment with only 10⁷ SRBC was without effect. BALB/c *nu/+* mice manifested no suppression, but a secondary IgG response after an analogous pretreatment with 10⁹ SRBC intraperitoneally. Induction of antigen-specific suppressor cells,[93] B-cell exhaustive differentiation, or blockade of receptors could explain the results.

In BALB/c nude mice given congeneic +/+ spleen cells with SRBC, the IgM PFC response appeared to be severely suppressed if the nude recipient had been pretreated with two high doses of SRBC (Table 2). The wide variations of the PFC counts indicated the complex situation of the adoptive transfer, the results were nevertheless significant. The bulk of the PFC response must have come from the transferred cells and an active suppressive mechanism (specific or nonspecific) must have been induced in the nude mouse spleens.[94] This suppression acted on direct (IgM), and not on indirect (IgG), PFC in experiments with primed donor (+/+) cells. Since the age of the recipients was 6 to 8 weeks, we doubted that the suppression would be affected solely by the nude recipient's cytotoxic/suppressor T cells and have suggested an effect of natural suppressors and/or macrophages in the recipient.[94] Interestingly, in microplate cultures of spleen cells from analogous +/+ and *nu/nu* (BALB/c) donors the suppressive effects of the *nu/nu* SRBC-pretreated ("tolerized") cells compared to nontreated *nu/nu* cells was marked only when the +/+ cells alone gave a high (140 to 240 IgM PFC per 10⁶ cells); with a low-responding +/+ spleen cell suspsnsion (25 IgM PFC/10⁶ cells) an enhancement was observed with cells of the "tolerized" *nu/nu* spleen. This suggested an interleukin-1-mediated effect[94] or a very complicated interaction of suppressors and natural suppressors[95] from both the +/+ and *nu/nu* spleens.[84]

In general, it appears that the unresponsive state in the nude mouse model may be a more complicated phenomenon than the specific tolerance state in euthymic animals.

We have described a model of oral tolerance induction to SRBC which leads in BALB/ c, *nu/+*, and +/+ mice to a complete specific unresponsiveness,[64] based possibly on T suppressor cells activated by intestinally processed antigen on antigen-presenting cells or even on intestinal epithelial cells.[96] These suppressor T cells obviously do emigrate into the general circulation.[97] This type of induction fails completely in BALB/c nude mice (2-month-

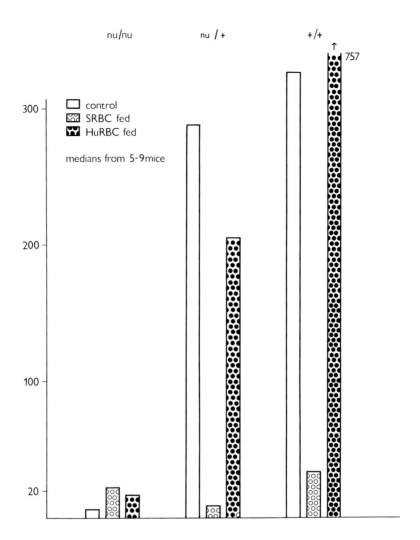

FIGURE 3. Influence of 30-day feeding with sheep erythrocytes (SRBC) or human erythrocytes (HuRBC) in drinking water on the spleen IgM PFC (per 10^6 cells) response to i.p. immunization with 3×10^7 SRBC (day 5). Columns represent medians from groups of 5 to 9 mice of BALB/c background. There was a highly significant difference ($p < 0.01$) between the middle and the outer columns in $nu/+$ and $+/+$ mice.

old) which show, on the contrary, a slight increase of IgM PFC in the spleen (Figure 3).[64] Oral tolerance induction during ontogeny presupposes a high occurrence of T cells in Peyer's patches and other components of the gut-associated lymphatic tissue.[98] This is very poorly developed in the nude mice, the enterocyte-lymphocyte interactions are almost missing[99] (Chapter 8) and, consequently, nude mice must cope with sensitization though the intestinal route in a way different from euthymic animals, perhaps by means of natural suppressors and macrophages.

Essential immunological consequences of the altered mechanisms of oral tolerance induction for IgG, IgE, and IgA responses, as well for the mononuclear phagocyte system (Chapter 7, Section II) are likely.

V. POLYCLONAL ACTIVATORS AND BACKGROUND IMMUNOGLOBULINS

Bacterial lipopolysaccharide (LPS) as a B-cell activator was expected to provoke a vigorous response in the nude mouse and it did, obviously thorugh its active component, lipid

A.[100-106] The mitogenic response was observed in spleen cells and thoracic duct lymphocytes, but not in cells from Peyer's patches.[105] This may be related to some exhaustive or nonspecific suppressive phenomenon or an altered anatomical disposition in the nude mouse gut-associated lymphatic tissues (GALT); addition of adherent cells and T cells increased the response of Peyer's patch cells.[105] The low response of nonenriched Peyer's patch cells is obviously linked with the strikingly scarce development of some components of GALT.[99]

However, in vivo reactivity of nude mice has been shown to be, in general, very inferior to in vitro reactivity of isolated spleen cells. Poor proliferation in the spleen was seen[107] and draining lymph nodes after s.c. introduction of LPS showed poor proliferation and differentiation of the responsive B-cell population.[99] The reaction was much more vigorous in euthymic littermate nodes.[99]

In the nude mouse spleens, suppressor cells of the mitogenic reaction were described,[107] however, in other experiments no effect of depletion of adherent cells and Thy 1[+] cells from a spleen cell suspension of nude mice (BALB/c, SPF) on the mitogenic response in vitro was found.[108] Nor could the response be changed by the addition of macrophages of splenic T cells from euthymic littermates.[108] It seems that LPS acts preferentially on a subpopulation of B cells occurring in the T areas of spleen and lymph nodes.[106]

Polyclonal activation by LPS or flagellin was described, but the specific anti-sheep red blood cells response remained in the IgM class.[109] Polyclonal activation in the absence of antigen has been demonstrated, in addition to xenogeneic erythrocytes, also for a number of haptens.[101,110,111] Increased antibody formation under LPS influence has been shown in a number of experiments in in vitro situations.[49,103,104,111,112] Again, little or no effect was found in vivo.[49,104] It was concluded that *nu/nu* mice may be deficient in a subpopulation of B cells which is responsive to both antigen and nonspecific B-cell activators and which is present in euthymic mice.[104] The possible defect is discussed in Section II. The mitogenic action and the antibody formation-stimulating effect of LPS may be separable, the latter representing rather a maturational signal for the responsive B cells.[113]

Antibody response to LPS *(E. coli)* is in nude mice identical to or higher than that in euthymic controls;[72,114] this could be demonstrated also in a bactericidal assay.[50]

T-cell mitogens PHA and concanavalian A do not provoke any response in nude mice in vivo[45] or in vitro.[103,114-116] With pokeweed mitogen which may act both on T and B cells, the situation is more complex and the results may be influenced by the epidemiological status of the experimental animals; both low responses[115-117] or no responses[103,114] of nude mouse spleen cells were recorded. Interestingly, nude mouse bone marrow cells (not necessarily lymphocytes) were demonstrated to respond to PHA in the same way as do control bone marrow cells and in an assay in which nude lymph nodes were unresponsive.[118] Pretreatment of LPS in vivo was found to induce a minute in vitro response of lymph node cells of nude mice (6 to 8 weeks of age) from a long-living outbred colony.[49]

Potent mitogens for nude spleen cells were described in lectin-binding proteins from leguminous seeds[119] which can be added to the complex list of B-cell stimulants.[4,119]

Also, a special effect of the T-cell mitogen PHA was described in cultured of nude mouse (C57Bl) spleen cells. There was no mitogenic action, but PHA did provoke interferon (type II) production which was identical in *nu/+* and *nu/nu* spleen cell cultures.[120] Concanavalin A stimulated only *nu/+* cells, not *nu/nu* cells, for interferon production and the positive response was sensitive to anti-Thy-1 treatment both in *nu/nu* and *nu/+* mice.[120]

This shows how complex the effect of polyclonal activators and mitogens may be in the nude model which does not provide "clean B cells", but, very likely, altered lineages of B cells interacting with changed macrophage, changed reticulum cell lines (Chapter 8, Section I) and variable numbers of pre-T and T cells (Chapter 4); and all this (in most experiments) in a not fully controlled epidemiological situation which may affect especially the in vivo responses.

The use of young nude mouse splenocytes as a B-cell population free of the modulating effects of T cells, e.g., in in vitro studies of the adenylate cyclase system[120a] may be more representative, but still the question remains whether one can have "B cells" in general, identical in both the euthymic and athymic state.

Polyclonal activation by bacterial products, antigenic pressures and, to some extent, also endogenous stimuli (such as antiidiotypic responses or reactions to other self-antigens) affect the level of immunoglobulins, the background immunoglobulin synthesis.

From the beginning of the nude mouse immunoglobulin studies there has been a consensus that in all nude mice of different strains IgM is normal or supranormal.[47,67,121-124] IgA was found to be low in most studies. In IgG sublcasses, there were many variations related to age and contamination or immunization. In general, greater differences were found between nudes and euthymic controls after immunization[121] and the levels of some subclasses, typically IgG_1, fell from the time of weaning to 2 months of life,[47,123] however, with marked individual variations. These results may have been influenced by the microbiological status of the experimental animals. In obviously well-kept SPF nudes of the CBA and BALB/c background it was determined by rocket electrophoresis[125] that at 6 weeks of age there was no significant difference in any class or subclass between *nu/nu* and *nu/+* animals, only the dispersion of the levels was significantly increased (except for IgM and IgG_1), and many individual nudes had undetectable quantities of IgG_1, IgG_{2A}, IgG_{2B}, and IgA. At 40 weeks, the nudes had (in addition to normal IgM) a higher level of IgG_1 and lower levels in other IgG sublcasses and IgA than *nu/+* mice. At 110 weeks, there was a decrease of IgG_1 both in *nu/nu* and *nu/+* mice, but *nu/nu* had markedly lower values for IgG_{2A}, IgG_{2B}, and IgA. IgM and IgG_2 were equal in both experimental groups. The IgG_1, marked individual variations occurred in the nudes.[125] The experiment was somewhat complicated by the fact that the 40-week age groups were kept in conventional or too conventional conditions 2 weeks prior to bleeding, the authors accept infection with mouse hepatitis virus as the explanation for the high IgG_1 in this age group of nudes. However, a high IgG_1 was found in different conditions in *nu/nu* mice of both conventional and germ-free stocks[126,127] and genetic predispositions of the background strain are suggested to be involved.[127] In the nudes, a restricted heterogeneity of serum immunoglobulins was found at 40 weeks of life,[125] the homogeneous Ig levels (especially IgG_1) accompanying reduced levels of heterogeneous immunoglobulins of the given subclass.[125] The increased occurrence of homogeneous Ig may be connected with a restricted clonal repertoire in the nudes as has been shown also for T cells (Chapter 4, Section II).

In BALB/c mice comparable to the animals of Mink et al.,[125] kept in a germ-free, SPF state, the organ distribution of the cells containing different Ig classes and subclasses was studied: minimal numbers of cIg^+ cells were found in Peyer's patches of *nu/nu* from 6 to 8 weeks, 40 weeks, and 100-week age groups. In nudes of a CBA and B10.LP background the numbers of cIg^+ cells in Peyer's patches was clearly higher at 8 weeks than at 40 weeks of age and $cIgA^+$ cells were the most frequent cells here.[129] Spleens of euthymic and athymic SPF or GF BALB/c mice contained a great part of all cIg^+ cells irrespective of their microbiological status and age, consequently dependent on endogenous stimulation.[128] Many of the positive cells contained both IgM and IgG, mostly IgG_2 immunoglobulins. In the bone marrow, cIg^+ cells (mostly IgM) increased greatly with age in both *nu/nu* and *nu/+* mice and more in the SPF than in the germ-free animals. $cIgA^+$ cells were found in higher numbers only in the bone marrow and mesenteric lymph nodes of the 100-week-old mice, both *nu/nu* and *nu/+*. In the distribution of all cIg cells there was little difference in both germ-free animal groups.[129]

In 6 to 10-week-old mice of the BALB/c background, it was found that there is little diffrerence in cIg^+ cells between $+/+$ and *nu/+* mice[130] and that the only site where $cIgA^+$ cells occur in *nu/nu* in marked numbers is the small intestine submucosa and mesenteric lymph nodes which may give some clue to the solution of the puzzling GALT status of nude mice. With the exception of cIgM cells, low levels of *nu/nu* cIg$^+$ cells were found in lymphatic organs as well as in the respiratory tree, parotid gland, and lactating mammary gland.[130]

IgE levels were elevated in individual nude mice in spite of their SPF state. In 3 out of 8 nudes the levels were higher than those of conventionally housed +/+ BALB/c mice.[131] Negligible serum levels were found in another study in BALB/c nudes, either noninfected or infected with a helminth (*Nippostrongylus brasiliensis*), 13 to 15 days of infection.[132] However, a considerable increase of IgE in the supernatant of nude mouse spleens cells could be obtained by LPS and interleukin 4 stimulation and surface IgE$^+$ cells were observed in these cultures. Also, IgG 1 and IgA secretion were induced in these nude mouse cell cultures.[132] In BALB/c and C57Bl/6 nude mice, *N. brasiliences* infection led to an increase of serum IgE measured by a radioimmunoassay from less than 1 ng/mℓ to 4 to 6 ng/mℓ at day 14 of infection; this was concomitant with an increase of all IgG subclasses, especially in C57Bl nudes.[133]

If single experimental situations were comparable, one could perhaps draw a curve showing the trend of improvement of IgG and IgA levels of the nude mice from the earliest days of their laboratory existence. Many B-cell functions seem to be strictly dependent on the microbial contaminations of the nude mouse colonies and exhaustive phenomena may be suggested in some B-cell profiles in conventional stocks, in addition to the possible defect of a B-cell lineage and in a minor deviation of migration and homing patterns which may be related to the T-deficient state.

REFERENCES

1. **Rygaard, J.,** *Thymus & Self, Immunobiology of the Mouse Mutant Nude,* F.A.D.L., Copenhagen, 1973.
2. **Osmond, D. G. and Nossal, G. J. V.,** Differentiation of lymphocytes in mouse bone marrow. I. Quantitative radioautographic studies of antiglobulin binding by lymphocytes in bone marrow and lymphoid tissues, *Cell. Immunol.,* 13, 117, 1974.
3. **Sprent, J.,** Circulating T and B lymphocytes of the mouse. I. Migratory properties, *Cell. Immunol.,* 7, 10, 1973.
4. **Kindred, B.,** Nude mice in immunology, *Prog. Allergy,* 26, 137, 1979.
5. **Sprent, J.,** Migration and lifespan of circulating B lymphocytes of nude (*nu/nu*) mice, in *Proc. 1st Int. Workshop on Nude Mice,* Rygaard, J. and Povlsen, C. O., Eds., G. Fischer, Stuttgart, 1974, 11.
6. **De Sousa, M. A. B., Parrott, D. M. V., and Pantelouris, E. M.,** The lymphoid tissues in mice with congenital aplasia of the thymus, *Clin. Exp. Immunol.,* 4, 637, 1969.
7. **Röpke, C. and Hougen, H. P.,** Turnover and lifespan of small lymphocytes in nude mice, in *Proc. 1st Int. Workshop on Nude Mice,* Rygaard, J. and Povlsen, C. O., Eds., G. Fischer, Stuttgart, 1974, 51.
8. **Hougen, H. P. and Röpke, C.,** Small lymphocytes in peripheral lymphoid tissues of nude mice. Lifespan and distribution, *Clin. Exp. Immunol.,* 22, 528, 1975.
9. **Parrott, D. M. V. and De Sousa, M. A. B.,** Thymus-dependent and thymus-independent populations: origin, migratory patterns and lifespan, *Clin. Exp. Immunol.,* 8, 663, 1971.
10. **Sprent, J. and Basten, A.,** Circulating T and B lymphocytes of the mouse. II. Lifespan, *Cell. Immunol.,* 7, 40, 1973.
11. **MacLennan, I. C. M. and Gray, D.,** Antigen-driven selection of virgin and memory B cells, *Immunol. Rev.,* 91, 61, 1986.
12. **Fulop, G. M. and Osmond, D. G.,** Regulation of bone marrow lymphocyte production. IV. Cells mediating the stimulation of marrow lymphocyte production by sheep red blood cells: studies in anti-IgM-suppressed mice, athymic mice, and silica treated mice, *Cell. Immunol.,* 75, 91, 1983.
13. **Paige, C. J., Kincade, P. W., Shinefeld, L. A., and Sato, V. L.,** Precursors of murine B lymphocytes. Physical and functional characterization and distinction from myeloid stem cells, *J. Exp. Med.,* 153, 154, 1981.
14. **Giri, J. G., Kincade, P. W., and Mizel, S. B.,** Interleukin 1-mediated induction of κ-light chain sythesis and surface immunoglobulin expression on pre-B cells, *J. Immunol.,* 132, 223, 1984.

15. **Koopman, W. J., Farrar, J. J., and Fuller-Bonar, J.,** Evidence for the identification of lymphocyte activating factor as the adherent cell-derived mediator responsible for enhanced antibody synthesis by nude mouse spleen cells, *Cell. Immunol.,* 35, 92, 1978.

16. **Osmond, D. G.,** Population dynamics of bone marrow B lymphocytes, *Immunol. Rev.,* 93, 103, 1986.

17. **Kubín, M., Holub, M., Mohelská, H., and Schlegerová, D.,** Experimental infection with *Mycobacterium kansasii* in athymic nude mice, *Exp. Pathol.,* 25, 233, 1984.

18. **Coffman, R. L.,** Surface antigen expression and immunoglobulin gene rearrangement during mouse pre-B cell development, *Immunol. Rev.,* 69, 5, 1982.

19. **Stein, H., Gerdes, J., and Mason, D. Y.,** The normal and malignant germinal centre, *Clin. Haematol.,* 11, 531, 1982.

20. **Jacobson, E. B. and Thorbecke, G. J.,** Secondary antibody response and germinal center development in nude mice reconstituted with thymus cells, in *Proc. 1st Int. Workshop on Nude Mice,* Rygaard, J. and Povlsen, C. O., Eds., G. Fischer, Stuttgart, 1974, 155.

21. **Kindred, B.,** T cell functions in nude mice: lack of secondary antibody response in vivo, *Exp. Cell Biol.,* 52, 17, 1984.

22. **Kindred, B. and Bösing-Schneider, R.,** Non-specific T-cell replacing factor fails to promote a secondary response in vivo, *Scand. J. Immunol.,* 14, 503, 1981.

23. **Baker, P. J., Reed, N. D., Stashak, P. W., Amsbaugh, D. F., and Prescott, B.,** Regulation of the antibody response to the type III pneumococcal polysaccharide. I. Nature of regulatory cells, *J. Exp. Med.,* 137, 1431, 1973.

24. **Reed, N. D., Manning, J. K., Baker, P. J., and Ulrich, J. T.,** Analysis of 'thymus-independent' immune responses using nude mice, in *Proc. 1st Int. Workshop on Nude Mice,* Rygaard, J. and Povlsen, C. O., Eds., G. Fischer, Stuttgart, 1974, 95.

25. **Benner, R., van Oudenaren, A., Björklund, M., Ivars, F., and Holmberg, D.,** 'Background' immunoglobulin production: measurement, biological significance and regulation, *Immunol. Today,* 3, 243, 1982.

26. **Haaijman, J. J., Slingerland-Teunissen, J., Benner, R., and van Oudenaren, A.,** The distribution of cytoplasmic immunoglobulin containing cells over various lymphoid organs of congenitally athymic (nude) mice as a function of age, *Immunology,* 36, 271, 1979.

27. **Gillette, R. W.,** Homing of labeled lymphoid cells in athymic mice: evidence for additional immunologic defects, *Cell. Immunol.* 17, 374, 1975.

28. **Parks, D. E., Doyle, M. V., and Weigle, W. O.,** Effect of lipopolysaccharide on immunogenicity and tolerogenicity of HGG in C57Bl/6J nude mice: evidence for a possible B cell deficiency, *J. Immunol.,* 119, 1923, 1977.

29. **Wortis, H. H., Burkly, L., Hughes, D., Roschelle, S., and Waneck, G.,** Lack of mature B cells in nude mice with x-linked immune deficiency, *J. Exp. Med.,* 155, 903, 1982.

30. **Griffith, A. L., Catsimpoolas, N., Dewanjee, M. K., and Wortis, H. H.,** Electrophoretic separation of radio-isotopically labeled mouse lymphocytes, *J. Immunol.,* 117, 1949, 1976.

31. **Palacios, R. and Leu, T.,** CCll: a monoclonal antibody specific for interleukin 3-sensitive mouse cells defines two major populations of B cell precursors in the bone marrow, *Immunol. Rev.,* 93, 125, 1986.

32. **Hayakawa, K., Hardy, R., Honda, M., Herzenberg, L. A., Steinberg, A., and Herzenberg, L. A.,** Lyt-1 B cells: functionally distinct lymphocytes that secrete IgM autoantibodies, *Proc. Natl. Acad. Sci. U.S.A.,* 81, 2494, 1984.

33. **Herzenberg, L. A., Stall, A. M., Lalor, P. A., Sidman, C., Moore, W. A., and Parks, D. R.,** Thy Ly-1 B cell lineage, *Immunol. Rev.,* 93, 81, 1986.

34. **Nisonoff, A., Ju, S.-T., and Owen, F. L.,** Studies of structure and immunosuppression of a cross-reactive idiotype in strain A mice, *Immunol. Rev.,* 34, 89, 1977.

35. **Mäkelä, O. and Karjalinen, K.,** Inherited immunoglobulin idiotypes of the mouse, *Immunol. Rev.,* 34, 119, 1977.

36. **Cancro, M. P., Sigal, N. H., and Klinman, N. R.,** Differential expression of an equivalent clonotype among BALB/c and C57Bl/6 mice, *J. Exp. Med.,* 147, 1, 1978.

37. **Nossal, G. S. V., Pike, B. L., Teale, J. M., Layton, J. E., Kay, T. W., and Battye, F. L.,** Cell fractionation methods and the target cells for clonal abortion of B-lymphocytes, *Immunol. Rev.,* 43, 184, 1979.

38. **MacLennan, I. C. M. and Gray, D.,** Antigen-driven selection of virgin and memory B cells, *Immunol. Rev.,* 91, 61, 1986.

39. **Cancro, M. P. and Klinman, N. R.,** B cell repertoire diversity in athymic mice, *J. Exp. Med.,* 131, 761, 1980.

40. **Quintáns, J. and Lefkovits, I.,** Precursor cells specific for sheep red cells in nude mice. Estimation of frequency in the microculture system, *Eur. J. Immunol.,* 3, 392, 1973.

41. **Stocker, J.,** Estimation of hapten-specific antibody-forming cell precursors in microcultures, *Immunology,* 30, 181, 1976.

42. **Stocker, J.,** Tolerance induction in maturing B cells, *Immunology,* 32, 283, 1977.

43. **Stocker, J.,** Functional maturation of B cells in vitro, *Immunology,* 32, 275, 1977.

44. **Pantelouris, E. M. and Flish, P. A.,** Responses of athymic ("nude") mice to sheep red blood cells, *Eur. J. Immunol.,* 2, 236, 1972.

45. **Wortis, H. H.,** Immunological responses of 'nude' mice, *Clin. Exp. Immunol.,* 8, 305, 1971.

46. **Reed, N. D. and Jutila, J. W.,** Immune responses of congenitally thymusless mice to heterologous erythrocytes, *Proc. Soc. Exp. Biol. Med.,* 139, 1234, 1972.

47. **Pritchard, H., Riddaway, J., and Micklem, H. S.,** Immune responses in congentally thymus-less mice. II. Quantitative studies of serum immunoglobulins, the antibody response to sheep erythrocytes and effect of thymus allografting, *Clin. Exp. Immunol.,* 13, 125, 1973.

48. **Kindred, B.,** The inception of the response to SRBC by nude mice injected with various doses of congenic or allogeneic thymus cells, *Cell. Immunol.,* 17, 277, 1975.

49. **Gershwin, M. E., Merchand, B., Gelfand, M. C., Vickers, I., Steinberg, A. D., and Hansen, C. T.,** The natural history and immuno-pathology of outbred athymic (nude) mice, *Clin. Immunol. Immunopathol.,* 4, 324, 1975.

50. **Holub, M., Hajdu, I., Jaroškóva, L., and Trebichavský, I.,** Lymphatic tissues and antibody-forming cells of athymic nude mice, *Z. Immunitaetsforsch.,* 146, 322, 1974.

50a. **Lafleur, L. and Mitchell, G. F.,** Differences in the immunological activities on antibody-secreting cell precursors in mouse spleen selected on the basis of antigen-binding capacity, *Eur. J. Immunol.,* 5, 648, 1975.

51. **Beattie, G., Lipsick, J., Lannom, R. A., Baird, S., Kaplan, N. O., and Osler, A. G.,** Induction of a T-cell-like response in athymic mice, in *Proc. 3rd Int. Workshop on Nude Mice,* Reed, N. D., Ed., G. Fischer, New York, 1982, 207.

52. **Fehninger, T. E., Martínez-Maza, O., Kanowith-Klein, S., and Ashman, R. F.,** Analysis of antigen-binding cell surface Ig profiles and Ig-secreting cells in mice carrying the nu allele: immune regulation abnormality in heterozygous *nu/+* mice, *J. Immunol.,* 128, 568, 1982.

53. **Holub, M., Hraba, T., and Madar, J.,** Specific unresponsiveness to sheep red blood cells visualized by levamisole in athymic nude mice, *Immunopharmacology,* 5, 129, 1982.

54. **Říhová, B. and Říha, I.,** Genetic regulation of antibody response to sheep red blood cells: isoelectric focusing analysis of sera of well responding strain A/J and poorly responding strain B10 mice, *Am. J. Reproduct. Immunol.,* 1, 164, 1981.

55. **Taniguchi, T., Suzuki, T., Malke, S., Nomoto, K., Hashimoto, K., Goda, A., and Takeye, K.,** Differences in antibody production to heterologous erythrocytes in conventional, specific pathogen free (SPF), germ free, and antigen free mice, *Microbiol. Immunol. (Jpn),* 22, 793, 1978.

56. **Andersson, J., Schreier, M. H., and Melchers, F.,** T-cell dependent B-cell stimulation is H-2 restricted and antigen dependent only at the resting B-cell level, *Proc. Natl. Acad. Sci. U.S.A.,* 77, 1612, 1980.

57. **Rosenberg, Y. J. and Chiller, L. M.,** Ability of antigen-specific helper cells to effect a class-restricted increase of total Ig-secreting cells in spleens after immunization with the antigen, *J. Exp. Med.,* 150, 517, 1979.

57a. **Vladutiu, A. O. and Rose, N. R.,** Cellular basis of the genetic control of immune responsiveness to murina thyroglobulin in mice, *Cell. Immunol.,* 17, 106, 1975.

58. **Říhová, B., Ulbrich, K., Větvička, V., and Kopeček, J.,** Biocompatibility of PEG-BSA polymers in inbred strains of mice, *Biomaterials,* 1988, in print.

59. **Větvička, V., Fornůsek, L., Říhová, B., and Kopeček, J.,** Properties of macrophages from low- and high-responder strains of mice. I. Effect of antigenic stimulation, *Folia Biol. (Prague),* 31, 20, 1985.

60. **Holub, M., Hajdu, I., Trebichavský, I., and Rossmann, P.,** Lack of plasma cell differentiation in athymic nude mice, in *Proc. 1st Int. Workshop on Nude Mice,* Rygaard, J. and Povlsen, C. O., Eds., G. Fischer, Stuttgart, 1974, 71.

61. **Holub, M., Jaroškóva, L., Hajdu, I., Říha, I., and Moticka, E. J.,** Enhancement of the immune response of genetically thymus-less mice by different cell populations, in *Microenvironmental Aspects of Immunity,* Jankovic, B. D. and Isakovic, K., Eds., Plenum Press, New York, 1973, 289.

62. **Kindred, B. and Weiler, E.,** The response to SRBC by nude mice injected with lymphoid cells other than thymus cells, *J. Immunol.,* 109, 382, 1972.

63. **Hajdu, I., Holub, M., and Trebichavský, I.,** The sequence of appearance of antibodies in mouse omentum plasma cells, *Exp. Cell Res.,* 75, 219, 1972.

64. **Tlaskalová-Hogenová, H. and Holub, M.,** Effect of fed xenogeneic red blood cells on the immune response of euthymic and athymic mice, in *Immune-Deficient Animals in Biomed. Res., Proc. 5th IWIDA,* Rygaard, J. et al., Eds., S. Karger, Basel, 1987, 101.

65. **Kölsch, E., Davies, A. J. S., and Leuchars, R.,** The immune response to phage fd in normal and thymus-deprived animals of a low responding inbred strain and genetically thymusless mice, *Eur. J. Immunol.,* 2, 541, 1972.

66. **Kindred, B. and Corley, R. B.,** Specificity of helper cells for different antigens, *Eur. J. Immunol.,* 8, 67, 1978.

67. **Crewter, P. and Warner, N. L.,** Serum immunoglobulins and antibodies in congenitally athymic (nude) mice, *Aust. J. Exp. Biol. Med. Sci.,* 50, 625, 1972.

68. **Finger, H., Hof, H., and Elekes, E.,** The adjuvant activity of *Bordetella pertussis* in mice with congenital aplasia of thymus, *Z. Immunitaetsforsch.,* 145, 460, 1973.

69. **Askonas, B. A., Davies, A. J. S., Jacobson, E. B., Leuchars, E., and Roelants, G. E.,** Thymus dependence of the antibody response to Maia squinado haemocyanin in mice, *Immunology,* 23, 791, 1972.

70. **Hale, M. L. and Hanna, E. E.,** Complementation of the anti-TNP PFC response of N:NIH nude mice from nude dams by spleen cells of nude mice from heterozygous dams, *Cell. Immunol.,* 47, 429, 1979.

70a. **Yrios, J. W. and Balisk, E.,** Immune response of athymic and euthymic germfree mice to *Campylobacter* ssp., *Infect. Immunol.,* 54, 339, 1986.

71. **Schott, C. F. and Merchant, B.,** Carrier-specific immune memory to a thymus-independent antigen in congenitally athymic mice, *J. Immunol.,* 122, 1710, 1979.

71a. **Rose, F. V. and Cebra, J. J.,** Isotype commitment of B-cells and dissemination of the primed state after mucosal contamination with *Mycoplasma pulmonis, Infect. Immunol.,* 49, 428, 1985.

72. **Manning, J. K., Reed, N. D., and Jutila, J. W.,** Antibody response to *Escherichia coli* lipopolysaccharide and type III pneumococcal polysaccharide by congenitally thymusless (nude) mice, *J. Immunol.,* 108, 1470, 1972.

73. **Di Pauli, R.,** Genetics of the immune response. I. Differences in the specificity of antibodies to lipo-polysaccharides among different strains of mice, *J. Immunol.,* 109, 394, 1972.

74. **Reed, N. D., Manning, J. K., and Rudbach, J. A.,** Immunologic responses of mice to lipopolysaccharide from *Escherichia coli, J. Infect. Dis.,* 128, S70, 1973.

75. **Aden, D. P. and Reed, N. D.,** In vitro immune response to lipopolysaccharide: thymus-derived cells not required, *Immunol. Commun.,* 2, 335, 1973.

76. **Marchalonis, J. J.,** Antibodies and surface immunoglobulins of immunised congenitally athymic (nu/nu) mice, *Aust. J. Exp. Biol. Med. Sci.,* 52, 535, 1974.

77. **Fidler, J. M.,** In vivo immune response to TNP hapten coupled to thymus-independent carrier lipopoly-saccharide, *Cell. Immunol.,* 16, 223, 1975.

78. **Chen, J. C. and Leon, M. A.,** The immune response to dextran in BALB/c mice. I. Modification of the 'thymus-independent' response by the T cell mitogen concanavalin A, *J. Immunol.,* 116, 416, 1976.

79. **Rüde, E., Wrede, J., and Gundelach, M. L.,** Production of IgG antibodies and enhanced resonse of nude mice to DNP-AE-dextran, *J. Immunol.,* 116, 527, 1976.

80. **Lake, J. P. and Reed, N. D.,** Regulation of the immune response to polyvinylpyrrolidone: effect of antilymphocyte serum on the response of normal and nude mice, *Cell. Immunol.,* 21, 364, 1976.

81. **Schuler, W., Lehle, G., Weiler, E., and Kölsch, E.,** Immune response against the T-independent antigen $\alpha(1 \rightarrow 3)$ dextran. I. Demonstration of an unexpected IgG response of athymic and germ-free-raised euthymic BALB/c mice, *Eur. J. Immunol.,* 12, 120, 1982.

82. **Manning, D. D. and Jutila, J. W.,** Immunosuppression of congenitally athymic (nude) mice with het-erologous anti-immunoglobulin heavy chain antisera, *Cell. Immunol.,* 14, 453, 1974.

83. **Bankhurst, A. D. and Warner, N. L.,** Surface immunoglobulins on the thoracic duct lymphocytes of the congenitally athymic (nude) mouse, *Aust. J. Exp. Biol. Med. Sci.,* 50, 661, 1972.

84. **Mitchell, G. F., Lafleur, L., and Andersson, J.,** Evidence for readily induced tolerance to heterologous erythrocytes in nude mice, *Scand. J. Immunol.,* 3, 39, 1974.

85. **Schrader, J. W.,** Induction of immunological tolerance to a thymus dependent antigen in the absence of thymus-derived cells, *J. Exp. Med.,* 139, 1303, 1974.

86. **Kindred, B.,** Specific unresponsiveness in nude mice given antigen before T cells, *Eur. J. Immunol.,* 5, 609, 1975.

87. **Etlinger, H. M. and Chiller, J. M.,** Induction of tolerance in athymic mice with an antigen which is highly immunogenic in euthymic mice, *Cell. Immunol.,* 33, 297, 1977.

88. **Bösing-Schneider, R. and Haug, M.,** Induction and abrogation of unresponsiveness in nude mouse cells, *J. Exp. Med.,* 144, 1458, 1976.

89. **Nossal, G. J. V. and Pike, B.,** Evidence for the clonal abortion theory of B-lymphocyte tolerance, *J. Exp. Med.,* 141, 904, 1975.

90. **Nossal, G. J. V., Pike, B. L., and Katz, D. H.,** Induction of B cell tolerance in vitro to 2,4-dinitro-phenyl coupled to a copolymer of D-glutamic acid and D-lysine (DNP-D-GL), *J. Exp. Med.,* 138, 312, 1973.

91. **Schrader, J. W.,** The in vitro induction of immunological tolerance in the B lymphocyte by oligovalent thymus-dependent antigens, *J. Exp. Med.,* 141, 967, 1975.

92. **Renoux, G. and Renoux, M.,** Thymus-like activities of sulphur derivatives on T-cell differentiation, *J. Exp. Med.,* 145, 466, 1977.

93. **Bösing-Schneider, R.,** Demonstration of antigen-specific suppressor cells in nude mice: a model for the induction of antigen-specific suppressor cells, *Cell. Immunol.,* 61, 245, 1981.

94. **Hraba, T., Madar, J., Šírová, M., Říha, I., and Holub, M.,** Factors affecting specific unresponsiveness of nude mouse spleen cells pretreated with high doses of SRBC, paper in preparation.

95. **Holda, J. H., Maier, T., and Claman, H. N.,** Murine graft-versus-host disease across minor barriers: immunosuppressive aspects of natural suppressor cells, *Immunol. Rev.,* 88, 87, 1985.

96. **Mowat, A. M.,** The regulation of immune responses to dietary protein antigens, *Immunol. Today,* 8, 93, 1987.

97. **Tomasi, T. B.,** Oral tolerance, *Transplantation,* 29, 353, 1980.

98. **Hanson, D. G., Vaz, N. M., Maia, L. C., Hornbrook, M. M., Lynch, J. M., and Roy, C. A.,** Inhibition of specific immune responses by feeding protein antigens, *Int. Arch. Allergy Appl. Immunol.,* 55, 526, 1977.

99. **Parrott, D. M. V. and de Sousa, M. A. B.,** B cell stimulation in nude (*nu/nu*) mice, in *Proc. 1st Int. Workshop on Nude Mice,* Rygaard, J. and Povlsen, C. O., Eds., G. Fischer, Stuttgart, 1974, 61.

100. **Andersson, J., Sjöberg, O., and Möller, G.,** Mitogens as probes for immunocyte activation and cellular cooperation, *Transplant. Rev.,* 11, 131, 1972.

101. **Sjöberg, O., Andersson, J., and Möller, G.,** Lipopolysaccharide can substitute for helper cells in the antibody response in vitro, *Eur. J. Immunol.,* 2, 326, 1972.

102. **Andersson, J., Melchers, F., Galanos, C., and Lüderitz, O.,** The mitogenic effect of lipopolysaccharide on bone marrow-derived mouse lymphocytes. Lipid A as the mitogenic part of the molecule, *J. Exp. Med.,* 137, 943, 1973.

103. **Watson, J., Epstein, R., Nakoinz, I., and Ralph, P.,** The role of humoral factors in the initiation of in vitro primary immune responses. II. Effects of lymphocyte mitogens, *J. Immunol.,* 110, 43, 1973.

104. **Parks, D. E., Doyle, N. V., and Weigle, W. O.,** Effect of lipopolysaccharide on immunogenicity and tolerogenicity of HGG in C57B1/6J nude mice: evidence for a possible B cell deficiency, *J. Immunol.,* 119, 1923, 1977.

105. **Kagnoff, M. F., Billings, P., and Cohn, M.,** Functional characteristics of Peyer's patch lymphoid cells. II. Lipopolysaccharide is thymus-dependent, *J. Exp. Med.,* 139, 407, 1974.

106. **Hanaoka, M. and Takigawa, M.,** Proliferation of B lymphocytes in the spleen of nude mice, *Proc. 2nd Int. Workshop on Nude Mice,* Nomura, T., Ohsawa, N., Tamaoki, N., and Fujiwara, K., Eds., G. Fischer, Stuttgart, 1977, 185.

107. **Smith, J. B. and Eaton, G. J.,** Suppressor cells in spleen from "nude" mice. Their effect on the mitogenic response of B lymphocytes, *J. Immunol.,* 117, 319, 1976.

108. **Takigawa, M. and Hanaoka, M.,** Role of T and adherent cells in in vitro response of nude mouse spleen cells to bacterial lipopolysaccharide, *Int. Arch. Allergy Appl. Immunol.,* 55, 131, 1977.

109. **Schrader, J. W.,** The mechanism of bone marrow-derived (B) lymphocyte activation. II. A second signal for antigen-specific activation provided by flagellin and lipopolysaccharides, *Eur. J. Immunol.,* 4, 20, 1974.

110. **Coutinho, A. and Möller, G.,** B cell mitogenic properties of thymus-independent antigens, *Nature (London) New Biol.,* 245, 12, 1973.

111. **Watson, J., Trenker, E., and Cohn, M.,** The use of bacterial polysaccharides to show that two signals are required for the induction of antibody synthesis, *J. Exp. Med.,* 138, 699, 1973.

112. **Bösing-Schneider, R.,** Differential effects of cyclic AMP on the in vitro induction of antibody synthesis, *Nature,* 256, 137, 1975.

113. **Quintáns, J. and Lefkovits, I.,** Clonal expansion of lipopolysaccharide-stimulated B lymphocytes, *J. Immunol.,* 113, 1373, 1974.

114. **Kearney, J. F. and Reade, P. C.,** Activation of thoracic duct lymphocytes from congenitally athymic 'nude' mice by mitogenic stimuli in vitro, *Austr. J. Exp. Biol. Med. Sci.,* 52, 207, 1974.

115. **Janossy, G. and Greaves, M. F.,** Lymphocyte activation. I. Response of T and B lymphocytes to phytomitogens, *Clin. Exp. Immunol.,* 9, 483, 1971.

116. **Vischer, T. L.,** Mitogenic factors produced by lymphocyte activation-effect on T and B cells, *J. Immunol.,* 109, 401, 1972.

117. **Gillette, R. W.,** Further evidence for the existence of B-lymphocyte sub-populations, *Cell. Immunol.,* 45, 26, 1979.

118. **Press, O. W. and Rosse, C.,** Thymic independence of bone marrow lymphocyte phytohemagglutinin (PHA) response demonstrated in nude mice, *Cell. Immunol.,* 28, 218, 1977.

119. **Gebauer, G., Schimpl, A., and Rüdiger, H.,** Lectin-binding proteins as potent mitogens for B lymphocytes from nu/nu mice, *Eur. J. Immunol.,* 12, 491, 1982.

120. **Kirchner, H., Fenkl, H., Zawatzky, R., Engler, H., and Becker, H.,** Dissociation between interferon production induced by phytohemagglutinin and concanavalin A in spleen cell cultures of nude mice, *Eur. J. Immunol.,* 10, 224, 1980.

121. **Salomon, J.-C. and Bazin, H.,** Low levels of some serum immunoglobulin classes in nude mice, *Eur. J. Clin. Biol. Res.,* 17, 880, 1972.

121a. **Wiemer, E. C., Griffor, M. C., and Scarpa, A.,** Antibody-induced cAMP accumulation in splenocytes from athymic nude mice, *FEBS Lett.,* 224, 33, 1987.

122. **Luzzati, A. L. and Jacobson, E. B.,** Serum immunoglobulin levels in nude mice, *Eur. J. Immunol.,* 2, 473, 1972.

123. **Bloemmen, J. and Eyssen, H.,** Immunoglobulin levels of sera of genetically thymusless (nude) mice, *Eur. J. Immunol.,* 3, 117, 1973.

124. **Bankhurst, A. D., Lambert, P. H., and Meischer, P. A.,** Studies on the thymic dependence of immunoglobulin classes of the mouse, *Proc. Soc. Exp. Biol. Med.,* 148, 501, 1975.

125. **Mink, J. G., Radl, J., van den Berg, P., Haaijman, J. J., Van Zwieten, M. J., and Benner, R.,** Serum immunoglobulins in nude mice and their heterozygous littermates during ageing, *Immunology,* 40, 539, 1980.

126. **Brogren, C. H., Warren, H. S., Nielsen, E., and Rygaard, J.,** Quantitative immunoelectrophoretic analysis of serum proteins and immunoglobulins in the serum and produced by spleen cell cultures of individual nude mice, in *Proc. 2nd Int. Workshop on Nude Mice,* Nomura, T., Ohsawa, N., Tamaoki, N., and Fujiwara, K., Eds., G. Fischer, Stuttgart, 1977, 157.

127. **Okudaira, H., Komagata, Y., Ghoda, A., and Ishizaka, K.,** Thymus-independent and dependent aspects of immunoglobulin synthesis and specific antibody formation in nude mice, in *Proc. 2nd Int. Workshop on Nude Mice,* Nomura, T., Ohsawa, N., Tamaoki, N., and Fujiwara, K., Eds., G. Fischer, Stuttgart, 1977, 167.

128. **van Oudenaren, A., Haaijman, J. J., and Benner, R.,** Frequencies of background cytoplasmic Ig-containing cells in various lymphoid organs of athymic and euthymic mice as a function of age and immune status, *Immunology,* 51, 735, 1984.

129. **Benner, R., van Oudenaren, A., Haaijman, J. J., Slingerland-Teunissen, J., Van der Kwast, Th.H., and Wolters, E. A. J.,** The influence of the thymus upon the number and class distribution of immunoglobulin containing cells in the bone marrow and other lymphoid organs of the mouse, in *Function and Structure of the Immune System,* Müller-Ruchholtz, W. and Müller-Hermelink, H. K., Eds., Plenum Press, New York, 1979, 133.

130. **Weisz-Carrington, P., Schrater, A. F., Lamm, M. E., and Thorbecke, G. J.,** Immunoglobulin isotypes in plasma cells of normal and athymic mice, *Cell. Immunol.,* 44, 343, 1979.

131. **Ito, K., Ogita, T., Suko, M., Mori, M., Kudo, K., Hayakawa, T., Okudaira, H., and Horiuchi, Y.,** IgE levels in nude mice, *Int. Archs. Allergy Appl. Immunol.,* 58, 474, 1979.

132. **Azuma, M., Hirano, T., Miyajima, H., Watanabe, N., Yagita, H., Enemoto, S., Furusawa, S., Ovary, Z., Kinashi, T., Honjo, T., and Okumura, K.,** Regulation of murine IgE production in SJA/9 and nude mice. Potentiation of IgE production by recombinant interleukin 4, *J. Immunol.,* 139, 2538, 1987.

133. **Lebrun, P. and Spiegelberg, H. L.,** Concomitant immunoglobulin E and immunoglobulin Gl formation in *Nippostrongylus brasiliensis*-infected mice, *J. Immunol.,* 139, 1459, 1987.

Chapter 6

STEM CELLS AND CONNECTIVE TISSUES

I. BONE MARROW STEM CELL POTENTIAL AND LEUKOCYTE NUMBERS

One of the few possibilities to establish unequivocally the basic defect of the *nu* mutation is the analysis of the mesenchymal (mesodermal) activity as reflected by the bone marrow stem cell potential. Of course, a reduced stem cell potential in the adult nude mouse may also be caused by a lack of thymic factors.[1] If such a defect, however, were also present in the euthymic heterozygous littermate (*nu/+*) and during fetal life, it would be a strong argument in favor of a primary mesenchymal defect caused by the *nu* gene. Such a defect in the *nu/+* heterozygote could be expected, since it has already been observed by Pantelouris that it shares leukopenia with the *nu/nu* homozygote.[2]

In fact, the first recording of the *nu/nu* and *nu/+* bone marrow cell pool-forming spleen colonies of myeloid and erythroid cells in lethally irradiated recipients (CFU/s) has already demonstrated that both have about the same potential, only a slight increase in the *nu/+* bone marrow proliferative capacity was revealed.[3] This work was done in mice of a closed but not inbred colony. In a study of CBA/J-backcrossed mice, we compared the CFU/s content of mice of the *nu/nu*, *nu/+*, and *+/+* genotype and found that the *nu* gene-bearing individuals have less than 20 CFU/s per 10^5 bone marrow cells, with the *+/+* mice at the expected levels of more than 30 CFU/s.[4] The *nu/nu* mouse bone marrow was shown to have a defective capacity to restore hemopoiesis, permanent chimerism, and immunological responsiveness in lethally irradiated recipients.[5] In this study no differentiation of *nu/+* (leukopenic) and *+/+* littermates was performed so that the CFU/s value of the nudes (10 to 11) compared with the mean of 14 to 15 CFU/s in a pool of estimated $^1/_3$ of *+/+* and $^2/_3$ of *nu/+* mice. This allowed for 10 to 11 CFU/s in *nu/+* littermates; an intrinsic defect in the proliferative capacity of nude mouse bone marrow stem cells was postulated.[5] In addition, a declining cellularity of the *nu/nu* bone marrow between 40 and 60 days of age was noted in mice of the first backcross to C3H, with a very short survival time;[5] we did not notice such a difference in the bone marrow cellularity of healthy mice.

An impediment in the development of precursor T lymphocytes and possibly other bone-marrow-derived cells was described in the nude mouse "environment"; a slower restoration with nude bone marrow cells was found when thymectomized irradiated and nude irradiated, allogeneic thymus-grafted recipients were compared.[6] In 1977, Loor suggested that the defective capacity of the *nu/nu* and *nu/+* bone marrow stem cell pool is "not necessarily a direct result of the *nu* mutation, but more likely a more or less direct consequence of a lack of some hormonal influence of the thymus . . . ". He thought that further analysis of thymus structures of the *nu/+* and *+/+* thymus may show some differences in secretory epithelial cells.[7]

We made a careful comparison of the cellularity of the *nu/+* and *+/+* thymus showing a quantitative reduction of the organ and a small increase of the proportion of medullary epithelial cells in *nu/+* mice.[8] At the same time, we have reinforced the notion that the number of circulating leukocytes and the stem cell potential is significantly lower in the nu gene-bearing mice of the CBA background[9] and we also obtained the same results in mice of the C57Bl and BALB/c background both in adults and in 17- and 19-day-old fetuses[9,10] (Figure 1). In the BALB/c mice, the difference between *nu/nu* and *nu/+* CFU/s number was significant too, but both values were only 16 and 37% of the *+/+* mice.

These results were obtained from transfers of femoral bone marrow cells into recipients irradiated with 8.0 Gy or more; colonies scored at day 8[9] or 11.[10] Less impressive figures

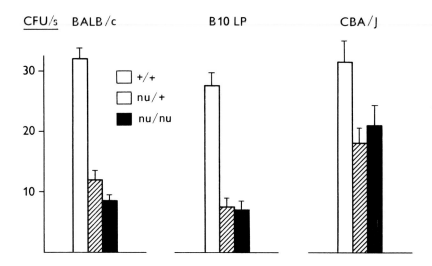

FIGURE 1.   Colony-forming units from 10^5 femoral bone marrow cells in the Till-McCulloch assay (means from 5 to 10 female mice aged 2 months, ± SEM). Recipients irradiated with 8.7 to 9.0 Gy, killed at day 8.

were obtained with the transfer of femoral bone marrow cells into 7.0 Gy-irradiated recipients. At day 8, the number of CFU/s (after correction for nonlinearity of the test) was 37,9 for pooled bone marrow cells of BALB/c $+/+$, 36,2 for *nu/nu* of an outbred, BALB/c-derived strain, and 36,5 for *nu/* $+$ of the outbred strain (results of Dr. E. Nečas). This outbred strain has peripheral white blood cell counts almost as high as BALB/c $+/+$; consequently, genetic factors must be considered in analyses of the *nu* gene-dependent stem cell potential. Using C57Bl/10 mice, recipients irradiated with 7.0 Gy, *nu/* $+$ CFU/s counts showed a great variability, but were lower than $+/+$ counts in 7 out of 11 experiments. (Dr. E. Nečas, paper in preparation).

The absence of T-cell factors[11] may deepen the stem cell defect in the *nu/nu* mouse, but we maintain that the conditions in the *nu/* $+$ hybrid cannot be explained by the reduction of the lymphatic tissue of the thymus, that the low stem cell potential expresses an unequivocal effect of the *nu* gene on the mesenchymal (mesodermal) derivatives and that this is a primary effect. The lower-than-normal stem cell potential of the *nu/* $+$ hybrid also rules out the possibility that the CFU/s content of the nude mouse hematopoietic centers could be virus-induced[12] or caused by the elevated numbers of *nu/nu* natural killer cells; NK cells have been implicated as regulators of hemopoiesis,[13-15] but their proportion in nude mouse tissues and blood (as shown by the presence of large granular lymphocytes) rises only in the postnatal development and it is about the same in the heterozygotes and $+/+$ mice.

The stromal cells of hematopoietic microenvironments play a crucial role in the control of stem cell differentiation and proliferation.[16] The putative mesenchymal defect may affect the bone marrow stromal cells as well. There are small differences in the bone marrow cell differential counts between $+/+$ and *nu/nu* mice;[9,17] the only consistent distinction in various strains of mice is the extremely low lymphoid cell content in the bone marrow of *nu/nu* mice, in addition to an increased proportion of very primitive ("reticulum") cells.[9] Since, however, we have found the lowered stem cell count of the *nu* gene-bearing mice also in the fetal liver on gestation day 17,[10] it seems that the migrating stem cells are affected indeed. Some quantitative reduction of the mesenchymal (mesodermal) cell supply may be sufficient to explain the defect both in the stem cell and stromal cell class: " . . . interactions between undifferentiated mesenchymal cells leading to regional specialization of inducing cells of the microenvironment may in turn be related to such parameters as cell-population

Table 1
NUMBER OF LEUKOCYTES IN 1 $\mu\ell$ OF TAIL VEIN BLOOD IN CBA/J MICE AGED 6 TO 8 WEEKS

Genotype (no. of animals)	All leukocytes	Lymphocytes		Monocytes	Neutrophils	Eosinophils, basophils
		Resting	Activated			
+/+—(9)	7350 ± 750	3200 ± 600	1650 ± 450	440 ± 90	1300 ± 360	760 ± 90
nu/+—(9)	2550 ± 800	1200 ± 450	600 ± 140	140 ± 30	520 ± 60	90 ± 10
nu/nu—(6)	2150 ± 550	300 ± 40	350 ± 40	160 ± 60	1090 ± 200	250 ± 60

Note: Means ± SEM.

density and aggregation, with further differentiation occurring once critical cell concentrations are achievd.''[18] We have stressed in the discussion of thymic dysgenesis that such a lower-than-critical concentration of mesenchymal cells may be the causative agent of the deviation of the epithelial anlage development (Chapter 3, Section V).

The stem cell potential is reflected in the white blood cell counts of *nu/nu*, *nu/+*, and +/+ mice. Not only lymphocytopenia which is most pronounced, but panleukopenia is routinely found when one compares the *nu/nu* white blood cell counts with the blood counts of normal, i.e., +/+ mice[4] and not with a mixture of leukopenic *nu/+* and normal +/+ littermates as done in the first analyses.[19]

Since in mice aged 1 to 3 months the proportion of peripheral blood lymphocytes in +/+ compared to *nu/nu* is about 3:1 and the proportion of neutrophils is about 1:2 to 2.5, it follows that there will be lymphocytopenia in all cases and absolute granulocytopenia in all cases where the total white blood cell count in the nudes is less than 50% of the +/+ mice. Rygaard has recorded only occasional differences in the number of granulocytes in his groups of the BALB/c, C3H, and C57Bl/6 background between nude and ''normal'' mice, his normal mice having a very low total white blood cell count.[17] We found in CBA/J,[20,21] C57Bl, and BALB/c mice,[8,9] a consistent difference between the normal +/+ and panleukopenic *nu/nu* and *nu/+* mice (Table 1).

The white blood cell count may be used for approximate determinations of heterozygous mice[2] only in colonies in good epidemiological condition with white blood cell count in 1$\mu\ell$ not rising above 10,000. We found that minor irritations like i.p. immunization with a corpuscular antigen evoke a marked leukocytosis lasting from 12 hr to 5 days after immunization in *nu/nu* mice and in *nu/+*, but not in +/+ mice;[21] consequently, in the period indicated there would be no difference between *nu/+* and +/+ mice. During infections such as *Pasterella pneumotropica* or infestation of the colony with *Trichomonas* and other parasites, the *nu/+* hybrids display a white blood cell count as high or higher than that in +/+ homozygotes (10 to 25,000) for a long period. In terms of hemolytic plaque-forming cells in a primary response to xenogeneic erythrocytes, the ''low-leukocyte'' mice[4] give lower responses than genetically-determined *nu/+* hybrids (Chapter 4, Section II) so that even some accidentally low leukocyte counts in +/+ mice cannot be excluded.

Interestingly, the differences in the total white blood cell count between normal and *nu* gene-bearing mice are present already in 17- to 19-day-old fetuses,[10] but the differential counts in fetuses are almost the same for all three genotypes;[10] only after the 1st postnatal week the proportion of lymphocytes declines in the nude mice with the proportion of monocytes and neutrophils increasing. In *nu* gene-bearing mice over 4 months of age the total white blood cell counts and the proportion of lymphocytes tend to decrease further. Lymphocyte counts may decline even more markedly in *nu/+* mice. In 2-year-old mice of the C3H/He background no differences between *nu/nu* and *nu/+* mice in these two parameters were noted.[22] The state of white blood cell counts in general is very much dependent on the epidemiological conditions of the colony and, in our experience, only minor age-related changes are found in real SPF colonies.

The number of colony-forming units in the *nu* gene-bearing mice can be temporarily corrected by one to three doses of levamisole,[9] an agent known to restore some defective immune functions by modulating, directly or indirectly, the intracellular cyclic GMP/cyclic AMP ratios.[23] Also, the white blood cell counts of *nu/nu* and *nu* + mice were elvated to the level of + / + littermates (C57 Bl/10 ScSn background) on day 5 after three s.c. injections of levamisole, but returned to the original values on day 12.[24] This shows that the hematopoietic defect of the *nu* gene-bearing mice has a common basic cause not residing in the thymus but in the compartments of stem and progenitor cells.

A deeper insight into the defect would be provided by closer approaches to the putative multipotential stem cells[25] which would also shed more light on the lymphoid series and possible defect in the T and B lineages.

The low levels of CFU/s established for the nude mice are reflected also in the erythroid lineage; the nudes have a mild anemia[26] which may be potentially important in considerations of their general metabolic profile (Chapter 9, Section II). Platelet production was found to be normal, more exactly about equal in *nu/nu* and *nu/* + which had a lower white blood cell count than the nudes.[26a]

II. CONNECTIVE TISSUES

Although the basic defects of the mouse mutant nude suggest some consequences in the cellular and extracellular components of connective tissues, the model remains almost unnoticed beyond the immunological boundaries.

Nevertheless, one group reports alterations in chondrocytes, osteocytes, and in the ground substance in BALB/c nude mice in unspecified conditions and compared to littermates.[27,28]

Osteocytes in the tibia diaphysis were in an actively osteolytic stage in 6-week-old nudes and their capsules displayed slightly decreased metachromatic staining and considerably decreased birefringence suggesting changes in the arrangement of acidic glycosaminoglycan chains.[27] Increased osteoclast activity was noticed in the metaphysis of the tibia.[28] The epiphyseal cartilage of the tibia in the nude mice of the same age had very narrow resting and maturation zones and premature mineralization in the proliferative zone. Here, the chondrocytes manifested degenerative changes.

The osteoclast activity may be attributed to an increased osteoclast-activating factor production in mononuclear phagocytes, including "activated peripheral blood leukocytes".[29]

No difference in multinucleate cell formation was found between B10.LP *nu/nu* and *nu/* + mice after glass coverslips implantation;[30] however, the cell covered area was much reduced at later stages (12 and 16 days after implantation) in the nudes,[30] showing a reduction of precursor cell immigration, proliferation, and ground substances formation in a chronic inflammatory lesion. This is paralleled by poor granuloma formation in different organs during a mycobacterial infection of nude mice.[31-33]

Some of the connective tissue alterations may be, however, at least in part attributed to incipient wasting in conventionally[34-36] reared nude mice which were found to develop autoimmune phenomena and degenerative changes; inapparent virus infections may be related to many pathological changes in the ground substance and basement membranes of connective tissue or of epithelial origin. Immune complex deposits in the basement lamina of renal glomeruli found in nude mice in conventional conditions are an outstanding example.[37,38]

Pantelouris suggested in the earliest days of nude mouse experimentation a parallel between senescence and nude mouse wasting, related to the very high IgM/IgG ratio and extending to the decreasing ratio of extractable to insoluble skin collagen and antinuclear factors.[34,39] The collagen changes were not demonstrable in SPF nude mice.[34]

Also, antinuclear factors are of the IgM class and it was clearly demonstrated that anti-double-stranded DNA antibodies in nudes are due to infections; germ-free BALB/c *nu/nu* had no significant autoantibody formation.[40] No autoimmune phenomena were observed in an SPF colony of outbred nude mice with an exceptionally long survival.[41]

Interestingly, some other vitus-associated effects were not demonstrated in *nu/nu* mice, e.g., the encephalomyocarditis virus was not diabetogenic in the nudes, as opposed to euthymic controls.[42] The defense of nude mice against unnatural pathogens (Chapter 7, Section II) may provide an explanation.

Only systematic studies on germ-free nude mice could provide an answer to whether some intrinsic factors related to thymic dysgenesis or to its cause do influence the state of connective tissues, basement laminas, collagens, and glycosaminoglycans.

III. MAST CELLS

The mast cell reflects the intensity of glycosoaminoglycan metabolism and connective tissue neoformation.[43,44] Their elevated numbers in cutaneous hypersensitivity reactions[45] may be attributed to the intensity of mesenchymal processes, with mast cells serving as accumulators of heparin and heparin-like compounds which have been secreted by their precursors and may be used later upon degranulation, together with heparin-bound vasoactive amins. The increase of mast cells in lymph nodes is antigen-provoked but not specifically related to the immune response.[46]

Interestingly, there are normal or elevated numbers of mast cells in the skin and lymphatic tissues of nude mice.[43,47,48] Their numbers increase with age and, in 6-month-old mice bearing the *nu* gene, i.e., also in heterozygotes, the number of mast cells in the popliteal lymph nodes is twice as high as that in normal (+/+) mice.[48] Also, in the lymph nodes of nudes with viral hepatitis, mast cells are more numerous.[48]

In skin grafts from mast-cell-deficient mice transferred to the back of nude recipients the number of mast cells differentiating from recipient bone marrow precursors is about normal.[49]

In skin grafts from A/H mice to CBA/J nudes resulting in permanent takes we have found high numbers of mast cells not only in the graft, but also in the surrounding recipient's connective tissue; in addition, low sulfated glycosoaminoglycans of the ground substance were abundant in the nude mouse recipient. The same observation was made in xenograft situation with chicken skin.[43]

Obviously, the local reaction to the graft lacking the efficient T-dependent components invokes higher involvement of mesenchymal tissuc rebuilding and barrier-forming processes. The same may be true of the elevated numbers of mast cells in the hairless skin of the nude and hairless (*hr/hr*) mice where thermoregulation imposes a considerable load of the dermal tissue metabolism.[50]

We also observed a much higher increase in the number of mast cells in the omenta of nude mice upon i.p. irritation, compared to euthymic mice.[43]

There is evidence that the nude mouse mast cells are normal as to their heparin and other sulfated glycosoaminoglycan content.[43]

In our view, the increase in the number of mast cells in the popliteal lymph nodes of *nu/+* mice as opposed to the +/+ mice[51] represents a hint that there is a slight deficiency in the immune reactivity fo the *nu/+* mice which is counteracted by nonspecific mechanisms whose obvious marker would be the presence of mast cells.

Mast cells in the intestinal and respiratory mucosae may represent a different type, a short-lived "lymphoid" mast cell, which is dependent on regulation by the T system.[52] It is important to note that the mucosal mast cells are also present in normal numbers in nude mice (as well as in nude rats, B rats, and eventually in a child with Di George syndrome).[53] The only difference found in nude mice is a lack of response of mucosal mast cells in the heavily deficient mucosal lymphatic apparatus to nematode infestation.[52] Also, the secretion of a mucosal mast cell protease during infection may be deficient in athymic animals.[54]

We did not note any difference in the occasional occurrence of basophils in *nu/nu* fetal or postnatal blood compared to the blood of euthymic littermates.

With the exception of mucosal mast cells, the mast cell system seems to be one of the sufficient and adequate mesenchymal cell systems in the athymic nude mouse which served in the last decade as an unequivocal disproof of the story on the thymic origin of mast cells.

REFERENCES

1. **Resnitzky, P., Zipori, D., and Trainin, N.,** Effect of neonatal thymectomy on hemopoietic tissue in mice, *Blood,* 37, 634, 1971.
2. **Pantelouris, E. M.,** Absence of thymus in a mouse mutant, *Nature,* 217, 370, 1968.
3. **Pritchard, H. and Micklem, H. S.,** Haemopoietic stem cell and progenitors of functional T-lymphocytes in the bone marrow of "nude" mice, *Clin. Exp. Immunol.,* 14, 597, 1973.
4. **Holub, M., Hajdu, I., Jaroškova, L., and Trebichavský, I.,** Lymphatic tissues and antibody-forming cells of athymic nude mice. *Z. Immunitaetsforsch.,* 146, 322, 1974.
5. **Zipori, D. and Trainin, N.,** Defective capacity of bone marrow from nude mice to restore lethally irradiated recipients, *Blood,* 42, 671, 1973.
6. **Splitter, G. A., McGuire, T. C., and Davis, W. C.,** The differentiation of bone marrow cells to functional T lymphocytes following implantation of thymus grafts and thymic stroma in nude and AT × BM mice, *Cell. Immunol.,* 34, 93, 1977.
7. **Loor, F.,** The abnormal differentiation of the T-lymphoid system in the congenitally athymic (nude) mouse, *Ann. Immunol. (Inst. Pasteur),* 128C, 719, 1977.
8. **Barták, A., Bokorová, M., Rychter, Z., and Holub, M.,** The thymus of the *nu/+* hybrid, *Folia Biol. (Prague),* 24, 419, 1978.
9. **Dolenská, S., Holub, M., and Mándi, B.,** Bone marrow stem cell potential in mice bearing the *nu* gene, *Folia Biol. (Prague),* 24, 421, 1978.
10. **Holub, M., Větvička, V., Fornůsek, L., and Paluska, E.,** Phagocytic cells of athymic nude mice in fetal life, in *Immune-Deficient Animals in Biomedical Research, Proc. 5th IWIDA,* Rygaard, J. et al., Eds., S. Karger, Basel, 1987, 59.
11. **Schrader, J. W. and Clark-Lewis, I.,** A T cell-derived factor stimulating multipotential hemopoietic stem cells: molecular weight and distinction from T cell growth factor and T cell-derived granulocyte-macrophage colony-stimulating factor, *J. Immunol.,* 129, 30, 1982.
12. **Bro-Jørgensen, K. and Knudtzon, S.,** Changes in hemopoiesis during the course of the acute LCM virus infection in mice, *Blood,* 49, 47, 1977.
13. **Cudkowicz, G. and Hochman, P. S.,** Do natural killer cells engage in regulated reaction against self to ensure homeostasis? *Immunol. Rev.,* 44, 13, 1979.
14. **Hansson, M., Kiessling, R., and Anderson, B.,** Human fetal thymus and bone marrow contain target cells for natural killer cells, *Eur. J. Immunol.,* 11, 8, 1982.
15. **Degliantoni, G., Perussia, B., Mangoni, L., and Trinchieri, G.,** Inhibition of bone marrow colony formation by human natural killer cells and by natural killer cell-derived colony-inhibiting activity, *J. Exp. Med.,* 161, 1152, 1985.
16. **Trentin, J. J.,** Hemopoietic inductive microenvironments, in *Stem Cells,* Cairnie, A. B., Lala, P. K., and Osmond, D. G., Eds., Academic Press, New York, 1966, 255.
17. **Rygaard, J.,** *Thymus & Self, Immunobiology of the Mouse Mutant Nude,* F.A.D.L., Copenhagen, 1973, 75.
18. **Metcalf, D. and Moore, M. A. S.,** Haemopoietic Cells, North-Holland, Amsterdam, 1971, 357.
19. **Wortis, H. H.,** Immunological responses of "nude" mice, *Clin. Exp. Immunol.,* 8, 305, 1971.
20. **Korčáková, L. and Holub, M.,** The response of peripheral lymphocytes of nude mice and leucopenic hybrids to antigen and lymphokine challenge, *Folia Biol. (Prague),* 24, 438, 1978.
21. **Korčáková, L., Holub, M., Nouza, K., and Dráber, P.,** Response of blood leucocytes to an intraperitoneal immunization in normal mice and leucopenic mice with the *nu* gene, *Folia Biol. (Praque),* 26, 176, 1980.
22. **Yunker, V. M., Gruntenko, E. V., and Moroskova, T. S.,** Leucocyte blood composition in mice C3H/ He *nu/nu,* C3H/He *nu/+* and C3H/He, *Folia Biol. (Prague),* 24, 437, 1978.
23. **Symoens, J. and Rosenthal, M.,** Levamisole in the modulation of the immune response: the current experimental and clinical state, *J. Reticuloendothel. Soc.,* 21, 175, 1977.

24. **Holub, M., Rychter, Z., and Machoninová, A.,** Induction of lymphatic tissue in the nude mouse dysgenetic thymus, in *Proc. 3rd Int. Workshop on Nude Mice,* Reed, N. D., Ed., G. Fischer, New York, 1982, 197.

25. **Visser, J. W. M., Bauman, J. G. J., Mulder, A. H., Eliason, J. F., and DeLeeuw, A. M.,** Isolation of murine pluripotent hemopoietic stem cell, *J. Exp. Med.,* 159, 1576, 1984.

26. **Bamberger, E. G., Machado, E. A., and Lozzio, B. B.,** Hematopoesis in hereditary athymic mice, *Lab. Anim. Sci.,* 27, 43, 1977.

26a. **Ebbe, S., Levin, J., Miller, K., Yee, T., Levin, F., and Phalen, E.,** Thrombocytopoietic response to immunothrombocytopenia in nude mice, *Blood,* 69, 192, 1987.

27. **Gyarmati, J., Jr., Mándi, B., Fachet, J., Matesz, K., and Varga, S.,** Functional structure of osteocytes in nude mice, *Hung. Rheumatol.,* Suppl., 21, 1983.

28. **Gyarmati, J., Jr., Mándi, B., Fachet, J., Varga, S., and Sikula, J.,** Alterations of the connective tissue in nude mice, *Thymus,* 5, 383, 1983.

29. **Yoneda, T. and Mundy, G. R.,** Prostaglandins are necessary for osteoclast activating factor production by activated peripheral blood leukocytes, *J. Exp. Med.,* 149, 279, 1979.

30. **Papadimitriou, J. M.,** The influence of the thymus on multinucleate giant cell formation, *J. Pathol.,* 118, 153, 1976.

31. **Ueda, K., Yamazaki, S., and Someya, S.,** Experimental mycobacterial infection in congenitally athymic "nude" mice, *J. Res Soc.,* 19, 77, 1976.

32. **Schlegerová, D., Kubín, M., and Holub, M.,** Lymphatic tissues of nude mice during early stages of *Mycobacterium kansasii* infection, *Folia Biol. (Prague),* 24, 428, 1978.

33. **Kubín, M., Holub, M., Mohelská, H., and Schlegerová, D.,** Experimental infection with *Mycobacterium kansasii* in athymic nude mice, *Exp. Pathol.,* 25, 233, 1984.

34. **Pantelouris, E. M.,** Premature autoimmune processes in nude mice, in *Proc. 1st Int. Workshop on Nude Mice,* Rygaard, J. and Povlsen, C. O., Eds., G. Fischer, Stuttgart, 1974, 235.

35. **Monier, J. C., Sepetjian, M., Czyba, J. C., Ortonne, J. P., and Thivolet, J.,** Spontaneous autoimmunization in nude mice, in *Proc. 1st Int. Workshop on Nude Mice,* Rygaard, J. and Povlsen, C. O., Eds., G. Fischer, Stuttgart, 1974, 243.

36. **Morel-Maroger, L. and Salomon, J.,** Autoimmune phenomena in nude mice, in *Proc. 1st Int. Workshop on Nude Mice,* Rygaard, J. and Povlsen, C. O., Eds., G. Fischer, Stuttgart, 1974, 251.

37. **Pelletier, M., Hinglais, N., and Bach, J. F.,** Characteristic immunohistological and ultrastructural glomerular lesion in nude mice, *Lab. Invest.,* 32, 388, 1975.

38. **Rossmann, P. and Holub, M.,** Renal lesion in nude mice, *Folia Biol. (Prague),* 24, 430, 1978.

39. **Pantelouris, E. M.,** Thymic involution and ageing, *Exp. Gerontol.,* 8, 169, 1973.

40. **Ogita, T., Okudaira, H., Tadokoro, K., Suko, M., Mizushima, Y., Gohda, A., and Horiuchi, Y.,** Antibody formation to double-stranded DNA in *nu/nu* and *nu/+* mice, *Int. Arch. Allergy Appl. Immunol.,* 57, 130, 1978.

41. **Gershwin, M. E., Merchant, B., Gelfand, M. C., Vickers, L., Steinberg, A. D., and Hansen, C. T.,** The natural history and immunopathology of outbred athymic (nude) mice, *Clin. Immunol. Immunopathol.,* 4, 324, 1975.

42. **Buschard, K., Rygaard, J., and Lund, E.,** The inability of a diabetogenic virus to induce diabetes mellitus in athymic (nude) mice, *Acta Pathol. Microbiol. Scand.(C),* 84, 299, 1976.

43. **Viklický, V. and Holub, M.,** Mast cells in skin grafts and omenta of nude mide, *Folia Biol. (Prague),* 24, 434, 1978.

44. **Viklický, V. and Poláčková, M.,** Specific and non-specific components in the effect of histocompatibility antigens in neonatal skin grafts on the host's immune response capacity, *J. Immunogenet.,* 1, 65, 1974.

45. **Dvorak, H. F. and Dvorak, A. M.,** Basophilic leukocytes in delayed hypersensitivity reactions in experimental animals and man, *Adv. Exp. Med. Biol.,* 28, 573, 1973.

46. **Wlodarski, K., Hancox, N. M., Zaleski, M., and Zaleska, G.,** The kinetics of mast cells in lymph nodes of immunized mice, *Immunology,* 24, 47, 1973.

47. **Wlodarski, K.,** Mast cells in the pinna of BALB/c 'nude' (*nu/nu*) and heterozygous (*nu/+*) mice, *Experientia,* 32, 1591, 1976.

48. **Wlodarski, K., Morrison, K., and Rose, N. R.,** Effect of *nu* gene on the number of mast cells in lymph nodes, *Scand. J. Immunol.,* 15, 105, 1982.

49. **Kitamura, Y., Shimada, M., Go, S., Matsuda, H., Hatanaka, K., and Seki, M.,** Distribution of mast-cell precursors in hematopoietic and lymphopoietic tissues of mice, *J. Exp. Med.,* 150, 482, 1979.

50. **Keller, R., Hess, M. W., and Riley, J. F.,** Mast cells in the skin of normal, hairless and athymic mice, *Experientia,* 32, 171, 1976.

51. **Straus, A. H., Nader, H. B., and Dietrich, C. P.,** Absence of heparin and heparin-like compounds in mast-cell-free tissues of animals, *Biochim. Biophys. Acta,* 717, 478, 1982.

52. **Ginsburg, H., Olson, E. C., Huff, T., Okudaira, H., and Ishizaka, T.,** Failure of mast-cell clonal growth in T cell-depleted cultures, in *The Immune System,* Vol. 2, Steinberg, C. M. and Lefkovits, I., Eds., S. Karger, Basel, 1981, 397.

53. **Mayrhofer, G. and Bazin, H.,** Nature of thymus dependency of mucosal mast cells. III. Mucosal mast cells in nude mice and nude rats, in B rats and in a child with the Di George syndrome, *Int. Archs. Allergy Appl. Immunol.*, 64, 320, 1981.

54. **Huntley, J. F., Newlands, G. F. J., Miller, H. R. P., McLauchlan, M., Rose, M. E., and Hesketh, P.,** Systemic release of mucosal mast cell protease during infection with the intestinal protozoal parasite, *Eimeria nieschulzi.* Studies in normal and nude rats, *Parasite Immunol.*, 7, 489, 1985.

Chapter 7

PHAGOCYTIC SYSTEMS AND NATIVE RESISTANCE

I. PHAGOCYTIC CELLS IN ONTOGENY

One of the essential problems of athymic life must be the defensive and regulatory systems which are roughly termed phagocytic and include both monocytes-macrophages and granulocytes of the neutrophil, possibly also of the eosinophil series from the metamyelocyte (in embryogenesis also myelocyte) stage on. The very nomenclature of these cellular systems makes the discussion of their meaning in normal and immunodeficient models somewhat hazy. The "mononuclear phagocyte system" is a term only a little better than "the macrophages" and a little worse than the effete "reticuloendothelial system" and the unborn "reticulohistiocytic system"; the trouble is that the cells, free or fixed, have many more functions besides phagocytosis and so any name hinting at this multiplicity would be more appropriate. (I never understood why the natural selection of scientific terms passed by "the histiocyte" which was endorsed by one of the representative international immunological conferences in 1959.[1]) We must stick to the accepted usage of mononuclear phagocyte system (MPS) in its original and revised form, comprising free and fixed macrophages, monocytes, interdigitating cells, "promonocytes", and precursor cells[2,3] among which the histologists' and pathologists' call "histiocyte" obviously belongs. It has to be remembered that the hematologist's progenitor stage which appears to be (unlike the highly phagocytic stage) positive for class II MHC antigens (Ia$^+$),[4,5] may not be confined to hematopoietic niches.

The MPS has multiple regulatory and secretory functions:[6] it may be viewed as "a huge, dispersed endocrine system"[7] the products of which may be classified into four major groups:[6]

1.   Products affecting extracellular and connective tissue proteins (lysosomal hydrolases, esterases, collagenase, plasminogen activator, finbronectin, etc.)
2.   Defense products (complement components, lysozyme, interferon).
3.   Biologically active products identical to — or additional to — interleukin 1 (lymphocyte-stimulating factor/s), granulocyte and macrophage colony-stimulating factor, mesenchymal growth factor, angiogenic factor)
4.   Small molecular weight compounds (prostaglandins, cyclic nucleotides, oxygen-derived products, thymidine).

It is obvious that the functional stage of MPS with all its potentials and humoral regulators has key importance in the development of the organism, especially of the organism affected by a basic disorder of the phylogenetically higher, lymphoid, immune system. The MPS is connected with the immune system by an array of reciprocal control mechanisms,[6] including antigen-independent lymphocyte-macrophage interactions.[6,8]

Not only the crucial role of MPS in the handling of antigens and infectious agents, but also its possible involvement in tissue growth, elimination of effete cells and tissue repair must be considered. Embryogenesis presents a specific problem, since MPS is concerned during this period mainly with the internal and intrinsic regulations, "amplifying requisite phagocytic functions" in different organs.[9]

An obvious need exists for functional macrophages in the earliest embryogenesis, from the moment of decay of the first worn-out cells; macrophages containing erythroblast nuclei and macrophages filled with cellular debris are found in the blood as soon as the yolk sac and embryonic circulations become joined.[10] Phagocytosis and other MPS functions play an integral part in all tissue and organ development, usually during invagination and separation processes; e.g., the yolk sac itself must be eliminated, pronephros and mesonephros replaced, the fetal cortical zone of adrenals must disappear around birth, many epithelial rudiments rebuilt; the development of fingers is conditioned by cellular death and phagocytic removal in the interdigital spaces; in general, morphogenesis proceeds as well by inductions and differentiations as by partial destructions and MPS interventions in exact space and time sequences. A specific mechanism of cellular death (apoptosis) is defined in the situations when the cell decay is a part of homeostatic regulation: expression of some sugar residues on the cell membrane promoting recognition and phagocytosis by MPS cells is the integral part of apoptosis.[11]

The stem cell-deficient nude (or *nu* gene-bearing) fetuses may develop at some stage a disbalance between the need of macrophages and the supply of their precursors; this may be corrected immediately by an enlargement of the macrophage-granulocyte progenitor compartment — MPS cells are obviously a self-regulating system.[12,13] But an increased metabolic rate and turnover within the MPS may last. More mature macrophage stages producing growth factors for mesenchymal cells and structures, such as fibroblast proliferation-stimulating factor,[14] angiopoietic factors,[15,16] endothelial cell proliferation, and migration and vascular smooth muscle stimulators[17-19] would be available in full compensation or overcompensation of the basic defects. A concomitant increase of the phagocytic capacities of MPS cells may be found during fetal life.

There are not enough data available on cellular phagocytic processes in rodent embryonic and fetal life. In general, the phagocytic performance of MPS — as judged from rat embryos — increases during intrauterine life; 22-day-old fetuses showed an increased ingestion rate of carbon particles in spleen and liver macrophages, when compared to 14-day-old fetuses.[20] This finding is in agreement with the observations in the more accessible pig[21] and sheep[10] fetuses; it was noted in the pig that in young fetuses the internalization of bacteria may not be associated with intracellular killing, i.e., during early intrauterine life phagocytosis is concerned mainly with the scavenger and not necessarily with the defensive function. In rat embryos, macrophages derived from local, subepidermal mesenchyme mature during the second half of fetal life. From day 12 on they have Fc and complement receptors and are capable of immune phagocytosis; they have discernible lysosomes from day 15 on.[22] In newborn — and obviously also in fetal — mice there is a defect in Ia$^+$ "phagocytes"[23] which are instrumental in antigen presentation whereas the phagocytic performance of Ia$^-$ spleen macrophages (or even Ia$^+$ spleen macrophages) appears to exceed adult levels.[24]

Using an in vitro phagocytosis assay with synthetic 2-hydroxyethylmethacrylate copolymer particles (HEMA) and blood MPS cells, we have found the phagocytic activity indices of monocytes (mean number of ingested particles per cell) to be about one third to one half of the values in adult blood, but the indices of fetal nude mice (gestation days 17 to 20) were invariably higher than the indices of *nu/+* or *+/+* mice[25,26] (Figure 1). This can be interpreted as the result of the higher MPS turn-over compensating the basic *nu* gene-caused defects: we imply that the stimulation may be present in tissue MPS cell as well; such a correlation exists in adult mice.

The enhanced phagocytic uptake in nude fetuses was found to be associated with a higher expression of some Fc receptors,[25,26] due to a higher stimulation of nude MPS cells. T cells present in the perinatal stage in the *nu/+* fetuses may produce a multipotential stem cell-stimulating factor,[27] but the direct macrophage/granulocyte progenitors seem not to be T-cell dependent. It was found in diffusion chamber cultures of adult mouse bone marrow cells that thymus cells added to T-cell-deficient cultures depress the generation of these progenitors.[28] On the other hand, a macrophage/granulocyte-colony stimulating factor was found in the nude mouse dysgenetic thymus (Chapter 8, Section IV). Also, there is a possibility that a link exists between the deep T-cell defect and the dissociation of the Ia$^+$

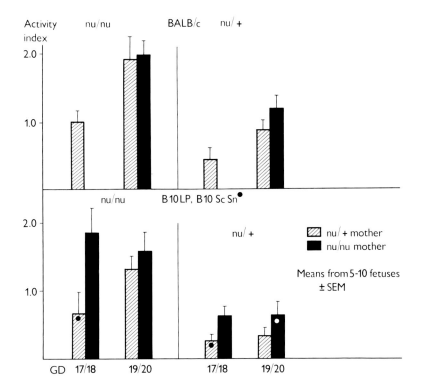

FIGURE 1.   Activity indices of monocytes (number of ingested HEMA particles per monocyte) in an in vitro phagocytosis test in withdrawn blood from *nu/nu* (left part) and *nu/+* (right part) fetuses on gestation days (GD) 17 to 20. BALB/c mice on the top, B10.LP or B10 ScSn on the bottom graphs. Significant differences ($p < 0.05$) between *nu/nu* and *nu/+* fetuses in all values except in 17/18 GD fetuses of *nu/+* mothers.

and cytotoxic (possibly phagocytic) activation pathway of MPS cells. Phagocytic cells present in neonatal mice were shown to lower the depression of Ia on macrophages[23] so that a circular process may be present in the nude fetuses until the onset of the postnatal microbial contamination.

The prenatal stimulation of *nu/nu* blood mononuclear phagocytes reflected by phagocytic uptake and Fc receptor expression was not found to persist in cells of the withdrawn blood of newborn mice[25] (Figure 2). With the microbial contamination of the litter the potential phagocytes may not be replaced in sufficient rates especially in the nude mice; the difference in the in vitro performance of nude *nu/+* and *+/+* blood MPS cells disappears and only in 18-day-old nude mice does the in vitro phagocytic uptake surpass again the same function of euthymic mice (Figure 2).

Peritoneal exudate and tissue (omental) macrophages of nude mice show a higher phagocytic uptake after only 40 days of life (Figure 4).

Obviously, the activated MPS cells migrate preferentially into the sites of the main microbial pressure, such as the intestinal system and lung and the seeding of precursors or local activation on other sites trail behind in the T-deficient mouse.

MPS cells provide a colony-stimulating activity for the expansion of the granulocyte/monocyte progenitor set[13] and, when stimulated, produce interleukin 1, a potent factor causing immediate neutrophil release from hematopoietic niches.[29] It is conceivable, then, that the nude MPS would drive the neutrophil granulocytes into higher phagocytic performance. However, there was no demonstrable difference in the phagocytic uptake of HEMA particles between nude and *nu/+* or *+/+* fetuses during intrauterine life (Figure 3).

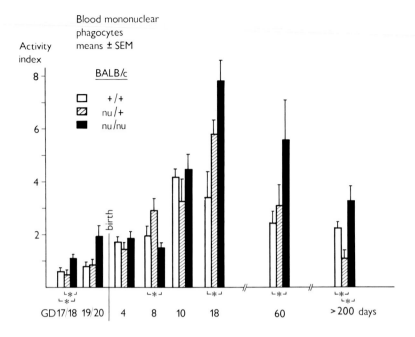

FIGURE 2.   Activity indices (as in Figure 1) in monocytes of mice of different age groups (5 to 14 mice per group). Significant differences ($p < 0.05$) are marked with asterisks.

After birth, the microbial contamination obviously causes a rapid increase of colony-stimulating factors (CSF). MPS cells are geared by the microbial contamination into an activated state and after about the 1st 10 days of life, drive the neutrophils into a state of increased Fc-receptor expression and consequently, high phagocytic potential. The increased pool of neutrophils released in the CSF and interleukin-1-linked process would modulate its own size by the resulting phagocytic inactivation of microbes — as in germ-free animals moved into a conventional environment.[30]

In the in vitro phagocytic assay, neutrophils of nude mice follow the blood MPS cells in a rapid increase of their phagocytic uptake; by day 18 they considerably surpass the same performance of blood neutrophils of *nu/+* and *+/+* littermates (Figure 3).

It should be reiterated that the only secretory function of the nude mouse dysgenetic thymus observed so far is the shedding of a promoting factor for the mononuclear phagocyte and granulocytes precursors (Chapter 3, Section V). The autoregulatory activity of MPS in the pre- and postnatal periods is obviously endorsed by a central thymic mechanism which may be even more pronounced than the support provided by the thymus and T-cell system in euthymic animals.

II. PHAGOCYTIC CELLS IN ADULT NUDE MICE

Although antimicrobial defense becomes the principal role of phagocytic cells in postnatal life, their secretory and regulatory functions in tissue growth, decay, and repair must be retained. In addition to the previously mentioned functions, interstitial or even exudate macrophages appear to influence the activity, including the endocrine activity, of neighboring or distant cells.[31-34] Both the defensive and the regulatory role of MPS cells are of paramount importance in the T-system-deficient, but perfectly viable and physiologically near-normal model.

The defensive role of nude mouse macrophages seems to be conditioned through activation by gut microflora; the defective IgA production[35] and the poorly developed gut-associated

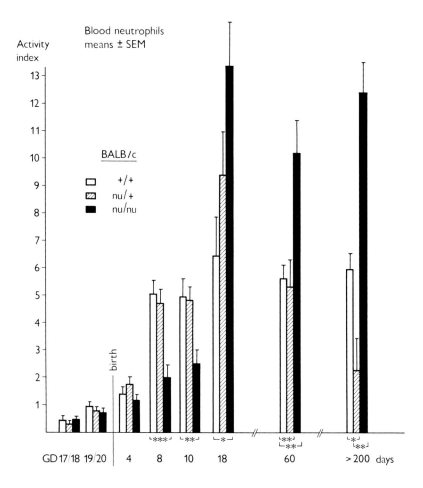

FIGURE 3.   Activity indices in neutrophils as in Figure 2. Significant differences are marked with asterisks: $p < 0.05*$, $p < 0.01**$, $p < 0.001***$.

lymphatic apparatus[36] allows nonspecific macrophage activators[7,37,38] to enter the internal environment. The activation is known to imply alteration of the enzymatic equipment of MPS cells,[39] enhancement of their receptor expression, phagocytosis, pinocytosis,[40] increase of their microbicidal potential against bacteria, protozoa, some viruses and fungi, and of their ability to destroy malignant cells.[7,39] In the nude mouse, the gut microflora pressure influences MPS cells which have been stimulated already during fetal life and show an increased tendency for phagocytic uptake (preceeding section); consequently the phagocytosis-triggered differentiation of some MPS cells into the state of "inflammatory" macrophages[41] may underlie the postnatal microbial activation of the bulk of nude mouse MPS cells.

A markedly increased phagocytosis and bactericidal activity of CBA nude mouse peritoneal macrophages was found in vitro, using 1 hr incubation with the facultative intracellular microbe *Listeria monocytogenes*.[42] In vivo elimination and killing of *Listeria* and *Brucella abortus* was considerably increased in nude mice from day 1 until day 21 or 30 of infection, i.e., the entire observation period.[42]

The enhanced bactericidal capacity was due mainly to splenic, hepatic, and other tissue-fixed macrophages. Increased phagocytosis, but lower bactericidal capacity of peritoneal phagocytes of nude mice was found after 35 min incubation with *Listeria* in another laboratory.[43] Clearance of *Salmonella typhimurium* from blood was 1000 times more effective

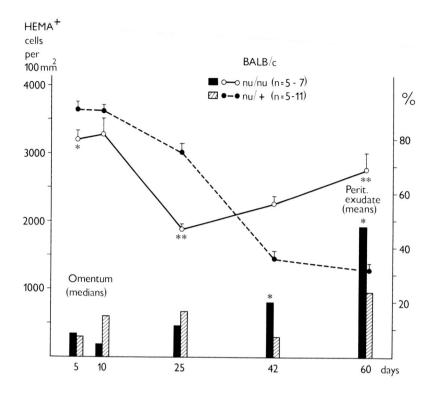

FIGURE 4.   Peritoneal exudate mononuclear phagocytes (top, curves) and omental phagocytic cells (bottom, columns) ingesting HEMA particles in vivo (20 min after i.p. injection).
Significant differences in single age groups are marked with asterisks: $p < 0.05*$, $p < 0.01**$.

at 3 hr after infection in nude mice, compared to euthymic controls; the killing of *Salmonellas*
and *Listerias* was elevated too; treatment with a phospholipidic bacterial extract enhanced
the uptake and digestion of bacteria in nude mice and in euthymic mice as well; the latter
showed a more pronounced effect.[44]

The high natural resistance of nude mice to *Listeria* infection was reported by many
laboratories.[42-48] The importance of activated macrophages in the process was proven directly
by experiments showing rapid growth of *Listerias* in nude mice after depletion of their
macrophages by various treatments.[45] Antibiotic elimination of the bulk of gut microflora
was shown to depress the high antibacterial activity of spleen and liver macrophages at 2
days after i.v. challenge with *Listeria*.[46] Also, thymic implants, grafted 5 weeks previously,
could abrogate the high resistance of random-bred BALB/c nude mice to *Listeria*.[46]

Variable results were obtained with peritoneal macrophages of nude mice. Their activation
seems to be less consistent and not detectable in some experimental conditions. The "lack
of sufficient local antigenic stimulation"[46] is one proposed explanation. Random-bred
BALB/c nude mice did not have "activated peritoneal macrophages" compared to *nu/+*
mice, when the cells were tested for phagocytosis and killing in vitro (45 min) of *Listeria*[46]
or for phagocytosis of sheep red blood cells.[47] Only increased percentage of macrophages
among resident or elicited peritoneal cells of nude mice was noted.[47] There was no indication
of activation of resident peritoneal macrophages of BALB/c nude mice in a tumoricidal
assay,[46] also, there was no marked difference in tumor cytostatis by nude or control resident
or elicited peritoneal macrophages; these cells activated by *Corynebacterium parvum* displayed a similar enhancement of their tumoricidal activity.[47] On the contrary, in a tumoricidal
assay using mouse tumor cells, peritoneal macrophages of C3H/HeN or BALB/c nude mice
were more cytotoxic than control cells and had also an enhanced response to chemotactic

stimuli[49] the responses of nude mouse peritoneal macrophages were quantitatively similar to the responses of activated peritoneal macrophages from normal mice infected with BCG. Most importantly, peritoneal macrophages harvested from germ-free nude mice did not show any in vitro tumoricidal activity.[49]

A comprehensive experiment using BALB/c nude mice and normal BALB/c mice established that elicited peritoneal macrophages of conventionally housed nude mice were more phagocytic for opsonized *Listeria* and showed after 4 hr of incubation a high level of kill; these cells also had a higher superoxide and hydrogen peroxide production. Reconstitution of these nude mice with thymus fragments 1 to 2 months previously or with splenic lymphocytes 2 days previously depressed the signs of macrophage activation.[50] When germ-free outbred nude mice were compared with microbiologically defined nude mice (exgerm-free, contaminated with a Gram-negative bacterial cocktail), the aforementioned macrophage functions were invariably higher in the contaminated group.[50] Peritoneal macrophages from exgerm-free nude mice (contaminated with a Gram-positive bacterial cocktail) gave no signs of enhanced bactericidal activity against *Listeria* after 2 hr of incubation unless they were elicited by proteose peptone.[51] Elicited neutrophils from germ-free and flora-defined nude mice were comparably bactericidal, but macrophages elicited from germ-free nudes were not active; there was no difference in bactericidia between nude mice and *nu/+* mice.[51] A slightly higher phagocytic uptake was found in peritoneal macrophages of germ-free nudes incubated with *Listerias* for 30 min, compared with the cells of germ-free or flora-defined *nu/+* mice.[51]

Germ-free *nu/nu* mice were reported to show more early clinical signs of disease when infected with mouse-adapted *Campylobacter* strains than their *nu/+* counterparts[52] this may have been caused by the *nu/nu* inability to produce specific secretory IgA which would prevent the penetration of bacteria into the intestinal epithelial cells; however, despite huge numbers of *Campylobacter* organisms in their intestinal tract and mesenteric lymph nodes, the infected nude mice did recover and were without pathological signs for up to 10 months,[52] obviously because of their phagocytic defense being stimulated during the infection.

This agrees in part with experiments on antiviral defense of nude mouse macrophages. Peritoneal macrophages of RNC nude mice raised in conventional conditions were resistant to vaccinia virus replication.[53] Macrophages taken from euthymic mice support virus growth as do macrophages from nude mice raised in germ-free conditions, or from nude mice which obtained a thymus graft 5 to 6 weeks previously.[53] Increased viricidal properties of peritoneal macrophages from nude mice raised in conventional conditions were also found with herpes simplex type 2 virus.[54]

Hence, the permanent or chronic activation of nude mouse macrophages is convincingly documented by the phagocytic uptake and to a lesser extent on cidal properties of the cells due to either oxidative or nonoxidative killing mechanisms. The activation appears to depend (1) on the presence of gut microflora which has a decisive enhancing effect on bactericidal activity and which is composed mainly of *Lactobacilli* and displays no differences from normal mice;[55] and influence of other inaparent bacterial or viral infections cannot be excluded; and (2) on the absence of postthymic cells, thymic cells and/or factors, released from a lymphatic thymus and affecting the differentiation and functional maturation of MPS cells, or, alternatively, producing some suppressive mechanisms of macrophage phagocytic potential. The degree of activation of nude MPS cells is obviously dependent on many environmental factors and conditions of the given mouse colony. Gross differences may thus become apparent in the results of different laboratories.

Activated macrophages play an important defensive role in a number of infections of nude mice, in addition to the well-analyzed *Listeria monocytogenes* and *Brucella abortus* experiments. As a rule, nude mice cope better with pathogens of other species than with natural mouse pathogens.[56,57] They are more successful with the initial stages of infections than with persistent infection: here the specific mechanisms for definitive elimination seem to be defective. As pointed out by Kindred,[57] only infects which a species can eliminate in time by a fully efficient immune apparatus — and not those which can be rapidly eliminated by an immune response of lower efficiency or range — will become natural pathogens of the species, the strain, or the mutant.

An impressive example of the unnatural infection is the influenza virus which is eliminated by nude mice MPS and other nonspecific systems successfully and within days.[58] On the other hand, the natural pathogen, mouse hepatitis virus, becomes the main danger of nude mouse colonies.[57] The nude mouse MPS defense seems to play a decisive role also in the rapid — but incomplete — elimination of fungi (*Candida albicans*[59]) and some protozoan parasites,[60] while the common murine flagellates *Hexamita muris* and *Giardia muris* infest nude mice to the extent that they were blamed for ''progressive wasting syndrome''.[61] Chronic infection develops in the genital tract of nudes after infection with the natural parasite *Chlamydia trachomatis;* this infection is resolved in heterozygotes within 20 days.[61a]

Kindred[57] draws an interesting conclusion that ''the T cell response (in euthymic mice) to viruses, as to protozoan and metazoan parasites, is most effective with natural pathogens; with virulent nonspecific pathogens, the T cell response leads to immunopathological damage and even earlier death''. Thus, the MPS-centered defense of the nude mice appears advantageous in evolutionarily nonestablished host-parasite situations.

The activation of the nude mice macrophages can be shown both in vivo and in vitro. The phagocytic uptake of synthetic (HEMA) particles or yeast particles by free peritoneal macrophages was found in more than 70% of peritoneal exudate macrophages in BALB/c nude mice, compared to 30% in $nu/+$ and $+/+$ BALB/c mice, 20 min after i.p. injection of the particles.[62] After 30 or 40 min, the percentage of phagocytosing macrophages was the same in all groups and the nude mouse macrophages were superior only in the number of particles ingested.[62] This shows that the resident peritoneal macrophages of SPF (but not germ-free) nude mice are in a permanent state of activation which can be matched by control macrophages only after direct stimulation. The same state was demonstrable in fixed macrophages in the omentum. Twice as many macrophages ingested the particles in the nude omenta 20 and 30 min after i.p. injection, after 40 min the differences between nude and euthymic mice disappeared.[62]

We have confirmed the finding[47] of a higher percentage of macrophages among all exudate cells in the nude mouse peritonea; their proportion decreased, however, 40 min after i.p. injection, at the time when the lower percentage of macrophages of euthymic mice started to rise.[62]

In vitro, the proportion of peritoneal macrophages ingesting HEMA particles after 60 min of incubation was more than 25 times higher in nude that in $nu/+$ or $+/+$ mice and the pinocytic activity of nude mouse peritoneal macrophages was 2.5 times higher. The activation of the nude mouse macrophages was documented by a markedly higher expression of Fc receptors for IgG_1 and of receptors for C3b and C5b components of complement;[62] these receptors are essential for the attachment and internalization phases of phagocytosis, respectively.

The same difference could be found also between blood professional phagocytes, monocytes, and neutrophils, of nude and control mice. A double or triple proportion of nude mouse neutrophils ingested HEMA particles in vitro, after 30 min incubation of full blood and the proportion of monocytes was also higher in most experiments.[63] Plasma exchange showed that the nude mouse leukocytes perform even better in the plasma of euthymic littermates. The state of the cells, including the neutrophils, was responsible for the performance, not a plasma factor; again, neutrophils of nude donors were found to have a higher expression of Fc receptors for IgG_1, IgG_{2A}, and IgG_{2B}. Nude mice monocytes were superior to control monocytes in ingesting HEMA particles via FC (IgG_1) receptors. Immunization or chronic infection caused an additional transitory increase of the percent of phagocytosing leukocytes. The numbers of active phagocytes rose to a greater extent in control, euthymic mice than in nude mice.[63]

Thymus tissue or T-lymphocyte transfer into nude mouse was shown to have both early (2 days) and late (5 to 8 weeks) depressive effects on the activated state of nude tissue or exudate MPS cells.[46,50,53] In blood professional phagocytes, we have found the early effect after transfer of thymic fragments subcutaneously. There was little change in the proportion of in vitro phagocytosing cells, but the number of HEMA particles ingested per monocyte or neutrophil dropped at day 3 after thymocyte transfer; 2 days later the high phagocytic uptake typical for nude mouse leukocytes reappeared[26] and was also found 2 weeks later. We reasoned[63] that the reconstitution of the nude mouse could lead to increased IgG synthesis and IgG isotypes belong to the most efficient opsonins; therefore, a possible depressive action of the thymocyte transfer would be obscured. In fact, 2 weeks upon transfer of cortisone-resistant thymocytes, the proportion of phagocytosing leukocytes and the number of HEMA particles ingested were further elevated.[63] However, at 1, 2 and even 16 months after transfer of cortisone-resistant thymocytes we have seen again a depression of phagocytic activity indices of leukocytes in vitro, especially in the monocytes. By this time, the ''late effect'' of normal thymic cells may have changed the whole immune status of the nude recipient.

There are no safe indications of a T-cell-mediated suppression of activated macrophages in the adult organism. On the contrary, the role of T cells in initiating macrophage activation is routinely assumed and shown to be mediated by lymphokines acting as differentiating signals, mitogens, and activators.[64-66] A number of small molecular weight macrophage metabolites such as prostaglandins were found to inhibit different T-cell functions, including lymphokine production:[6] as well as Ia expression on macrophages (accessory cells);[67] this may complicate the conditions of thymus transfer to nude mice. In our view, the late effect of thymus reconstitution of nude mice on their MPS cell status is most likely due to a slow repopulation of thymus-dependent areas of the gut-associated lymphatic tissues and subsequent shielding-off the influence of gut microflora, resulting, in several steps, in a decrease of the gut microflora pressure on MPS. The early transient depression of the phagocytic functions may be explained by lymphokines released by the transferred T cells and influencing the expression of Ia antigens on MPS cells.[68] Lymphokine-induced differentiation of Ia$^+$ low phagocytic macrophages[69] may alter the phagocytic performance of the whole population of MPS cells. Nonreconstituted nude mice were found to be deficient in generations of Ia$^+$ antigen-presenting macrophages.[69-72] The Ia-inducing lymphokine may be identical to gamma interferon[73] and its production was deficient in nude mouse spleen cell cultures of *Listeria*-immunized mice with the *Listeria* antigen.[72] In cultures of normal or thymectomized mice its production could be abolished by pretreatment of the spleen cells with anti-Thy 1.2 antibody and complement.[72] In this respect the nude mice (BALB/c) were inferior in the generation of Ia$^+$ peritoneal exudate macrophages to neonatally thymectomized BALB/c mice[72] showing that the phenomenon may be conditioned by the presence of thymus during fetal development or, alternatively, by a deeper extrathymic defect of Thy-1 expression in the nude mouse.

It has been asserted that the two important characteristics of the ''macrophage activation'', Ia expression and cytocidal capacity, are in some situations and both in vivo and in vitro clearly dissociated within a given macrophage population.[74] For instance, interferon gamma-induced tumour cell killing was rapid and transient in culture, and, on the contrary, Ia expression increased more slowly and was longer-lasting.[74,75] Beryllium sulfate or LPS elicited in vivo macrophages with a high Ia expression but no cytotoxicity, Concanavalin A and live *Listeria* microbes elicited macrophages with elevated both Ia and cytocidal properties;[74] both traits were expressed mainly in the same macrophage population.[74] Important immunoregulating functions of these multifaceted MPS cells were proposed, e.g., in the control of excessive T-cell proliferation[74] in euthymic models; how complex is the macrophage role in the athymic environment remains to be found. Nude mouse granuloma macrophages with burdens of intracellular *Mycobacterium leprae* bacilli cannot be activated by interferon gamma for tumoristatic activity, superoxide radical formation, or Ia expression.[75a]

MPS cells are important or most important regulators of precursor cell compartments expansion, acting, probably by interleukin-1 release, on cells like fibroblasts and endothelia which then produce hematopoietic growth factors.[76] Low doses of IL 1 have been shown in vitro to directly stimulate granulocyte-macrophage colonies (G/M-CFU), especially esterase-rich macrophage colonies.[77] This is another example of the circular process of self-expanding MPS cell pools in the nude mice.

As mentioned in Chapter 3, Section V and Section I, this chapter, even the thymic support for the precursors of mononuclear phagocytes and granulocytes is present in the nude mouse. In postnatal development, the stimulatory effects of the gut microflora may play an additional role. Therefore, it is not surprising that Wilson et al.[78] have found in nude mice of N:NIH(s) background elevated quantities of progenitors for monocyte-granulocyte pathways (colony forming units in methylcellulose supported culture system) and of progenitors for other mesenchymal cells (plaque-forming units in culture, mostly fibroblastic). Significant elevation in relative and absolute numbers of colony- and plaque-forming units were recorded from the bone marrow and spleen of 6-week-old *nu/nu* mice, compared to *nu/+* controls.[78]

In summary, the nude mouse phagocytic system, comprising both tissue and exudate MPS cells and blood leukocytes, may be interpreted as one of the sufficient factors of defense and of tissue regulation. The stem cell defect and lack of thymic and T-cell influence in prenatal and postnatal ontogeny appears to be responsible for a peculiar type of differentiation of MPS cells and their subsets as well as for their stimulation. The postnatal activation of MPS cells and neutrophils is due also to the gut microflora and its factors. The effectiveness of the phagocytic defense is fully adequate to cope with infects which are not natural pathogens of the species.

Some characteristics of nude mouse mononuclear phagocyte systems are surveyed in Table 1.

In broader biological terms, the plasticity of the MPS is able to assure a balanced development and defense of the organism affected by a basic disorder of the thymic system; "macrophages" in this animal model are in a way a self-sufficient connection between "the universe of epitopic self-nonself determinants.[79]

Table 1
PROPERTIES OF NUDE MOUSE MONONUCLEAR PHAGOCYTES

Precursor supply	Normal or increased (CFU-G, M)
Ia expression	Lower than normal; lower response to inductive factors, lower production of inductive factors
Fc receptor expression C receptor expression	On a higher proportion of monocytes and peritoneal macrophages of young adult non-germ-free mice
Mechanism of activation	Postnatally—stimuli from gut microflora and autoregulatory expansion of precursor sets by mature macrophages
Phagocytosis	Both ingestion and killing of some tested bacteria enhanced, especially in tissue and blood mononuclear phagocytes; high rate and extent of internalization of synthetic particles appearing postnatally first in blood, later in tissues (exudates); function dependent on the epidemiological status of animals
Viricidia, tumoricidia	Enhanced against some viruses (nonnatural pathogens); enhanced against some mouse tumors

REFERENCES

1. **Holub, M.,** Report of the Symposium Committee concerning the nomenclature of cells responsible for the immune reactions, in *Mechanisms of Antibody Formation, Proc. Soc. Prague,* Holub, M. and Jarošková, L., Eds., Academic Press, New York, 1960, 23.
2. **van Furth, R., Cohn, Z. A., Hursch, J. G., Humphrey, J. H., Spector, W. G., and Langevoort, H. L.,** The mononuclear phagocyte system: a new classification of macrophages, monocytes and their precursor cells, *Bull. W. H. O.,* 46, 845, 1972.
3. **van Furth,** Current view on the Mononuclear Phagocyte System, *Immunobiology,* 161, 178, 1982.
4. **Broxmeyer, H. E.,** Relationship of cell-cycle expression of Ia-like antigenic determinants on normal and leukemia human granulocyte-macrophage progenitor cells to regulation in vitro by acidic isoferritins, *J. Clin. Invest.,* 69, 632, 1982.
5. **Broxmeyer, H. E.,** Association of the sensitivity of mouse granulocyte-macrophage progenitor cells to inhibition by acidic isoferritins with expression of Ia antigens for I-A and I-E/C subregions during DNA synthesis, *J. Immunol.,* 129, 1002, 1982.
6. **Unanue, E.,** The regulatory role of macrophages in antigenic stimulation. II. Symbiotic relationship between lymphocytes and macrophages, *Adv. Immunol.,* 31, 1, 1981.
7. **Nelson, D. S.,** Macrophages: progress and problems, *Clin. Exp. Immunol.,* 45, 225, 1981.
8. **Lipsky, P. E. and Rosenthal, A. S.,** Macrophage-lymphocyte interactions: antigen-independent binding of guinea pig lymph node lymphocytes by macrophages, *J. Immunol.,* 115, 440, 1975.
9. **Douglas, S. D.,** Mononuclear phagocytes and tissue regulatory mechanisms, *Dev. Comp. Immunol.,* 4, 7, 1980.
10. **Al Salami, M., Simpson-Morgan, M. W., and Morris, B.,** Haemopoiesis and the development of immunological reactivity in the sheep fetus, in *Immunology of the Sheep,* Morris, B. and Miyasaka, M., Eds., Editiones Roche, Basel, 1985, 19.
11. **Duvall, E. and Wyllie, A. H.,** Death and the cell, *Immunol. Today,* 7, 115, 1986.
12. **Kurland, J. I., Pelus, L. M., Ralph, P., Bockman, R. S., and Moore, M. A. S.,** Induction of prostaglandin E synthesis in normal and neoplastic macrophages: role of colony-stimulating factor(s) distinct from effects on myeloid progenitor cell proliferation. *Proc. Natl. Acad. Sci. U.S.A.,* 76, 2326, 1979.
13. **Cline, M. J. and Golde, D. W.,** Cellular interactions in haematopoiesis, *Nature,* 277, 177, 1979.
14. **Leibovich, S. J.,** Production of macrophage-dependent fibroblast-stimulating activity (M-FSA) by murine macrophages, *Exp. Cell Res.,* 113, 47, 1978.

15. **Polverini, P. J., Cotran, R. S., Gimbrone, M. A., Jr., and Unanue, E. R.,** Activated macrophages induce vascular proliferation, *Nature,* 269, 804, 1977.

16. **Holub, M., Jarošková, L., Fischer, H., and Viklický, V.,** Neoformation of lymphatics in the mouse omentum, in *Function and Structure of the Immune System,* Müller-Ruchholz, W. and Müller-Hermelink, H. K., Eds., Plenum Press, New York, 1979, 427.

17. **Greenburg, G. B. and Hunt, T. K.,** The proliferative response in vitro of vascular endothelial and smooth muscle cells exposed to wound fluids and macrophages, *J. Cell Physiol.,* 97, 353, 1978.

18. **Martin, B. M., Gimbrone, M. A., Jr., Unanue, E. R., and Cotran, R. S.,** Stimulation of nonlymphoid mesenchymal cell proliferation by a macrophage-derived growth factor, *J. Immunol.,* 126, 1510, 1981.

19. **Polverini, P. J. and Leibovich, S. J.,** Induction of neovascularization and nonlymphoid mesenchymal cell proliferation by macrophage cell lines, *J. Leukocyte Biol.,* 37, 279, 1985.

20. **Reade, P. C. and Casley-Smith, J. R.,** The functional development of the reticuloendothelial system. II. The histology of blood clearance by the fixed macrophages of fetal rats, *Immunology,* 9, 61, 1965.

21. **Dlabač, V., Miler, I., Kruml, J., Kovářů, F., and Leon, M. A.,** The development and mechanism of bactericidal activity of sera and phagocytosis in pig fetuses and germfree newborn piglets, in *Development Aspects of Antibody Formation and Structure,* Šterzl, J. and Říha, I., Eds., Academia, Prague, 1970, 105.

22. **Takahashi, K., Takahashi, H., Naito, M., Sato, T., and Kojima, M.,** Ultrastructural and functional development of macrophages in the dermal tissue of rat fetuses, *Cell Tissue Res.,* 232, 539, 1983.

23. **Snyder, D. S., Lu, C. Y., and Unanue, E. R.,** Control of macrophage Ia expression in neonatal mice — role of a splenic suppressor cell, *J. Immunol.,* 128, 1458, 1982.

24. **Inaba, K., Masuda, T., Miyama-Inaba, M., Aotsuka, Y., Kura, F., Komatsubara, S., Ido, M., and Muramatsu, S.,** Ontogeny of 'macrophage' function. III. Manifestation of high accessory cell activity for primary antibody response by Ia$^+$ functional cells in newborn mouse spleen in collaboration with Ia$^-$ macrophages, *Immunology,* 47, 449, 1982.

25. **Holub, M., Větvička, V., Fornůsek, L., and Chalupná, J.,** Phagocytic uptake of synthetic particles in blood leukocytes of fetal and newborn athymic nude mice, *Immunol. Lett.,* 8, 93, 1984.

26. **Holub, M., Větvička, V., Fornůsek, L., and Paluska, E.,** Phagocytic cells of athymic nude mice in fetal life, in *Immune-Deficient Animals in Biomedical Research, Proc. 5th IWIDA,* Rygaard, J. et al., Eds., S. Karger, Basel, 1987, 59.

27. **Schrader, J. W. and Clark-Lewis, I.,** A T cell-derived factor stimulating multipotential hemopoietic stem cells: molecular weight and distinction from T cell growth factor and T cell-derived granulocyte-macrophage colony-stimulating factor, *J. Immunol.,* 129, 30, 1982.

28. **Benestad, H. B. and Strom-Gundersen, I.,** Thymic hormones and syngeneic T-lymphocytes are not required for leukopoiesis in an in vivo culture system for mouse bone marrow cells, *Exp. Hematol.,* 12, 319, 1984.

29. **Kampschmidt, R. F.,** The numerous postulated biological manifestations of interleukin-1, *J. Leukocyte Biol.,* 36, 341, 1984.

30. **Bealmear, P.,** Host defense mechanisms in gnothobiotic animals, in *Immunologic Defects in Laboratory Animals,* Vol. 2, Gershwin, M. E. and Merchant, B., Eds., Plenum Press, New York, 1981, 261.

31. **Dayer, J. M., Passwell, J. H., Schneebenger, E. E., and Krane, S. M.,** Interactions among rheumatoid synovial cells and monocytes-macrophages: production of collagenase-stimulating factor by human monocytes exposed to concanavalin A or immunoglobulin Fc fragments, *J. Immunol.,* 124, 1712, 1980.

32. **Kirsch, T. M., Friedman, A. C., Vogel, R. L., and Flickinger, G. L.,** Macrophages in corpora lutea of mice: characterization and effects on steroid secretion, *Biol. Reprod.* 25, 629, 1981.

33. **Yee, J. B. and Hutson, J. C.,** Effect of testicular macrophage-conditioned medium in Leydig cells in culture, *Endocrinology,* 116, 2682, 1985.

34. **Filkins, J. P. and Yelich, M. R.,** Mechanism of hyperinsulinemia after reticuloendothelial system phagocytosis, *Am. J. Physiol.,* 242(E), 115, 1982.

35. **Crewter, P. and Warner, N. L.,** Serum immunoglobulins and antibodies in congenitally athymic (nude) mice, *Aust. J. Exp. Biol. Med. Sci.,* 50, 625, 1972.

36. **Guy-Grand, D., Griscelli, C., and Vassali, P.,** Peyer's patches, gut IgA plasma cells and thymic function: study in nude mice bearing thymic grafts, *J. Immunol.,* 115, 361, 1975.

37. **Gordon, S., Unkeless, J. C., and Cohn, Z. A.,** Induction of macrophage plasminogen activator by endotoxin stimulation and phagocytosis, *J. Exp. Med.,* 140, 995, 1974.

38. **Gospos, C., Freudenberg, N., Bank, A., and Freudenberg, M. A.,** Effect of endotoxin-induced shock on the reticuloendothelial system. Phagocytic activity and DNA-synthesis of reticuloendothelial cells following endotoxin treatment, *Beitr. Pathol.,* 161, 100, 1977.

39. **Karnovsky, M. L. and Lazdins, J. K.,** Biochemical criteria for activated macrophages, *J. Immunol.,* 121, 809, 1978.

40. **Cohn, Z. A.,** The activation of mononuclear phagocytes: fact, fancy, and future, *J. Immunol.,* 121, 813, 1978.

41. **Baggiolini, M., Schnyder, J., Dewald, B., Bretz, U., and Payne, T. G.,** Phagocytosis-stimulated macrophages. Production of prostaglandins and SRS-A, and prostaglandin effects on macrophage activation, *Immunobiology,* 161, 369, 1982.

42. **Cheers, C. and Waller, R.,** Activated macrophages in congenitally athymic "nude" mice and in lethally irradiated mice, *J. Immunol.,* 115, 844, 1975.

43. **Zinkernagel, R. M. and Blanden, R. V.,** Macrophage activation in mice lacking thymus-derived (T) cells, *Experientia,* 31, 591, 1975.

44. **Fauve, R. M. and Hevin, B.,** Résistance paradoxale des souris thymoprivés à l'infection par *Listeria monocytogenes* et *Salmonella typhimurium* et action immunostimulante d'un extrait bactérien phospholipidique (EBP), *C.R. Acad. Sci. Paris (D),* 279, 1603, 1974.

45. **Nomoto, K., Shimotori, S., Muraoka, S., Miyake, T., Taniguchi, T., Takeya, K., Suzuki, T., and Goda, A.,** Analysis of protective immunity to various microorganisms by the use of nude mice, in *Proc. 2nd Int. Workshop on Nude Mice,* Nomura, T., Ohsawa, N., Tamaoki, N., and Fujiwara, K., Eds., G. Fischer, Stuttgart, 1977, 113.

46. **Nickol, A. D. and Bonventre, P. F.,** Anomalous high native resistance of athymic mice to bacterial pathogens, *Infect. Immun.,* 18, 636, 1977.

47. **Johnson, W. J. and Balish, E.,** Macrophage function in germ-free, athymic (*nu/nu*), and conventional-flora (*nu/+*) mice, *J. RES Soc.,* 28, 55, 1980.

48. **Emmerling, P., Finger, H., and Hof, H.,** Cell-mediated resistance to infection with *Listeria* monocytogenes in nude mice, *Infect. Immun.,* 15, 382, 1977.

49. **Meltzer, M. S.,** Tumoricidal responses in vitro of peritoneal macrophages from conventionally housed and germ-free nude mice, *Cell. Immunol.,* 22, 176, 1976.

50. **Sharp, A. K. and Colson, M. J.,** The regulation of macrophage activity in congenitally athymic mice, *Eur. J. Immunol.,* 14, 102, 1984.

51. **Czuprynski, C. J. and Brown, J. F.,** Phagocytes from flora-defined and germ-free athymic nude mice do not demonstrate enhanced antibacterial activity, *Infect. Immun.,* 50, 425, 1985.

52. **Yrios, J. W. and Balish, E.,** Pathogenesis of *Campylobacter* spp. in athymic and euthymic germ-free mice, *Infect. Immun.,* 53, 384, 1986.

53. **Rama Rao, G., Rawls, W. E., Perey, D. Y. E., and Tompkins, W. A. F.,** Macrophage activation in congenitally athymic mice raised under conventional or germ-free conditions, *J. RES Soc.,* 21, 13, 1977.

54. **Mogensen, S. C. and Anderson, H. K.,** Role of activated macrophages in resistance of congenitally athymic nude mice to hepatitis induced by herpes simplex virus type 2, *Infect. Immun.,* 19, 792, 1978.

55. **Herweg, C. and Kunstyr, I.,** Intestinal microflora of the nude mice, *Folia Biol. (Prague),* 24, 444, 1978.

56. **Mitchell, G. F. and Holmes, M. C.,** Nude mice in the study of susceptibility and responses to infection with metazoan and protozoan parasites, in *Proc. 3rd Int. Workshop on Nude Mice,* Reed, N. D., Ed., G. Fischer, New York, 1982, 1.

57. **Kindred, B.,** Deficient and sufficient immune systems in nude mice, in *Immunologic Defects in Laboratory Animals,* Vol. 1, Gershwin, M. E. and Merchant, B., Eds., Plenum Press, New York, 1981, 215.

58. **Wyde, P. R., Couch, R. B., Mackler, B. F., Cate, T. R., and Levy, B. M.,** Effects of low- and high-passage influenza virus infection in normal and nude mice, *Infect. Immun.,* 15, 221, 1977.

59. **Cutler, J. E.,** Acute systemic candidiasis in normal and congenitally thymic-deficient (nude) mice, *J. RES Soc.,* 19, 121, 1976.

60. **Mitchell, G. F.,** Studies on immune responses to parasite antigens in mice. V. Different susceptibilities of hypothymic and intact mice to *Babasia rodhaini, Int. Arch. Allergy Appl. Immunol.,* 53, 385, 1977.

61. **Boorman, G. A., Lina, P. H. C., Zurcher, C., and Nieuwerkerk, H. T. M.,** *Hexamita* and *Giardia* as a cause of mortality in congenitally thymus-less (nude) mice, *Clin. Exp. Immunol.,* 15, 623, 1973.

61a. **Rank, R. G., Soderberg, L. S. F., and Barron, A. L.,** Chronic chlamydial genital infection in congenitally athymic nude mice, *Infect. Immun.,* 48, 847, 1985.

62. **Větvička, V., Fornůsek, L., Holub, M., Zídková, J., and Kopeček, J.,** Macrophages of athymic nude mice: Fc receptors, C receptors, phagocytic and pinocytic activities, *Eur J. Cell Biol.,* 35, 35, 1984.

63. **Holub, M., Fornůsek, L., Větvička, V., and Chalupná, J.,** Enhanced phagocytic activity of blood leukocytes in athymic nude mice, *J. Leukocyte Biol.,* 35, 605, 1984.

64. **Mackaness, G. B.,** Delayed hypersensitivity and the mechanism of cellular resistance to infection, *Prog. Immunol.,* 1, 413, 1971.

65. **Unanue, E. R.,** Cooperation between mononuclear phagocytes and lymphocytes in immunity, *N. Engl. J. Med.,* 303, 977, 1980.

66. **Sorg, C.,** Modulation of macrophage functions by lymphokines, *Immunobiology,* 161, 352, 1982.

67. **Oppenheim, J. J., Kovacs, E. J., Matsushima, K., and Durum, S. K.,** There is more than one interleukin 1, *Immunol. Today,* 7, 45, 1986.

68. **Steinman, R. M., Nogueira, N., Witmer, M. D., Tydings, J. D., and Mellman, I. S.,** Lymphokine enhances the expression and synthesis of Ia antigens on cultured mouse peritoneal macrophages, *J. Exp. Med.,* 152, 1248, 1980.

69. **Tzehoval, E., De Baetselier, P., Feldman, M., and Segal, S.,** The peritoneal antigen-presenting macrophage: control and immunogenic properties of distinct subpopulation, *Eur. J. Immunol.,* 11, 323, 1981.

70. **Lu, C. Y., Peters, E., and Unanue, E. R.,** Ia-bearing macrophages in athymic mice: antigen presentation and regulation, *J. Immunol.,* 126, 2496, 1981.

71. **Holub, M., Jarošková, L., Hajdu, I., Říha, I., and Moticka, E. J.,** Enhancement of the immune response of genetically thymus-less mice by different cell populations, in *Microenvironmental Aspects of Immunity,* Janković, B. D. and Isaković, K., Eds., Plenum Press, New York, 1973, 289.

72. **Koga, T., Mitsuyama, M., Wanatabe, Y., Yoshikai, Y., and Nomomoto, K.,** Macrophage Ia expression in athymic mice versus neonatally thymectomized mice, *Immunobiology,* 171, 67, 1986.

73. **Schreiber, R. D., Hicks, L. J., Celeda, A., Buchmeier, N. A., and Gray, P. W.,** Monoclonal antibodies to murine γ-interferon which differentially modulate macrophage activation and antiviral activity, *J. Immunol.,* 134, 1609, 1985.

74. **Friedman, A. and Beller, D. I.,** Simultaneous expression of Ia and cytocidal activity by macrophages, and the consequences for antigen presentation, *Immunology,* 61, 435, 1987.

75. **Sher, M. G., Unanue, E. R., and Beller, D. I.,** Regulation of macrophage populations. III. The immunologic induction of exudates rich in Ia-bearing macrophages is a radiosensitive process, *J. Immunol.,* 128, 447, 1982.

75a. **Sibley, L. D. and Krahenbuhl, J. L.,** Defective activation of granuloma macrophages from *Mycobacterium leprae* -infected nude mice, *J. Leukocyte Biol.,* 43, 60, 1988.

76. **Bagby, G. C.,** Production of multilineage growth factors by hematopoietic stromal cells: an intercellular regulatory network involving mononuclear phagocytes and interleukin-1, *Blood Cells,* 13, 147, 1987.

77. **Gallicchio, V. S., Watts, T. D., and Della Puca, R.,** Synergistic action of recombinant-derived murine interleukin-1 on the augmentation of colony stimulating activity on murine granulocyte-macrophage hematopoietic stem cells in vitro, *Exp. Cell Biol.,* 55, 83, 1987.

78. **Wilson, F. D., Gershwin, M. E., Shifrine, M., and Graham, R.,** Increased clonegenic (CFU-C, PFU-C) populations from bone marrow and spleen of nude mice, *Dev. Comp. Immunol.,* 1, 373, 1977.

79. **Varesio, L., Landolfo, S., Giovarelli, M., and Forni, G.,** The macrophage as the social interconnection within the immune system, *Dev. Comp. Immunol.,* 4, 11, 1980.

Chapter 8

LYMPHATIC TISSUES AND CELLULAR IMMUNE REACTIONS

I. LYMPHATIC TISSUES

Nude mice have lived up to the expectations about the outlook of peripheral lymphatic tissues in the "athymic" state. The T-dependent areas like the splenic periarteriolar sheath, lymph node paracortex, and interfollicular tissue and domes in the gut-associated lymphatic tissue (GALT) were devoid of lymphocytes or, in the case of the spleen, contained scarce lymphoid cells and blast cells especially on days following immunization.[1-3] The germinal centers, a reactive structure most popular in the era of the first nude mouse studies, were absent even after administration of a thymus-independent antigen like *Shigella* endotoxin[4] or *Pneumococcus* polysaccharide.[3] These activators did not provoke basic changes in the lymphatic organs, there was only some increased lymphocyte traffic and homing and consequently, more defined postcapillary venules with higher endothelia.[3,4] In spite of the lack of true germinal centers with the typical structure and centrocyte-centroblast population, the localization of ^{125}I-labeled polymerized flagellin or bovine serum albumin (BSA) in the primary follicles of draining and remote lymph nodes, and total antigen capture in lymphatic tissues were normal.[5] This means that the interdigitating cells and follicular dendritic cells retaining antigen in antigen-antibody complexes for prolonged periods of time[6,7] were present and functional.

The essence of lymphatic tissue is the interaction of the reticulum cells with trafficking or settling lymphoid cells and the structural memory of these interactions; consequently, the main question of the nude mouse lymphatic tissue is the presence and nature of the dendritic cells. The lymphocyte and macrophage populations (Chapters 4, 5, and 7) follow their spatial organization, their antigen-presenting capacity and, eventually, are modulated by their humoral factors.[8]

In a comprehensive study of ICR mice, Groscurth gives a clear delineation of the present state of knowledge of the reticulum *in situ* and its ontogeny.[9-11] The picture may be analogous in all lymphatic tissues without epithelial stromal components.

In the mesenteric lymph node of ICR mice the first supporting framework is formed by primitive reticular cells which may be the last piece of the preimmunological legacy of Maximow's primitive mesenchymal cells.[12] These cells must be considered the main component of the primordium of the organ; their processes are connected with desmosome-like structures[10] suggesting a local derivation. Primitive reticular cells attain within the first postnatal week the ultrastructural features of fibroblastic reticular cells forming the reticular fibrils and, in the outer cortex, of dendritic reticular cells which later concentrate as a delicate network supporting the follicles, their long branching processes occasionally still connected by desmosomes.[9] Dendritic reticular cells form a very dense mesh in the germinal centers and the intercellular slits between their intertwined processes are filled with a characteristic electron-dense material.[10]

This is the B-cell microenvironment of the outer cortex of lymph nodes or of the splenic follicles where different stages and lineages of B cells are activated or reactivated (Chapter 5, Section II). In BALB/c *nu/nu* mice (6- to 8-week-old) the ultrastructural distinction in this area consists of fewer branching processes of the dendritic cells and only occasional formation of the mesh of intertwined processes characteristic of germinal centers[11] (Figures 1 and 2). The relative paucity of the dendritic cell network can be corrected by thymus implantation in the newborn or adult period.[11]

Dendritic cell concentration and dendritic network development may be influenced in the

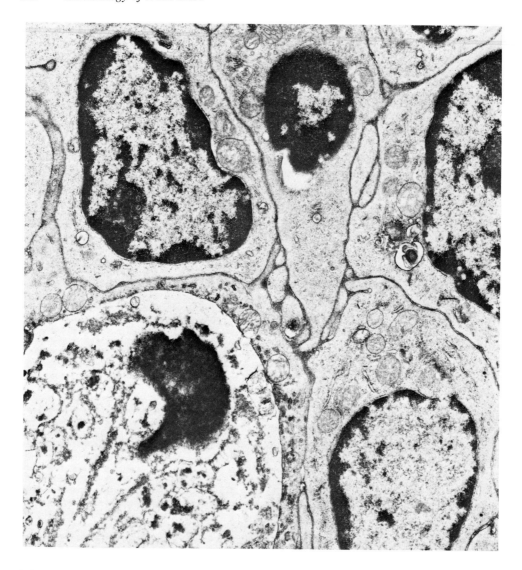

FIGURE 1.   Mesenteric lymph node of a normal BALB/c mouse, female, aged 2 months: follicular llarea in the outer cortex with the characteristic dark intercellular spaces formed by branching processes of follicular dendritic cells, with embedded lymphoid cells, one of them decaying (bottom left). (Transmission electron microscope; magnification × 14,500; P. Rossmann.)

last 3 to 4 days of intrauterine life by thymic factors and hence the nude subnormal development may be due to thymic dysgenesis, well marked on these days (Chapter 3, Section V). However, in view of the possible primary defect in mesenchymal cell accumulation, proliferation, and critical mass formation (Chapter 6, Section I; Chapter 3, Section V) it cannot be excluded that the follicular dendritic cells (FDC) are just another example of that primary mesenchymal defect. It can be corrected by thymus implantation, but this may mean more cellular interactions also within the peripheral lymphatic tissues than a mere supplementation of helper or amplifier T cells and thymic hormones.

In different lymph nodes other than mesenteric, the follicles, i.e., the areas supported by the FDC, tend to become hypertrophic,[13] possibly as a compensatory mechanism for the subnormal efficiency of antigen trapping which in this way is quantitatively normalized.[5] In mice with a combined immune defect known to support surprising numbers of Thy-1[+]-

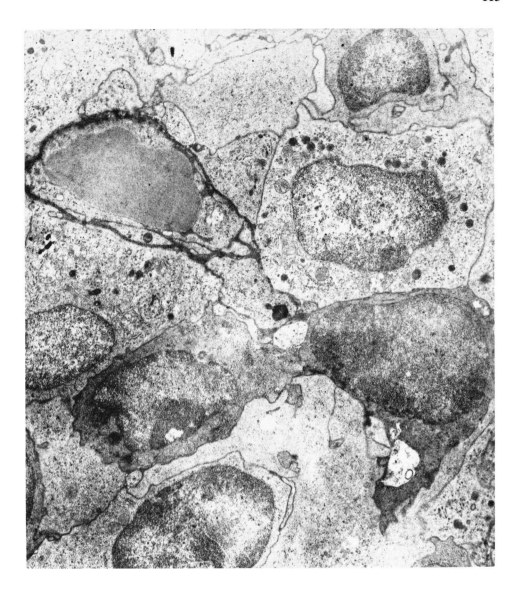

FIGURE 2. Mesenteric lymph node of a BALB/c nu/nu, female, aged 2 months: follicular area in the outer cortex analogous to Figure 1. The labyrinthine mesh formed by follicular dendritic cells processes and filled with dark material is less developed, lymphoid cells in different regressive stages and with increased numbers of lysosome-like particles in the cytoplasm. (Transmission electron microscope; magnification × 10,500, P. Rossmann.)

and IL-2-producing cells later in life,[14,15] the follicles are undeveloped and replaced only by a dense lymphocytic rim under the subcapsular sinus in the cervical, branchial, and axillary nodes.[16]

It may be suggested that, in this case, the disordered and defective cortical development and the disorder in the organization and numbers of FDC is also caused by some B-cell defect[17] which is combined with the nude mouse FDC paucity and which has little to do with thymic regulation.

In nude rat lymph nodes where the germinal center formation is subnormal, but not absent, FDC appear to be ultrastructurally identical to FDC of control rats. However, the concentration of immune complex deposits was lower in the follicles of nude rats and it was speculated that this reflects at least a maturational difference of FDC; in the nude rat, FDC would express less C3 or Fc receptors.[18a]

The second reticulum component of the lymphatic tissues is the family of interdigitating cells (IDC). These cells dominate the lymph node paracortex (deep cortex), the splenic periarteriolar sheath, the interfollicular area, and subepithelial compartments of Peyer's patches[8,18,19] and other T-dependent areas. They occur under the disguise of veiled cells and Langerhans cells in the lymph and nonlymphatic tissues.[20] They are obviously a part of the mobile pool of mononuclear phagocytes backed by bone marrow precursors[9,20] and settling in the T areas of lymphatic tissues. In the mesenteric lymph nodes of ICR mice, IDC precursor cells with a monocyte-like ultrastructure appear in the paracortex in the vicinity of postcapillary venules immediately after birth, before follicular dendritic cells could differentiate in the cortex.[10] This may be related[10] to the fact that the first lymphocytes immigrating postnatally into the lymph nodes seem to belong to the T lineage.[21] These cells may be missing in the nude mice.

In normal ICR mice, IDC dominate within the first postnatal week the middle and inner third of the lymph node cortex and this area becomes rapidly populated by lymphocytes so that after 2 weeks the IDC-lymphoid cell population constitutes the adult picture of the lymph node paracortex[10] (Figure 3).

In nude mice (BALB/c) at 6 weeks of age the IDC do not seem to be different in ultrastructure and quantity from those in euthymic mice;[10,11] the only difference being the missing close contacts and cytoplasmic invaginations with the scarce lymphocytes of the area.[11] According to a cytochemical marker (α-naphthylacetate esterase), these lymphocytes are not T cells, or not normal T cells.[22] Immunohistochemically (using a polyclonal anti-mouse brain serum), "a few" positive, presumably Thy 1$^+$, lymphoid cells were described in the paracortex of the mesenterial nodes of BALB/c nude mice aged 8 to 10 weeks.[23] The same occasional appearance of positive cells of the T lineage was recorded in all the other T areas; periarteriolar sheath of the spleen, interfollicular area of Peyer's patches,[23] and subepithelial zones of Peyer's patches. Analogous cells have been shown conclusively in mice of about the same age to be immature T cells,[11,24] albeit some small proportion of Thy 1$^+$ strongly positive cells without the TL marker could not be excluded in the tissues and in circulation, including thoracic duct lymph.[24,25]

Using double labeling with anti-Thy 1 and anti-Lyt 2 or L3T4 markers, small numbers of cytotoxic/suppressor or helper T cells were found in Peyer's patch domes of BALB/c *nu/nu* mice aged 8 or 16 weeks (females, probably conventional rearing conditions).[27a] These differentiated T cells were vastly outnumbered by immature, only Thy-1-positive cells.[27a]

It cannot be said that the IDC family is normal in the nudes. It is rather more abundant than in euthymic mice. Langerhans cells can be readily found in the dermis and epidermis of nude mice[26] and in the subcapsular sinus and paracortical area of cervical and axillar lymph nodes.[27] Here they may accumulate and modulate into the IDC mesh, raising with time the volume of the whole area[27,28] (Figures 4 and 5). A morphometric study in BALB/c nudes, kept in a well-controlled SPF state and 5 weeks old, established[27] that the

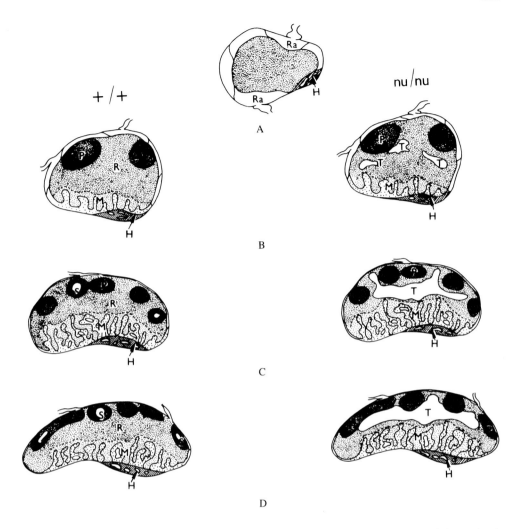

FIGURE 3. Schematic representation of the postnatal development of the mesenteric lymph node in a euthymic and *nu/nu* mouse. (A) newborn, (B) 2 weeks, (C) 5 weeks, (D) 12 weeks. (Ra) marginal sinus, (H) hilus, (P, S) primary, secondary (germinal center) corical follicle, (R) paracortex, (M) medulla, (T) reticular area, filled with interdigitating cells and few lymphocytes in the nu/nu mouse. (From Müntener, M., Groscurth, P., and Kistler, G., *Beitr. Pathol.*, 155, 56, 1975. With permission.)

absolute and relative weight of the cervical and axillary nodes is higher in the nudes than in control *nu/+* mice, the volume of the cortical, paracortical, and medullary parts larger, and the number of paracortical Langerhans cells per unit area 4 times higher in the nudes, the number of IDC 6.6 times higher.[27] This was stated already by Rygaard.[1] It puts an end to the long-lived controversy of whether the reticular paracortex in the nudes only seems larger because of the paucity of lymphocytes[23] or indeed is larger.[1,16,29]

The IDC family is obviously not dependent on thymus and T cells in transit or in residence. The IDC family seems to be an independent auxiliary system in the "athymic" state. The extent of the IDC-dominated T areas in the nude lymph nodes is variable in different anatomical locations. It attains maximal proportions in 6- to 8-week old mice in general, with the exception of the mediastinal lymph nodes where an altogether changed architecture occurs and IDC areas tend to form a core of the trabeculae or cords (Chapter 3, Section VI, Figure 15).

The seeming contradiction of reticulum development in the lymphatic tissues of the athymic

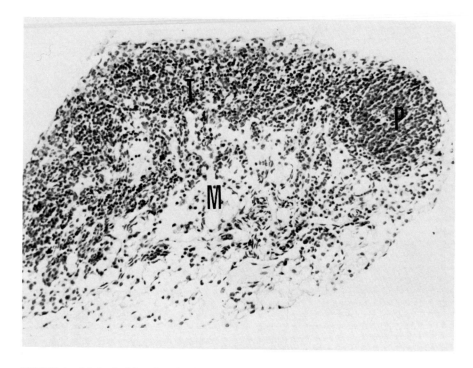

FIGURE 4.   Mediastinal lymph node of a 3-week-old CBA/J *nu/nu* male. At this age, mediastinal nodes are considerably larger in *nu/nu* than in euthymic mice and contain numerous lymphocytes in the paracortical area (T). The medulla is very large and the cortex is represented by one follicle only (P). (Hem. -eos.; magnification × 120.)

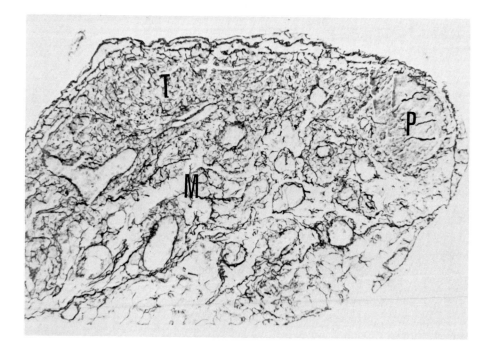

FIGURE 5.   The same lymph node as in Figure 4, after silver impregnation disclosing the rich reticulum in the T area. (Gömöry, hem. poststain; magnification × 120.)

mouse (well developed IDC in T areas, underdeveloped FDC in B areas) is compatible with the fact that IDC are derived from mononuclear phagocyte progenitors which are normal or supranormal in the nude mouse (Chapter 7) FDC from the presumably defective primitive mesenchyme. This may represent a logical compensatory mechanism for the heavily deficient T cell and only partially deficient B-cell lineage supply. The germinal center formation, so deeply deficient in nude mice, in spite of the fact that ''the majority of lymphocytes within the centers are of B-cell origin''[29a] can be explained by taking into account also the stroma.

In general, the B areas (splenic follicles, lymph node cortical follicles, follicles in Peyer's patches and medullary cords of lymph nodes) are densely populated by sIgM B lymphocytes and analogous cells are also scattered in T areas.[13,23,29] Plasma cells are found in some medullary cords while others are mainly lymphocytic.[13,16] Occasional blastic- and plasma cells were described also in the paracortical portions of the lymph nodes.[23]

The development of ''high endothelial'' venules in the nudes follow the pattern seen in euthymic mice.[30] On day 4 after birth the first lymphocytes in diapedesis through the venules become apparent and the endothelia increase their ribosomal and mitochondrial content and their rough endoplasmic-Golgi complex system. The only difference in the nudes is a conspicuous proportion of granulocytes migrating through the venule walls.[30] Also, typical high endothelial venules occur in the nudes deep in the medullary cords.[16] This suggests an altered (widened) area of lymphocyte recirculation connected with the altered relations of T and B lymphocyte populations and subpopulations (Chapters 4 and 5). Also, the splenic periarteriolar sheath extends and forms irregular projections into the follicular areas. In 9- to 12-week-old adult BALB/c nudes the major part of the white pulp was found to be irregularly dispersed in the red pulp.[31]

Interestingly, the GALT seems to be more affected by the low supply of recirculating lymphocytes and there is no conspicuous IDC accumulation and hypertrophy of the T areas such as that which occurs in the lymph nodes.[1,4,23,32] Also, the repopulation after thymus cell transfer from adult ''syngeneic'' donors was minimal and slow, compared to other tissues.[33] The altered homing conditions described in nude mice[34] may be especially pronounced here, and the IDC precursors, e.g., veiled cells, may proceed from the gut wall into the mesenteric lymph nodes[19] without contributing to the hypertrophy of the area just as in the nodes. The defective GALT obviously has some bearing for the postnatal activation of mononuclear phagocytes (Chapter 7) and for the induction of oral tolerance.[35]

Also, the number of lymphoid cells, mostly small lymphocytes, situated within the epithelial cells of the small intestine mucosa is reduced in athymic mice.[35a] These lymphocytes are especially frequent over the Peyer's patches. They are believed to be mostly thymus independent[36a] and involved in the immune responses against antigens occurring in the intestinal lumen.[37a] Characteristic groups of lymphocytes in Peyer's patches epithelium are present in small numbers in nude (BALB/c, 3 months old) mice.[35a]

The development of lymphatic tissue can be directly followed in the mouse omentum.[36] The number of local (temporarily settled) precursors of B lymphocytes appeared to be lower in the nude mouse omenta than in control BALB/c omenta,[37] however, the number of omental macrophages was markedly higher in the nudes (B10 Sc Sn) aged 2 months (as documented also in Chapter 7, Section I, Figure 1) and upon i.p. immunization with SRBC the number of dense lymphatic areas (pseudofollicles) was significantly higher in *nu/nu* than in *nu/+* mice (days 3 to 8).[37-39] Intraperitoneal immunization also provokes neoformation of lymphatic vessels and sprouting of blood capillaries.[38,39] The angiogenetic process is conditioned by macrophages and/or activated macrophage-released factors[39] and on a spatial arrangement of Ia[+] dendritic cells which correspond to IDC precursors.[20,40] Special ''pendant lymphatic nodules'' (PLN) originate on the basis of capillary loops; IDC and fibroblastic reticulum cells form their supporting network and peritoneal exudate macrophages their surface lining.[40] As to surface markers, PLN correspond to lymph node tissue,[40] but represent only a temporary

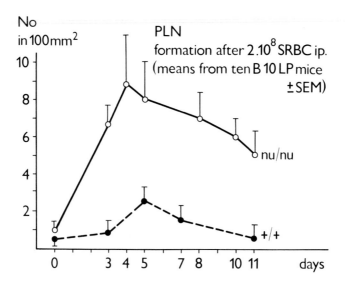

FIGURE 6.   Absolute numbers of pendant lymphatic nodules (PLN) in a unit area of the omentum in B10.LP *nu/nu* and +/+ mice. PLN originate on the basis of a loop or direct outgrowth of a newly formed lymphatic vessel and grow mainly by apposition of exudate cells.

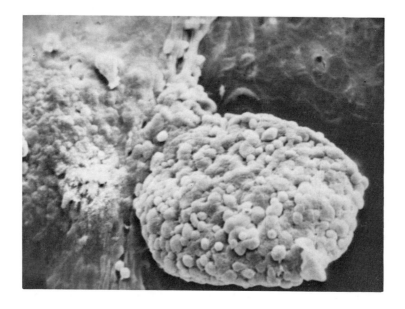

FIGURE 7.   A small PLN (see Figure 6) formed within 7 days after i.p. immunization in the omentum of a 17-day-old B10.LP *nu/nu* mouse. PLN is covered by exudate macrophages with a few lymphocytes. (Scanning electron microscope; magnification × 550, O. Kofroňová.)

structure on the omentum.[39,40] Formation of these PLN is markedly enhanced in the nude mice (BALB/c and C57Bl), both quantitatively (Figure 6) and in the kinetics of stromal and lining cell differentiation (Figures 7 through 10). Macrophages prevail and a lesser tendency for mesotheliazation is visible in the nudes.

This shows that the processes of tissue differentiation, including vascularization, which

119

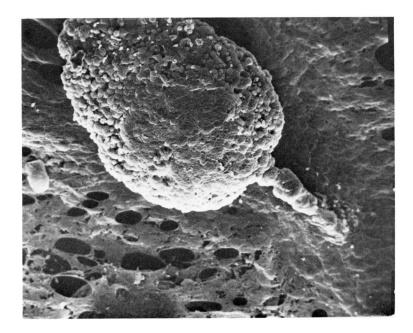

FIGURE 8.   A large PLN formed within 10 days after i.p. immunization in a 75-day-old
B10.LP *nu/nu* mouse. The central area of the nodule and its stalk are covered by flat,
mesothelium-like cells. (Scanning electron microscope; magnification × 250, O. Kofroňová.)

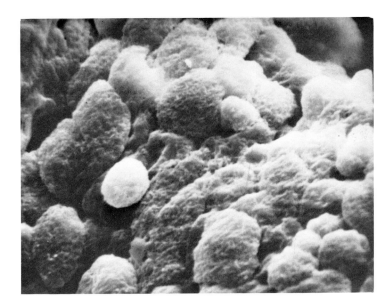

FIGURE 9.   A detail from PLN in Figure 7. The surface is formed by macrophages
with abundant ruffling membranes and one small lymphocyte. (Scanning electron
microscope; magnification × 2500, O. Kofroňová.)

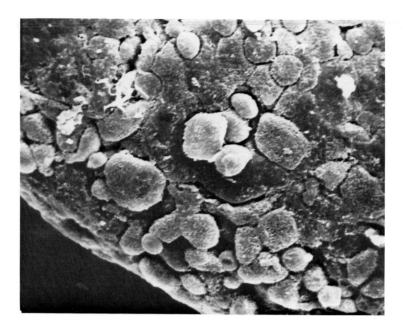

FIGURE 10.   A detail from a PLN formed in the omentum of an 18-day-old B10.LP
+/+ mouse, 7 days after i.p. immunization (analogous area to Figure 9). The surface
is mostly overgrown by mesothelia with poor settling of exudate macrophages. (Scanning
electron microscope; magnification × 1250, O. Kofroňová.)

are based on the migration streams of precursors of the mononuclear phagocyte family are
not deficient in the nude mouse; on the contrary, they seem to represent a quantitative
compensatory mechanism of the qualitatively deficient T and B lymphoid cell interactions.

In nude mice reconstituted with thymocytes, thymic implants, or thymic hormones and
T-replacing factors, the state of lymphatic tissues reflects the incomplete efficiency of the
procedure.[41-47] Kindred[45] summarizes the experience: "In general, reconstituted nude mice
mount responses with magnitude intermediate between the responses of normals and those
of nonreconstituted nudes, but they rarely reach normal levels. The numbers of Thy-1 positive
cells may approach normal . . ."[45] but the architecture of secondary lymphatic organs
displays attenuated anomalies at all times.[47] Kindred remarks that a T-cell-reconstituted
mouse is far from being just a skin-covered culture bottle, "but rather a complex, structured
organism;"[45] this is reflected by the lymphatic organs and often neglected by immunologists.

A close scrutiny was devoted to the germinal centers which were present, but scarce in
most reconstituted nudes.[1,48-50] Germinal centers could be induced in nude mice 5 months
after injection of viable or killed thymus cells; after only 2 weeks some recipients had small
or prominent germinal centers in their spleens and axillary lymph nodes.[48] The system used
implied graft-vs.-host reactions upon transfer of viable cells[48] as did most transplantation
systems at the early times of nude mouse experimentation. In reconstituted nude mice the
T-dependent areas of lymph nodes and spleens did not attain a normal lymphoid cellularity
even in individuals developing germinal centers.[33,48] Meanwhile, it was clearly shown that
allogeneic thymic lymphocytes disappear from the spleen of nude hosts after 7 days, semiallogeneic lymphocytes after about 3 weeks, and only "syngeneic lymphocytes" (recipients
were from an eighth or sixth backcross to either BALB/c or C57Bl/6 strains) are detectable
for months in young nude mice.[51]

In the system of organ transfer between noncompatible thymus donors and nudes, "full
population" of T areas in some spleens and some lymph nodes was described 43 days after
grafting,[3] without any relation to the eventual restoration of germinal centers.[3]

H-2 compatibility is in general not necessary in reconstitutions of nude mice with neonatal thymuses;[44] repopulation of the T areas was described in this situation repeatedly[1,49] and proceeded slowly, sometimes corresponding with the increase of Thy-1-positive cells in lymphatic organs.[52] Also, reconstitution with cultured thymic grafts led to an increase of lymphocytic populations in T-dependent areas.[53] There was always lack of correspondence between Thy-1-positive cells and T-cell functions and a conspicuous individual variation among the nude recipients.[45] Precultured syngeneic or allogeneic thymus grafts (mainly epithelial) provoked ''rich'' lymphocytic populations in splenic periarteriolar sheaths and lymph node paracortex of some BALB/c *nu/nu* recipients;[43,46] the effect was visible after 3 to 8 months, again, as in the case of the thymocyte transfer,[48] this was the time when the dysgenetic thymus of the nude recipient could also have been altered by the humoral factors shed from the transplanted thymic epithelia,[43] or influenced by the congeneic thymic lymphocytes (Chapter 3, Section VI, Figure 16). Unfortunately, the attention of almost all authors of reconstitution studies was centered on the state of the peripheral lymphatic tissues and the implanted thymic fragments.

In functional terms, reconstitution with thymus grafts is usually less efficient than that with large numbers of congeneic T cells.[45] It is likely that the allogeneic thymic fragments have mainly a humoral effect, since also xenogeneic thymuses (rat,[54] bovine[55]) have been shown to produce some functional improvement in some recipients (responses to T mitogens, skin transplant rejection, responses to allo- and xenoantigens in mixed leukocyte cultures[54,55]).

Thymus hormones in repeated injections providing a high actual concentration of the active principle in the recipient were shown to give some functional improvement[56,57] and some increase of lymphocytic and blastic populations in T areas of peripheral lymph nodes were described immediately after three doses of a thymosin preparation.[58] Secretion from thymus implanted in a diffusion chamber was inadequate.[59,60]

T-cell-replacing factors were more effective with nude lymphoid cells in vitro, as were the thymic hormones in most experiments.[61,62] In vivo, the T-cell-replacing factors had to be injected into the nudes at least 3 days before antigen to provoke some functional response,[45,63] but there are no reports of the effect on lymphatic organs. In our experience, a ''lymph node activating factor'' derived from cultures of allogeneic (B10 and B10D2) lymph node cells caused an increase of dense lymphatic tissue in cortical and paracortical areas and appearance of small light centers, possibly incipient germinal centers in follicles of popliteal lymph nodes of BALB/c mice of all three (+/+ , *nu/+* , *nu/nu*) genotypes.[64]

In all reconstitutions the reality in the recipient mouse, in single lymphatic tissues and even single units of lymphatic tissues[47] may be influenced especially at later times by the nude host reactions; these represent an enhanced development found in normal nudes which would live long enough[14] (Chapter 4). The high individual variability of reconstituted mice both in functional and structural terms, and the equal effectivity of congeneic vs. allogeneic thymus transfer[45] point in this direction.

The situation was clearly dissected by the experiments performed by Zingernagel et al.[65] and provided evidence that ''precursor T cell in nude mice can acquire restriction specificity and immunocompetence independently of a conventional, functional, H-2 compatible thymus if exposed to an allogeneic fetal (newborn) thymus that contains functional thymocytes of the donor type.''[65]

The role played by the structural, stromal peculiarities of the nude recipients may influence the cellular traffic in the lymphatic organs and contribute to the basic functional differences between in vivo and in vitro reconstitutions. As mentioned above, even 13 months after a newborn thymus implantation there were signs of increased lymphocyte traffic (transformation of lymph node medullary cord venules into high endothelial venules, subnormal differentiation of plasma cells in the cords, subnormal occurrence of germinal centers, formation of lymphocyte clusters characteristic of the nude mouse lymph node medulla, and the vicinity of high endothelial venules in the paracortex).[47]

Inasmuch as the nude mouse is not a skin-covered culture bottle, the reconstitutions are not reconstitutions. From the linguistic aspect, reconstitution means "to build up again by putting back together the original parts or elements". Thymuses and thymocytes are not original parts and elements which one would put back. They have never been in the nude mouse whose defenses cannot be built up again, but supplemented, substituted, or improved.

The main reason of most T cell or thymus transfers may be rather to "anticipate or accelerate the natural course of the nude mouse disease",[66] more exactly of the nude mouse solution of the consequences of the thymic defect. The bulk of the effect would be due to triggering of the host T-cell differentiation which occurs spontaneously up to the interleukin-2-regulated events,[14,15] provided the mouse lives long enough (Chapter 4). This process is of course strictly dependent on the state of nude mouse central and peripheral microenvironments. The relative differentiation block[66] in nude mouse T-cell population can be overcome by an intervention which has clearly only a triggering effect: 1 to 5×10^6 human peripheral blood T lymphocytes, irradiated with 2500 rad, injected i.p., induced several months lasting T-cell functions in 5- to 8-week-old BALB/c *nu/nu* mice, including IgM and IgG responses to SRBC or ovalbumin, lectin responsiveness, and strong Thy 1 expression in splenic cells.[66] Only a narrow cell dose range was effective, larger cell numbers induced resistance to subsequent treatments and thymocytes or IL-2-producing leukemic T cells did not trigger the nude mouse T-cell differentiation, whereas a non-IL-2-producing leukemic T cell did. The nature of the triggering action was unexplored and lymphatic tissues were not examined, but it is obvious that the T-cell areas in peripheral lymphatic organs and the dysgenetic thymus have been involved.

II. CELL-MEDIATED IMMUNE REACTIONS

The first and almost last direct experimental evidence for the absence of delayed-type hypersensitivity in nudes comes from the Pritchard and Micklem study showing that oxazolone sensitization does not provoke lymphocyte proliferation in the draining lymph node, nor infiltration of the ear subcutaneous tissues after challenge.[67] No hypersensitivity was also obtained with hepatitis B virus antigen,[68] fowl globulin,[69] and antigens of allogeneic cells.[70]

All this would, of course, considerably change many phenomena during chronic infections by microbial or protozoal agents. However, there was some specific response in the macrophages derived from inactivated *Mycobacterium kansasii*-sensitized nude mice (C57Bl, aged 6 to 10 weeks), as judged by migration inhibition in the presence of antigen.[71]

During some infections, an adjuvant or stimulatory activity of the pathogen may be in operation; in a mycobacterial infection there was a conspicuous lymphocyte repopulation of the T areas of lymphatic tissues, in addition to IDC (epitheloid cells?) increase.[71] This coincides with the low hypersensitivity component manifested during mycobacterial and related infections by low granuloma formation and decreased incidence of necrotic foci.[71-74] Granuloma formation is lacking also in nude mice infected with *Listeria monocytogenes*.[99] Also, probably due to low levels of effector lymphocytes and to the impossibility of further enhancement of the antibacterial activity of nude mouse macrophages (Chapter 7) recombinant gamma interferon could not cure chronic listeriosis in NMRI *nu/nu* mice.[100] In *Mycobacterium leprae* infections, frequently studied on nude mice, the reversal reaction is believed to be associated with development of delayed hypersensitivity; in fact, adoptive transfer of splenocytes from *nu/+* mice vaccinated with *M. leprae* and/or BCG induced reversal reaction in infected nudes.[101] On the other hand, chronic polymyositis induced in mice by coxsackievirus Bl, cannot be provoked in *nu/nu* mice unless they are supplemented with spleen cells of normal mice.[102]

To summarize, the situation may not be without an advantage for the nude, more or less

T-deficient mouse[45] which seems to be inferior to euthymic mice only in the late, chronic phase of the infective processes.[45,71,74]

Of course, the most attractive deficiency of the nude mouse has been, since its discovery, its allo- and xenotransplantation reaction, something which has been considered "a failure to reject" and which is, more realistically, a decreased potential to fulfill the rejection reaction.

The first full functional defect described in the nude mice, one would say in "the early nude mice", was the lack or inadequacy of transplantation reaction against xenografts, including human.[75,76] The nude mouse has been found to tolerate not only allogeneic mouse skin[77-80] but also the skin of almost exotic xenogeneic sources down to bird, lizard, and snake skin,[1,81] so that feathered nude mice have almost become a trademark, albeit the transplantations may not be that successful in other and more recent nude mouse colonies.

Bovine thymus grafts were found to reconstitute the nude mouse tissues and responses if they came from embryonic, not 4- to 6-month-old calves.[82] The success of the xenograft is obviously dependent not only on the nude mouse defense, but also on the viability of the transferred tissue.

In xenotransplantations of chicken skin, we have seen at least a 50-day survival and feather growth on the graft in C57Bl/10 ScSn nude mice, provided the skin came from newly hatched chicken.[83] However, the nude recipient was all but anergic, there was a massive reaction in the draining lymph nodes, including accumulation of lymphocytes in the T areas, forming cuffs around postcapillary venules, and finally secondary follicle formation.[83] There was also a marked reaction around the graft which included mast cell accumulation in the early stage.[83]

Allogeneic and xenogeneic skin grafts induce cytotoxic antibodies in nude recipients.[84-86] The antibodies switched from the IgM to IgG class in nude mice of all backgrounds tested (C57Bl/6, B10.LP, C3H, and BALB/c).[86] A secondary response could be obtained if the first graft was removed before the appearance of IgG antibodies,[86] the concomitant presence of both the graft and the antibodies of the IgG class led to a specific unresponsiveness.[86] The concentration of cytotoxic antibodies formed by the nudes was sufficient to cause the rejection of the graft after administration of rabbit complement.[87,88] It was suggested that — in this type of response — the nude mouse complement may be inefficient.[88,89]

Even if the allo- and xenotransplantation reaction of the nude recipient were inadequate, the situation is complicated, especially in tumor transplantations, by the fact that the recipient, influenced by the neoplasm in many respects, provides the stroma and demarcation[90,91] which may not be in all instances a limiting, but also a supporting, factor. The transplanted tissue provokes angiogenesis in general by factors shed by activated macrophages.[103] Specific factors have been characterized in neoplastic tissues,[104] but also some organotypic angiogenesis resulting in fenestrated capillaries in normal human thyroid tissue transferred to *nu/nu* recipients was recorded.[105] Vessels of human skin transplanted onto Swiss nude mice lose, after anastomosis with the host circulation, their endothelia within weeks; murine endothelia replace the original lining and produce finally a murine basement membrane.[105a] It was conclusively shown that human sarcomas transplanted to nude mice produce collagens of interstitial matrices mostly of human origin whereas human carcinomas have exclusively murine stromas after a brief period of composite human-mouse collagen types.[106] The nude mouse stroma of a human malignant tissue was found to turn eventually into a murine sarcoma itself.[91,107,108] This may also help to explain the presence of a putative mouse oncovirus in long-term human osteosarcoma xenotransplant in nude mice of an undefined colony.[92] The mechanism by which the nude host fibroblast turns into neoplastic cells is unknown, however, spontaneous transfection of host cells by human tumor DNA has been reported in experiments with implantation of human lung cancer cell lines established in nude recipients.[109]

Improvement of transplantability of human tumors to nude mice is dependent on a comprehensive knowledge of the *nu/nu* main lines of defense. Direct and local enhancement of tumoricidal activity of nude mouse peritoneal macrophages by different human melanomas was recorded.[110] Interestingly, a poorly tumorigenic cell line provoked a higher and longer lasting tumoricidal activity increase than a highly tumorigenic line[110] suggesting that macrophages are in some situations the crucial mechanism in nude host defense. The mononuclear phagocyte system is very hard to control in the nude mouse, antimacrophage agents have been found in one of the early studies to be either lethal or highly toxic.[111] Also, NK cells (Chapter 4, Section III) will play a decisive role in the nude mouse reactions against NK-sensitive implants.[112]

Construction of hybrid nude mice may be a better and more practical way[112] than attempts to decrease the *nu/nu* defenses by irradiation and splenectomy which were found to increase considerably the number of takes.[113] An important improvement in transplantability of human tumors would be the orthotopic propagation instead of the easy subcutaneous route or of the implantation under the kidney capsule; even fresh human lung tumors could be propagated with a high success rate by the intrabronchial implantation.[114]

The vast amount of literature on the use of nude mice in oncology is reflected in the IWIDA publications, in the Fogh-Giovanella volumes, and in the specialized surveys listed in Chapter 1, Table 1.

The growth of nonmalignant transplants other than skin is limited in most cases[93,94] and also benign tumors fail to live through the nude mouse transplant reaction.[95,96] However, some tissue residues can be found as late as 15 weeks after transplantation[95] as also can allogeneic cells after thymus cell transfer in some situations,[97] but not in all experimental settings.[51] Also, fetal xenografts of endocrine tissues were found to take and produce their specific factors for prolonged periods of time.[98] Implanted human pancreatic islets produced normoglycemia in diabetic nude mice for 30 days.[114a] Autonomous growth and metabolism was observed in xenografts of organs, such as toxic cat goiters.[115]

Again, the limits of success of tissue transplantation into nude mice depend rather on the nature and viability of the graft itself than on the variable ability of different nude recipients to fulfill the rejection.

An important insight into the nude mouse transplantation barrier was obtained from transfers of congeneic spleen memory cells: whereas 5- to 6-week-old BALB/c nude mice were permissive, 25- to 32-week-old nudes completely abolished the thymus-dependent memory; helper T cells (L3T4$^+$) activation of a B-cell barrier was postulated in aging mice.[115a]

A most interesting question of the immunoregulatory functions in the T-cell-deficient nude mice during pregnancy, e.g., of host-vs.-graft reaction in allogeneic or semiallogeneic pregnancies was attacked by Clark and associates. A local nonspecific suppression of the maternal immune response exists and is associated with the presence of small granulated non-T-lymphocytes in the decidua. These cells block the generation of cytotoxic T lymphocytes in several model situations.[116,117] The suppressive factor was obtained also from the decidua of allopregnant CD1 nude mice.[117] In intraspecies pregnancies (*Mus caroli* embryos in *Mus musculus* uteri) nude mice selectively discriminated against the foreign embryos earlier in pregnancy than +/+ females.[118]

The nude mouse allogeneic pregnancies testify that there are very essential situations where classical cytotoxic T cells are not the key factor[118] and that paraimmunological mechanisms, especially in cell-mediated immunity, may be more important than we have believed so far.

REFERENCES

1. **Rygaard, J.,** *Thymus & Self, Immunobiology of the Mouse Mutant Nude,* F.A.D.L., Copenhagen, 1973, 65.
2. **de Sousa, M. A. B., Parrott, D. M. V., and Pantelouris, E. M.,** The lymphoid tissues in mice with congenital aplasia of the thymus, *Clin. Exp. Immunol.,* 4, 637, 1969.
3. **de Sousa, M. A. B., Pritchard, H., and Parrott, D. M. V.,** An analysis of some morphological features of the lymphoid system in nude mice, in *Proc. 1st Int. Workshop on Nude Mice,* Rygaard, J. and Povlsen, C. O., Eds., G. Fischer, Stuttgart, 1974, 119.
4. **Parrott, D. M. V. and de Sousa, M. A. B.,** B cell stimulation in nude (*nu/nu*) mice, in *Proc. 1st Int. Workshop on Nude Mice,* Rygaard, J. and Povlsen, C. O., Eds., G. Fischer, Stuttgart, 1974, 61.
5. **Mitchell, J., Pye, J., Holmes, M. C., and Nossal, G. J. V.,** Antigens in immunity. Antigen localization in congenitally athymic nude mice, *Aust. J. Exp. Biol. Med. Sci.,* 50, 637, 1972.
6. **Veerman, A. J. P. and van Ewijk, W.,** White pulp compartments in the spleen of rats and mice. A light and electron microscopic study of lymphoid and non-lymphoid cell types in T- and B-areas, *Cell Tissue Res.,* 156, 417, 1975.
7. **Chen, L. L., Adams, J. C., and Steinman, R. M.,** Anatomy of germinal centers in mouse spleen, with special reference to "follicular dendritic cells", *J. Cell Biol.,* 77, 148, 1978.
8. **Friebss, A.,** Interdigitating reticulum cells in the popliteal lymph node of the rat, *Cell Tissue Res.,* 170, 43, 1976.
9. **Groscurth, P.,** Non-lymphatic cells in the lymph node cortex of the mouse. I. Morphology and distribution of the interdigitating cells and the dendritic reticular cells in the mesenteric lymph node of the adult ICR mouse, *Pathol. Res. Pract.,* 169, 212, 1980.
10. **Groscurth, P.,** Non-lymphatic cells in the lymph node cortex of the mouse. II. Postnatal development of the interdigitating cells and the dendritic reticular cells, *Pathol. Res. Pract.,* 169, 235, 1980.
11. **Groscurth, P.,** Non-lymphatic cells in the lymph node cortex of the mouse. III. Interdigitating cells and dendritic reticular cells in the mesenteric lymph node of the homozygous "nude" (*nu/nu*) mouse, *Pathol. Res. Pract.,* 169, 255, 1980.
12. **Maximow, A.,** Bindegewebe and blutbildende Gewebe, in *Handbuch der mikroskopischen Anatomie des Merschen,* Vol. 2 (Part 1) v. Moellendorff, W., Ed., J. Springer, Berlin, 1927, 232.
13. **Sainte-Marie, G. and Peng, F.-S.,** Structural and cell population changes in the lymph nodes of the athymic nude mouse, *Lab. Invest.,* 49, 420, 1983.
14. **Bamat, J., Sordat, B., Lees, R. K., Zaech, P., Ceredig, R., and MacDonald, H. R.,** Development and localization of T-like cells in the nude mouse, *Exp. Cell Biol.,* 52, 25, 1984.
15. **MacDonald, H. R., Lees, R. M., Glasebrook, A. L., and Sordat, B.,** Interleukin 2 production by lymphoid cells from congenitally athymic (*nu/nu*) mice, *J. Immunol.,* 129, 521, 1982.
16. **Sainte-Marie, G. and Peng, F.-S.,** Lymph nodes of the N:NIH(s)II-*nu/nu* mouse, *Lab. Invest.,* 52, 631, 1985.
17. **Palacios, R. and Leu, T.,** CC11: a monoclonal antibody specific for interleukin 3-sensitive mouse cells defines two major populations of B cell precursors in the bone marrow, *Immunol. Rev.,* 93, 125, 1986.
18. **Veerman, A. J. P. and van Ewijk, W.,** White pulp compartments in the spleen of rats and mice. A light and electron microscopic study of lymphoid and nonlymphoid cells in T- and B-areas, *Cell Tissue Res.,* 156, 417, 1975.
18a. **Mjaaland, S. and Fossum, S.,** The localization of antigen in lymph node follicles of congenitally athymic nude rats, *Scand. J. Immunol.,* 26, 141, 1987.
19. **Sminia, T., Wilders, M. M., Janse, E. M., and Hoefsmit, E. C. M.,** Characterization of non-lymphoid cells in Peyer's patches of the rat, *Immunobiology,* 164, 136, 1983.
20. **Hoefsmit, E. C. M., Duijvestijn, A. M., and Kamperdijk, E. W. A.,** Relation between Langerhans cells, veiled cells, and interdigitating cells, *Immunobiology,* 161, 255, 1982.
21. **Joel, D. D., Hess, M. W., and Cottier, H.,** Magnitude and pattern of thymic lymphocyte migration in neonatal mice, *J. Exp. Med.,* 135, 907, 1972.
22. **Mueller, J., Brun del Re, G., Buerki, H., Keller, H.-U., Hess, M. W., and Cottier, H.,** Nonspecific acid esterase activity: a criterion for differentiation of T and B lymphocytes in mouse lymph nodes, *Eur. J. Immunol.,* 5, 270, 1975.
23. **Hoffmann-Fezer, G., Rodt, H., and Thierfelder, S.,** Immunohistochemical identification of T- and B-lymphocytes delineated by the unlabeled antibody enzyme method. II. Anatomical distribution of T- and B-cells in lymphoid organs of nude mice, *Beitr. Pathol.,* 161, 17, 1977.
24. **Roelants, G. E., Loor, F., von Boehmer, H., Sprent, J., Hägg, L.-B., Mayor, K. S., and Rydén, A.,** Five types of lymphocytes ($Ig^- \Theta^-$, $Ig^- \Theta^{+weak}$, $Ig^- \Theta^{+strong}$, $Ig^+ \Theta^-$ and $Ig^+ \Theta^+$) characterized by double immunofluorescence and electrophoretic mobility. Organ distribution in normal and nude mice, *Eur. J. Immunol.,* 5, 127, 1975.

25. **Roelants, G. E., Mayor, K. S., Hägg, L.-B., and Loor, F.,** Immature T lineage lymphocytes in athymic mice. Presence of TL, lifespan and homeostatic regulation, *Eur. J. Immunol.,* 6, 75, 1976.

25a. **Ermak, Th. H. and Owen, R. L.,** Phenotype and distribution of T lymphocytes in Peyer's patches of athymic mice, *Histochemistry,* 87, 321, 1987.

26. **Hunter, J. A. A., Fairley, D. J., Priestley, G. C., and Cubie, H. A.,** Langerhans cells in the epidermis of athymic mice, *Br. J. Dermatol.,* 94, 119, 1976.

27. **Maruyama, T., Hasegawa, T., Kobayashi, F., Tanaka, S., and Uda, H.,** High incidence of Langerhans cells in lymph nodes of athymic nude mice: an ultrastructural and morphometric study, *J. Leukocyte Biol.,* 35, 441, 1984.

28. **Sakuma, H., Kasajima, T., Imai, Y., and Kojima, M.,** An electron microscopic study on the reticuloendothelial cells in the lymph nodes, *Acta Pathol. Jpn.,* 31, 449, 1981.

29. **Holub, M., Hajdu, I., Jarošková, L., and Trebichavský, I.,** Lymphatic tissues and antibody-forming cells of athymic nude mice, *Z. Immunitaetsforsch.,* 146, 322, 1974.

29a. **Thorbecke, G. and Lerman, S. P.,** Germinal centers and their role in immune responses, *Adv. Exp. Biol.,* 73A, 83, 1976.

30. **van Deurs, B. and Röpke, C.,** The postnatal development of high-endothelial venules in lymph nodes of mice, *Anat. Rec.,* 181, 659, 1975.

31. **Müntener, M., Groscurth, P., and Kistler, G.,** Histogenese des Immunsystems der "nude" Maus. III. Postnatale Entwicklung von Lymphknoten und Milz: eine Lichtmikroskopische Studie, *Beitr. Pathol.,* 155, 56, 1975.

32. **Guy-Grand, D., Griscelli, C., and Vassali, P.,** Peyer's patches, gut IgA plasma cells and thymic function: study in nude mice bearing thymic grafts, *J. Immunol.,* 115, 361, 1975.

33. **Jacobson, E. B., Caporale, L. H., and Thorbecke, G. J.,** Effect of thymus cell injections on germinal center formation in lymphoid tissues of nude (thymusless) mice, *Cell. Immunol.,* 13, 416, 1974.

34. **Gillette, R. W.,** Homing of labeled lymphoid cells in athymic mice: evidence for additional immunologic defects, *Cell. Immunol.,* 17, 374, 1975.

35. **Tlaskalová-Hogenová, H. and Holub, M.,** Effect of fed xenogeneic red blood cells on the immune response of euthymic and athymic mice, in *Immune-Deficient Animals in Biomedical Research, Proc. 5th IWIDA,* Rygaard, J. et al., Eds., S. Karger, Basel, 1987, 101.

35a. **Rell, K. W., Lamprecht, J., Siciński, P., Bem, W., and Rowiński, J.,** Frequency of occurrence and distribution of the intra-epithelial lymphoid cells in the follicle-associated epithelium in phenotypically normal and athymic nude mice, *J. Anat.,* 152, 121, 1987.

36. **Holub, M., Hajdu, I., Trebichavský, I., and Jarošková, L.,** Formation of lymphoid cells from local precursors in irradiated mouse omenta, *Eur. J. Immunol.,* 1, 465, 1971.

36a. **Abe, K. and Ito, T.,** Qualitative and quantitative morphologic study of Peyer's patches of the mouse after neonatal thymectomy and hydrocortisone injection, *Am. J. Anat.,* 151, 227, 1978.

37. **Jarošková, L., Trebichavský, I., Tučková, L., Jankásková, D., and Holub, M.,** The omental immune apparatus of athymic nude mice, *Folia Biol. (Prague),* 24, 432, 1978.

37a. **Collan, Y.,** Characteristics of non-epithelial cells in the epithelium of normal rat ileum, *Scand. J. Gastroenterol.,* 7(18), 3, 1972.

38. **Holub, M. and Polanová, E.,** The response of omental lymphatics to antigenic stimulation, in *Lymphology, Proc. 6th Int. Congr. of Lymphology,* Málek, P. and Bartoš, V., Eds., Thieme, Stuttgart, 1978, 264.

39. **Holub, M., Jarošková, L., Fischer, H., and Viklický, V.,** Neoformation of lymphatics in the mouse omentum, in *Function & Structure of the Immune System,* Müller-Ruchholtz, W. and Müller-Hermelink, H. K., Eds., Plenum Press, New York, 1979, 427.

40. **Holub, M., Kofroňová, O., Mohelská, H., and Ludvík, L.,** Ultrastructure of pendant lymphatic nodules — a novel type of lymphatic tissue, *Czech. Med.,* 1987, in print.

41. **Loor, F., Kindred, B., and Hägg, L. B.,** Incomplete restoration of T-cell reactivity in nude mice after neonatal allogeneic thymus grafting, *Cell. Immunol.,* 26, 29, 1976.

42. **Loor, F.,** The abnormal differentiation of the T-lymphoid system in the congenitally athymic (nude) mice, *Ann. Immunol. Inst. Pasteur,* 128C, 719, 1977.

43. **Hong, R., Schulte-Wissermann, H., Tarrett-Toth, E., Horowitz, S. D., and Manning, D. D.,** Transplantation of cultured thymic fragments. II. Results in nude mice, *J. Exp. Med.,* 149, 398, 1979.

44. **Jacobsen, G. K., Rygaard, J., and Povlsen, C. O.,** Immunological reconstitution of tumor-transplanted and thymus-grafted nude mice, *Exp. Cell Biol.,* 49, 148, 1981.

45. **Kindred, B.,** Deficient and sufficient immune systems in the nude mouse, in *Immunologic Defects in Laboratory Animals,* Gershwin, M. E. and Merchant, B., Eds., Plenum Press, New York, 1981, 215.

46. **Manning, J. K. and Hong, R.,** Transplantation of cultured thymic fragments: results in nude mice. IV. Effect of amount of thymic tissue, *Thymus,* 5, 407, 1983.

47. **Sainte-Marie, G., Peng, F.-S., and Pelletier, M.,** Morphological anomalies in the lymph nodes of 13-month-old thymus-grafted nude mice, *Thymus,* 8, 77, 1986.

48. **Jacobson, E. B. and Thorbecke, G. J.,** Secondary antibody response and germinal center development in nude mice reconstituted with thymus cells, in *Proc. 1st Int. Workshop on Nude Mice,* Rygaard, J. and Povlsen, C. O., Eds., G. Fischer, Stuttgart, 1974, 155.

49. **de Souza, M. A. B. and Pritchard, H.,** The cellular basis of immunological recovery in nude mice after thymus grafting, *Immunology,* 26, 769, 1974.

50. **Kindred, B. and Sordat, B.,** Lymphocytes which differentiate in an allogeneic thymus. II. Evidence for both central and peripheral mechanisms in tolerance to donor strain tissues, *Eur. J. Immunol.,* 7, 437, 1977.

51. **Piguet, P.-F. and Vassalli, P.,** Failure of allogeneic thymocytes to survive in nude mice, *Eur. J. Immunol.,* 10, 12, 1980.

52. **Loor, F. and Kindred, B.,** Differentiation of T-cell precursors in nude mice demonstrated by immunofluorescence of T-cell membrane markers, *J. Exp. Med.,* 138, 1044, 1973.

53. **Wortis, H. H.,** Pleiotropic effects of the nude mutation, *Birth Defects Orig. Artic. Ser.,* XI(1), 528, 1975.

54. **Manning, J. K. and Hong, R.,** Transplantation of cultured thymic fragments: results in nude mice. V. Reconstitution with xenogeneic (rat) thymic tissue, *Scand. J. Immunol.,* 19, 403, 1984.

55. **Rygaard, J., Andersen, D. H., Friis, C. W., and Aagaard, J.,** Morphology and functional changes in nude mice grafted with embryonic and adult bovine thymus, *Folia Biol. (Prague),* 24, 426, 1978.

56. **Ikehara, S., Hamashima, Y., and Matsuda, T.,** Immunological restoration of both thymectomised and athymic nude mice by a thymus factor, *Nature,* 258, 335, 1975.

57. **Ikehara, S., Matsuda, T., and Hamashima, Y.,** Restoration of T functions by a thymus factor in nude mice, in *Proc. 2nd Int. Workshop on Nude Mice,* Nomura, T., Ohsawa, N., Tamaoka, N., and Fujiwara, K., Eds., G. Fischer, Stuttgart, 1977, 265.

58. **Thurman, G. B., Silver, B. B., Hooper, J. A., Giovanella, B. C., and Goldstein, A. L.,** In vitro mitogenic responses of spleen cells and ultrastructural studies of lymph nodes from nude mice following thymosin administration in vivo, in *Proc. 1st Int. Workshop on Nude Mice,* Rygaard, J. and Povlsen, C. O., Eds., G. Fischer, Stuttgart, 1974, 105.

59. **Stutman, O.,** Inability to restore immune functions in nude mice with humoral thymic function, *Fed. Proc. Fed. Am. Soc. Exp. Biol.,* 33, 736, 1974.

60. **Jutila, J. W., Reed, N. D., and Isaak, D. D.,** Studies on the immune response of congenitally athymic (nude) mice. Immunodeficiency in man and animals, *Birth Defects Orig. Artic. Ser.,* XI (1), 522, 1975.

61. **Ikehara, S., Hamashima, Y., and Matsuda, T.,** Immunological restoration of both thymectomised and athymic nude mice by a thymus factor, *Nature,* 258, 335, 1975.

62. **Ikehara, S., Matsuda, T., and Hamashima, Y.,** Restoration of T cell functions by a thymus factor in nude mice, in *Proc. 2nd Int. Workshop on Nude Mice,* Nomura, T., Ohsawa, N., Tamaoka, N., and Fujiwara, K., Eds., G. Fischer, Stuttgart, 1977, 265.

63. **Kindred, B., Bösing-Schneider, R., and Corley, R. B.,** In vivo activity of a nonspecific T cell-replacing factor, *J. Immunol.,* 122, 350, 1979.

64. **Korčáková, L. and Holub, M.,** Lymph node activating factor from mixed cultures of allogeneic lymphoid cells: effect on the lymph nodes of euthymic and athymic mice, *Allerg. Immunol. (Leipzig),* 23, 287, 1977.

65. **Zingernagel, R. M., Althage, A., Waterfield, E., Kindred, B., Welsh, R. M., Callahan, G., and Pincetl, P.,** Restriction specificities, alloreactivity, and allotolerance expressed by T cells from nude mice reconstituted with H-2-compatible or -incompatible thymus grafts, *J. Exp. Med.,* 151, 376, 1980.

66. **Dosch, H.-M., White, D., and Grant, C.,** Reconstitution of nude mouse T cell function in vivo: IL 2 independent effect of human T cells, *J. Immunol.,* 134, 336, 1985.

67. **Pritchard, H. and Micklem, H. S.,** Immune response in congenitally thymus-less mice. I. Absence of response to oxazolone, *Clin. Exp. Immunol.,* 10, 151, 1972.

68. **Roberts, I. M., Bernard, C. C., Vyas, G. M., and Mackay, I. R.,** T-cell dependence of immune response to hepatitis B antigen in mice, *Nature,* 254, 606, 1975.

69. **Miller, J. F. A. P., Vadas, M. A., Whitelaw, A., and Gamble, J.,** Role of major histocompatibility complex gene products in delayed-type hypersensitivity, *Proc. Natl. Acad. Sci. U.S.A.,* 73, 2486, 1976.

70. **Smith, F. and Miller, J. F. A. P.,** Delayed type hypersensitivity to allogeneic cells in mice. I. Requirements for optimal sensitization and definition of the response, *Int. Arch. Allergy Appl. Immunol.,* 58, 285, 1979.

71. **Kubín, N., Holub, M., Mohelská, H., and Schlegerová, D.,** Experimental infection with *Mycobacterium kansasii* in athymic nude mice, *Exp. Pathol.,* 25, 233, 1984.

72. **Schlegerová, D., Kubín, M., and Holub, M.,** Lymphatic tissues in nude mice during early stages of *Mycobacterium kansasii* infection, *Folia Biol. (Prague),* 24, 428, 1978.

73. **Sher, N. A., Chaparas, S. D., Greensberg, L. E., Merchant, E. B., and Vickers, J. H.,** Response of congenitally athymic (nude) mice to infection with *Mycobacterium bovis* (strain BCG), *J. Natl. Cancer Inst.,* 54, 1419, 1975.

74. **Ueda, K., Yamazaki, S., and Someya, S.,** Experimental mycobacterial infection in congenitally athymic nude mice, *J. RES Soc.,* 19, 77, 1976.

75. **Rygaard, J. and Povlsen, C. O.,** Heterotransplantation of a human malignant tumor to "nude" mice, *Acta Pathol. Microbiol. Scand.,* 77, 758, 1969.

76. **Rygaard, J.,** Immunobiology of the mouse mutant "nude", *Acta Pathol. Microbiol. Scand.,* 77, 761, 1969.

77. **Kindred, B.,** Immunological unresponsiveness of genetically thymus-less (nude) mice, *Eur. J. Immunol.,* 1, 59, 1971.

78. **Pantelouris, E. M.,** Observations on the immunobiology of nude mice, *Immunology,* 20, 247, 1971.

79. **Wortis, H. H.,** Immunological responses of 'nude'mice, *Clin. Exp. Immunol.,* 8, 305, 1971.

80. **Pennycuik, P. R.,** Unresponsiveness of nude mice to skin allografts, *Transplantation,* 11, 417, 1971.

81. **Manning, D. D., Reed, N. D., and Schaffer, C. F.,** Maintenance of skin xenografts of widely divergent phylogenetic origin on congenitally athymic (nude) mice, *J. Exp. Med.,* 138, 488, 1973.

82. **Rygaard, J., Andersen, D. H., Friis, C. W., and Aagaard, J.,** Morphology and functional changes in nude mice grafted with embryonic and adult bovine thymus, *Folia Biol. (Prague),* 24, 426, 1979.

83. **Viklický, V. and Holub, M.,** Mast cells in skin grafts and omenta of nude mice, *Folia Biol. (Prague),* 24, 434, 1978.

84. **Rygaard, J.,** Skin grafts in nude mice. I. Allografts in nude mice of three different backgrounds (BALB/c, C3H, C57Bl), *Acta Pathol. Microbiol. Scand. (A),* 82, 80, 1974.

85. **Rygaard, J.,** Skin grafts in nude mice. II. Rat skin grafts in nude mice of three genetic backgrounds (BALB/c, C3H, C57Bl). The effect after preparation by thymus grafts, *Acta Pathol. Microbiol. Scand. (A),* 82, 93, 1974.

86. **Capel, P. J. A., Lems, S. P. M., and Koene, R. A. P.,** Antibody response to allogeneic and xenogeneic skin grafts in nude mice, in *Proc. 3rd Int. Workshop on Nude Mice,* Reed, N. D., Ed., G. Fischer, New York, 1982, 275.

87. **Gerlag, P. G. G., Capel, P. J. A., Berden, J. H. M., and Koene, R. A. P.,** Antibody response and skin graft rejection in the nude mouse, *Transplant. Proc.,* 9, 1179, 1977.

88. **Koene, R. A. P., Gerlag, P. G. G., Jansen, J. L. J., Hagemann, J. F. H. M., and Wijdeveld, P. G.-A. B.,** Rejection of skin grafts in the nude mouse, *Nature,* 251, 69, 1974.

89. **Koene, R. A. P., Gerlag, P. G. G., Hagemann, J. F. H. M., van Haelst, U. J. G., and Wijdeveld, P. G.-A. B.,** Hyperacute rejection of skin allografts in the mouse by the administration of alloantibody and rabbit complement, *J. Immunol.,* 111, 520, 1973.

90. **Slagel, D. E., Bevins, W. B., and Beasley, J. J.,** Phenotypic character of serially heterotransplanted tumors in athymic mice, in *Proc. 3rd Int. Workshop on Nude Mice,* Reed, N. D., Ed., G. Fischer, New York, 1982, 589.

91. **Beattie, G. M., Knowles, A. F., Jensen, F. C., Baird, S. M., and Kaplan, N. O.,** Induction of sarcomas in athymic mice, *Proc. Natl. Acad. Sci. U.S.A.,* 79, 3033, 1982.

92. **Kodousek, R., Pospíšil, J., Poučková, P., Krajčí, D., Kodet, R., Stejskal, J., Čiampor, F., and Rajčány, J.,** Virus identification in xenograft of human osteosarcoma in athymic nude (*nu/nu*) mice, *Čs. Patol.,* 23, 93, 1987.

93. **Giovanella, B. C. and Stehlin, J. S.,** Assessment of the malignant potential of cultured cells by injection in "nude" mice, in *Proc. 1st Int. Workshop on Nude Mice,* Rygaard, J. and Povlsen, C. O., Eds., G. Fischer, Stuttgart, 1974, 279.

94. **Stiles, C. D., Desmond, W., Chuman, L. M., Sato, G., and Saier, M. H.,** Growth and control of heterologous tissue culture cells in the congenitally athymic nude mouse, *Cancer Res.,* 36, 1353, 1976.

95. **Shimosato, Y., Kameya, T., Nagai, K., Hirohashi, S., Koide, T., Hayashi, H., and Nomura, T.,** Transplantation of human tumors in nude mice, *J. Natl. Cancer Inst.,* 56, 1251, 1976.

96. **Ohsawa, N., Ueyama, Y., Morita, K., and Kondo, Y.,** Heterotransplantation of human functioning tumors to nude mice, in *Proc. 2nd Int. Workshop on Nude Mice,* Nomura, T., Ohsawa, N., Tamaoki, N., and Fujiwara, K., Eds., G. Fischer, Stuttgart, 1977, 395.

97. **Kindred, B. and Loor, F.,** Survival and activity of congeneic and allogeneic thymus cell suspensions in nude mice, *Cell Immunol.,* 16, 432, 1975.

98. **Fortmeyer, H. P.,** Thymusaplastische Maus (nu/nu), Thymusaplastische Ratte (rnu/rnu), *Haltung Zucht, Versuchsmodelle,* Paul Parey, Berlin, 1981, 53.

99. **Heymer, B., Hof, H., Emmerling, P., and Finger, H.,** Morphology and time course of experimental listeriosis in nude mice, *Infect. Immunol.,* 14, 832, 1976.

100. **Hof, H.,** Failure of recombinant murine γ-interferon to cure chronic listeriosis in nude, athymic mice, *Thymus,* 10, 247, 1987.

101. **Shannon, E. J., Chehl, S., Job, C. K., and Hastings, R. C.,** Adoptively transferred reactivity to *M. leprae* in nude mice infected with *M. leprae, Clin. Exp. Immunol.,* 70, 143, 1987.

102. **Ytterberg, S. R., Mahowald, M. L., and Messner, R. P.,** Coxsackievirus B 1-induced polymyositis. Lack of disease expression in *nu/nu* mice, *J. Clin. Invest.,* 80, 499, 1987.

103. **Koch, A. E., Polverini, P. J., and Leibovich, S. J.,** Induction of neovascularisation by activated human monocytes, *J. Leukocyte Biol.,* 39, 233, 1986.

104. **Fett, J. W., Strydom, D. J., Lobb, R. R., Alderman, E. M., Bethune, J. L., Riordan, J. F., and Vallee, B. L.,** Isolation and characterization of angiogenin, an angiogenic protein from human carcinoma cells, *Biochemistry,* 24, 5480, 1985.

105. **Mölne, J., Jörtsö, E., Smeds, S., and Ericson, L. E.,** Vascularization of normal human thyroid tissue transplanted to nude mice, *Exp. Cell Biol.,* 55, 104, 1987.

105a. **Demarchez, M., Hartmann, D., and Prunieras, M.,** An immunohistological study of the revascularization process in human skin transplanted onto the nude mouse, *Transplantation,* 43, 896, 1987.

106. **Duprez, A., Guerret, S., Vignaud, J.-M., Plenat, F., Hartmann, D., and Grimaud, J.-A.,** The interstitial matrix of human carcinomas and sarcomas transplanted to the nude mouse: immunolocalization of some human and murine components, *Cell. Molec. Biol.,* 33, 647, 1987.

107. **Goldberg, D. M. and Pavia, R. A.,** In vivo horizontal oncogenesis by a human tumor in nude mice, *Proc. Natl. Acad. Sci. U.S.A.,* 79, 2389, 1982.

108. **Sparrow, S., Jones, M., Billington, S., and Stace, B.,** The in vivo malignant transformation of mouse fibroblasts in the presence of human tumour xenografts, *Br. J. Cancer,* 53, 793, 1986.

109. **Gupta, V., Rajaraman, S., Gadson, P., and Costanzi, J. J.,** Primary transfection as a mechanism for transformation of host cells by human tumor cells implanted in nude mice, *Cancer Res.,* 47, 5194, 1987.

110. **Benomar, A., Gerlier, D., and Doré, J.-F.,** In vivo activation of mouse macrophages by human melanoma cells, *J. Natl. Cancer Inst.,* 79, 131, 1987.

111. **Jaffrey, B. J., Lair, S. V., Hudson, J. W., Lozio, B. B., Machado, E. A., and Chase, D. C.,** Heterotransplantation of human neoplasms, *J. Oral Surgery,* 37, 16, 1979.

112. **Kojima, T., Maruo, K., Hioki, K., and Endo, S.,** Genetic improvement of nude mice for cancer research, in *Immune-Deficient Animals in Biomedical Research, Proc. 5th IWIDA,* Rygaard, J. et al., Eds., S. Karger, Basel, 1987, 18.

113. **Sudo, K.,** Improvement of transplantability of human neoplastic cells to nude mice, *Jpn. J. Exp. Med.,* 57, 189, 1987.

114. **McLemore, T. L., Liu, M. C., Blacker, P. C., Gregg, M., Alley, M. C., Abbott, B. J., Shoemaker, R. H., Bohlman, M. E., Litterst, C. C., Hubbard, W. C., Brennan, R. H., McMahon, J. B., Fine, D. L., Eggleston, J. C., Mayo, J. G., and Boyd, M. R.,** Novel intrapulmonary model for orthotopic propagation of human lung cancers in athymic nude mice, *Cancer Res.,* 47, 5132, 1987.

114a. **Ricordi, C. and Scharp, D. W.,** Reversal of diabetes in nude mice after transplantation of fresh and 7-day-cultured (24°C) human pancreatic islets, *Transplantation,* 45, 994, 1988.

115. **Peter, H. J., Gerber, H., Studer, H., Becker, D. V., and Peterson, M. E.,** Autonomy of growth and of iodine metabolism in hyperthyroid feline goiters transplanted onto nude mice, *J. Clin. Invest.,* 80, 491, 1987.

115a. **Moll, H. and Bösing-Schneider, R.,** The transplantation barrier of nude mice, *Immunobiology,* 177, 23, 1988.

116. **Clark, D. A., Slapsys, R. M., Croy, B. A., and Rossant, J.,** Immunoregulation of host-versus-graft responses in the uterus, *Immunol. Today,* 5, 111, 1984.

117. **Clark, D. A., Chaput, A., Walker, C., and Rosenthal, K. L.,** Active suppression of host-vs-graft reaction in pregnant mice. VI. Soluble suppressor activity obtained from decidua of allopregnant mice blocks the response to IL 2, *J. Immunol.,* 134, 1659, 1985.

118. **Clark, D. A., Croy, B. A., Rossant, J., and Chaouat, G.,** Immune presensitization and local intrauterine defences as determinants of success or failure of murine interspecies pregnancies, *J. Reprod. Fert.,* 77, 633, 1986.

Chapter 9

HAIRLESSNESS AND METABOLIC COMPENSATIONS

I. THE SKIN

Compared with the abundant literature on mouse hairlessness, there are surprisingly few reports of what is wrong with the skin of the nude mouse. Flanagan did notice the first abnormality in 6-day-old nudes: bent and coiled hair failed to penetrate the epidermis. He concluded that there is an abnormal, imperfect keratinization of hair in the follicles;[1] the usual amount of sulfhydryl groups was missing in developing hair follicles.[1]

According to our material (BALB/c, C57B1/10.LP, C3H, CBA/J, and C57B1/10 ScSn nude mice) fetuses of both athymic or euthymic mothers have a few curly vibrissae from intrauterine day 16 on. Around birth, nude mice can be — with a high probability — diagnosed by the paucity of their vibrissae.[2] Up to the 2nd week of life, nude mice are macroscopically hairless, later they develop cyclically short and poor hair cover over the head, around the neck, and on the front legs, especially over the back.

Histologically, BALB/c nudes have poorly developed hair follicles at birth, with the exception of the follicles and bulbs of the vibrissae.[3] Within the first week, however, the hair follicles and bulbs rapidly develop and every follicle in the dermis has a small and curly hair. By 8 days, degenerative changes are visible and by 10 to 20 days the follicles between the bulb and the sebaceous gland regress and hairs are mostly fragmented or missing in conspicuously dilated hair canals.[3] Later, the small and curly hairs reappear in some areas and their follicles and bulbs seem to be normal, apparently regenerated. The degenerative process initiated by the dilatation of the hair canal is further marked by proliferation of squamous cells and large amounts of keratin debris in the dilated canals and by pycnosis of epithelial cells in some bulbs.[3] In the regressing bulbs and follicles hair disappears first from the proximal portion and later from the canal. In the skin on the back there are usually no hair follicles left in the adult nudes.[3]

The hair growth cycles and wave patterns are analogous in the nudes (C57B1/6 Icr background) and in their haired littermates.[4] The hair growth wave started on the throat and collar and proceeded caudally. In the nudes there was an almost constant interval between hair growth cycles (11 to 19 days), in the haired littermates this interval was prolonged after thc third cycle. Duration of single cycles increased in the nudes from 3 to 5 days (second cycle) to 36 to 38 days (fifth cycle) and in the haired littermates the prolongation of the third and subsequent cycles was much more pronounced (134 days for the fifth cycle). The increased frequency of hair cycles in the nudes could not be altered by implantation of normal thymuses.[4]

The development of vibrissae as a tactile sense organ is connected with complicated nerve fibers ending in and around the follicles, each sinus hair is represented in the somato-sensory cortex of the brain by a neuronal aggregation (''barrel''). Interestingly, in the nude and hairless (hr/hr) mice the barrels representing labial hair are diminished in numbers, the number of hair follicles, however, is normal.[5]

The condition of the nudes cannot be described as hairlessness, but rather as a recurrent loss of hair due to imperfect keratinization in the hair shaft. In an extensive and comprehensive study of comparative histology of hairlessness in mice and the genetics of the defect, as it was conceived in 1931,[6] the nude mutation cannot be identified in any of the categories, except for the poorly documented ''hairlessness of undetermined genetic nature''.[6] In the modern list of mouse gene effects (Chapter 2), very few references are given to the structural and biochemical basis of different types of hairlessness and in fact very little analytical and

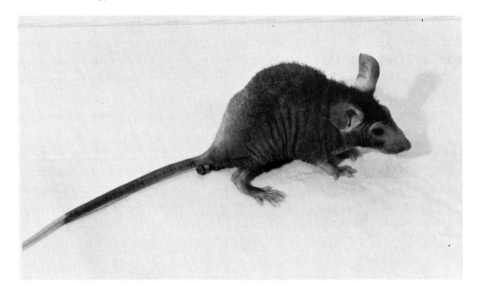

FIGURE 1.   A 'haired' nude mouse; C57B1/10.LP male, 2-month old, after six doses of cyclosporin A (80 mg/kg) per os.

comparative work exists. In any case, it cannot be excluded that the mutant nude was already here in 1931 and even the first report from 1850 may well deal with three specimens of this mutant, two dying — "apparently from cold" — in an old grape vase, the third one escaping . . . [7].

Keratinization in the nude mouse hair follicles could be improved by oral administration of 80 mg/kg of cyclosporin A for 10 days; its discontinuation caused the newly formed hair to break again at skin level after 3 to 4 days[8] (Figure 1). The same effect was achieved even with 10 mg/kg; no difference in numbers of hair follicles was found in the treated vs. control nude mice.[8a]

The same effect, possibly a direct biochemical action on keratin formation, was seen in the patchy hairless mutant "naked", but not in the hairless (*hr/hr*) mutant where the hair defect is deeper and keratin cysts are formed in the hair follicles.[8] One of the few biochemical approaches to the hair defect in mice was undertaken in the naked mutant[9] and it may be inferred from the cyclosporin A effect that it also has some bearing for the nude defect.

The naked mutant has been known since 1927. Mice homozygous for this dominant gene have almost no hair and nails and most individuals die within 10 days after birth. Heterozygotes (N/+) have hair breaking off near the root in successive waves proceeding in a cranio-caudal direction, causing patchy depilation. New successive waves of hair growth follow the depilation process. Analysis of hair from black and white naked heterozygotes and normal homozygotes (NS-FR strain) has shown a low tyrosine and glycine content of the "naked" hair (deficiency of the HG proteins), associated with a significantly lower phenylalanine content and an increase of the relative amounts of leucine, lysine, and proline.[9] Since the murine hair contains in normal individuals more tyrosine than any animal hair so far investigated[9] and the HG proteins are located in the intercellular membrane complex,[9] it may well be that some types of hair dysplasias in mice are caused by the HG proteins deficiency and that these types include the nude mouse and its keratins.

The cyclosporin A effect shows that in the case of hair formation the ectodermal defect of nude mice can be corrected. In the dysgenetic thymus of the nude mouse the same doses of cyclosporin A induced in our experiments the disappearance of cysts and shrinking of the organ into epithelial acini and ducts reminiscent of the embryonic state of the dysgenetic thymus. This suggests an effect of the drug on thymic epithelial cells (Figure 1, also Chapter 3, Figures 8 and 13).

Such an effect was reported in normal mouse thymuses which undergo a marked reduction of the medulla and of the numbers of the keratin-positive medullary epithelial cells after prolonged feeding with cyclosporin A.[9a]

The hairlessness is not due to the thymic defect. As quoted by Kindred, it was demonstrated that a tetraparental (allophenic) mouse produced by fusion of a nude and a normal early embryo had a thymus, but only patchy hair growth.[10] A supportive piece of evidence comes from the fact that the nude skin remains hairless when grafted on to normal mice and vice versa.[11]

The basic, primary defect affecting the hair growth remains the enigmatic ectodermal abnormality, probably a single enzyme defect. This defect may have a marked influence on the status of the nude mouse epidermis.

In a biochemical study of the nude mouse epidermis in comparison with the epidermis of the hr/hr mutant, Brysk and collaborators probed the epidermal glycoproteins with concanavalin A.[12] The FITC-labeled lectin bound well to all strata of *nu/nu* and *hr/hr* epidermis with the exception of the stratum corneum. When, however, different populations of keratinocytes were isolated and analyzed by gel electrophoresis, cells of the stratum corneum also were labeled by concanavalin A and substantial differences between *nu/nu* and *hr/hr* keratinocytes appeared, connected with changes of glycoprotein distribution during keratinization. The most striking difference was the absence of a glycoprotein with a molecular weight of 40,000 in the *nu/nu* stratum corneum.[12] This glycoprotein is a dominant feature in the epidermis of *hr/hr* mice and of man.[12] This shows that the nude epidermis is altered, albeit the alteration is not histologically evident.

There is a higher threshold in the nude epidermis for the induction of proliferation by the tumor promoter 12-*O*-tetradecanoyl phorbol 13-acetate; the low responsiveness is present even in the nude skin grafted to heterozygous littermates.[13] Consequently, the low responsiveness which may explain the decreased incidence of epithelial tumors resides in the epidermis itself and is not due to some humoral factors. Ultraviolet radiation provokes squamous cell carcinomas in nude mice skin, in thymus-reconstituted nude mice skin, and in nude mouse skin transplanted to normal mice much faster than in the skin of euthymic controls.[13a] Obviously, the nude mouse skin permits transmission of larger doses of radiation to the basal cell layers and this is the dominant factor in this type of carcinogenesis.

Dissociated epidermal cells of the nude mouse express the Thy 1 marker in higher numbers than epidermal cells from euthymic controls (BALB/c).[14] This may be interpreted as a sign of enhanced cell-to-cell contacts of less mature cells during tissue growth and differentiation. The rate of renewal of epidermal cells in the nude mouse skin has been found to be somewhat higher and the mitotic duration a little shorter than those in the skin of the hairless (*hr/hr*) mouse.[15] Again, this shows the thymus-independent nature of the nude mouse skin condition resulting in massive enlargement and keratinization of the nude mouse epidermis.[16]

The occurrence of Ia positive cells, mainly the migrating Langerhans cells, is qualitatively normal in the nude mouse skin.[17,18] The same is true of the interdigitating cells of lymphatic tissues which may be closely related to the skin Langerhans cells (Chapter 8, Section I). Also, the influx of Langerhans cell precursors from the nude mouse bone marrow seems to be sufficient.[19] Curiously, the influx of nude mouse Langerhans cell precursors into grafted euthymic littermate's (BALB/c background) skin triggers the expression of the Ia marker on all epidermal cells of the graft; the same occurs in both parabiotic partners when the pair consists of a *nu/+* and a *nu/nu* individual and in the nude mouse given *nu/+* spleen cells and even after normal mouse serum inoculation.[19] In addition to an unknown difference in the nude mouse and euthymic mouse microenvironments (including different levels of immunoglobulins) these results suggest again that the keratinocytes closely parallel the thymic epithelial cell potentials and that the nude mouse keratinocytes may not be dissimilar to keratinocytes of the normal epidermis in terms of the expression of MHC class II (Ia) antigens.

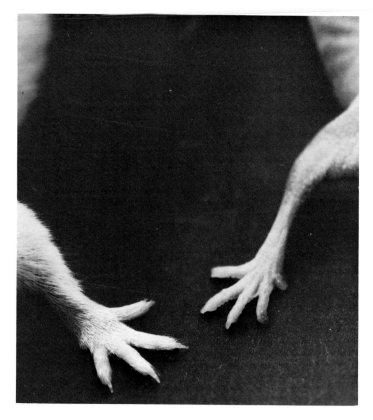

FIGURE 2.   On the right, shortened and blunt claws on the foreleg of a BALB/c
nu/nu male, aged 2 months. On the left, the foreleg of the euthymic littermate.

In general, keratinocytes may share the differentiation pathway, as witnessed by surface antigen expression, with thymic epithelial cells as suggested from human data by Haynes[20] and others at least for the upper epidermal cells and Hassall's corpuscles;[21] also, some alpha-keratin components are shared by upper epidermal cells and thymus stromal epithelia.[22] In view of the relative thymus independence of the skin immunological status and its associated lymphoid tissues (SALT)[23] it is particularly intriguing to remember the possible, but so far unexplored, immunological role of the SALT in the thymusless animal. Lymphocyte differentiating and activating factors different from known thymic hormones like thymosin, thymopoietin, and thymulin were found in human epidermal cell cultures[24] and in murine keratinocyte lines.[25] The keratinocyte factor may be closely related, if not identical, to interleukin 1.[26] This is of special significance in view of the activated state of the nude mouse mononuclear phagocyte system (Chapter 7).

The murine epidermis also contains a special kind of bone marrow-derived cells with dendritic morphology which do not express Ia, but express Thy 1, T_3, and the gamma chain of the T-cell receptor thus resembling a subpopulation of immature thymic and peripheral lymphoid cells.[26a,27a]

No qualitative differences were discernable between euthymic and athymic NMRI mice in the interepithelial cells (mainly Langerhans cells) of the oral mucosa.[27]

The only skin-associated structure of the nude mouse, other than hair, which may show some alteration are the claws; Flanagan has described their deformation.[1] We have seen in mice of the BALB/c, C57B1, and C3H background minor changes in all individuals over 1 month of age. They affect only the forelegs where the claws of the third and fifth finger are bent, shortened, or forked (Figure 2). In 1-week-old nudes these claws are short and blunt. We did not see any gross anomalies in the development of teeth of the nude individuals.

Nor are there alterations of skin-associated glands including preputial sebaceous glands of the males. Keratinization of the skin and ducts proceeds here normally in a striking difference with hair keratinization, and the lipid secretory product of these glands has an identical composition by gas chromatography with that of normal mice.[28]

Taken together, the result of the nude mutation is imperfect keratinization in the hair shaft in the skin with only minor alterations of other ectodermal derivatives. The status of keratinocytes and other epidermal cells seems to be close to normal, especially in the ability to express Ia antigens which may have some bearing to the solution of the consequences of the thymic dysgenesis.

II. METABOLIC RATES AND DEVIATIONS

Paying attention to broader physiological questions of the life of nude mice was in the tradition of the Pantelouris laboratory.[29] Flisch measured the metabolic rates of the nude mice, their haired littermates, and other hairless mice (sha/sha) which are without any immunologic symptomatology. The metabolic rates of nu/nu and sha/sha mice were at ambient temperatures of 18 and 25°C higher than the metabolic rates at 35°C.[29] The elevated metabolic rate of nu/nu mice, consequently, was a normal reaction coping with the great heat loss through the hairless skin and not necessarily connected with athymia or other defects. Also, the respiratory quotient increased in nu/nu, compared to a constant value in haired littermates, at 8 weeks of age and approached 1.0 in the wasting stage suggesting the exhaustion of fat reserves.[29]

Nude mice had, consequently, about one third higher total food intake at environmental temperatures between 21 and 26°C, compared to haired nu/+ mice of the same strain.[30] Improvement of the hygienic standard not only of the environment (e.g., large-scale laminar flow system, sterilized bedding), but also of the food (irradiated instead of autoclaved diet) increases the growth rates of the nude mice and prolongs their life-span.[31]

One of the principal consequences of the high food intake in the nude is their changed lipid metabolism. We have found the following values in C57B1/10.LP mice/(aged $2^1/_2$ months, kept SPF at 26°C), fasted overnight: $+/+$ mice serum triglycerides 0.383 mmol/ℓ, nu/nu mice 0.203 (means from five mice in each group). For cholesterol the relation was opposite: $+/+$ 2.83, nu/nu 3.55 mmol/ℓ.[32] Mice of one C57B1 strain were found to have high cholesterol levels and a high tendency to atherosclerotic lesions after an atherogenic diet.[33] Therefore, we also tested nudes of the BALB/c background which is of the low cholesterol group.[33] In nonfasting mice, $+/+$ had 0.98 mmol/ℓ of serum triglycerides, compared to 0.735 mmol/ℓ in nontreated nu/nu, and 0.331 mmol/ℓ of human tumor-bearing nu/nu (all values are means from five mice). The cholesterol levels were 3.178 mmol/ℓ (in $+/+$) vs. 3.878 mmol/ℓ (normal nudes) and 4.823 mmol/ℓ (tumor-bearing nudes).[32] Cold adaptation (nonshivering thermogenesis, Chapter 10, Section II) resulted in nude mice of both B10.LP or BALB/c background in very low levels of serum and liver triglycerides.

It follows that the serum cholesterol levels are higher in most nude mice and increased further during xenogeneic tumor development. High caloric demands of the nude mouse at all temperatures below the thermoneutrality zone lead to mobilization of triglycerides from adipocyte stores, followed by an increased level of free fatty acids in blood. The production of very-low-density lipoproteins in the liver is increased and utilized as the energy substrate. A higher concentration of low-density lipoproteins where triglycerides are replaced by cholesterol esters results. Low-density lipoproteins supply cholesterol to extrahepatic parenchymal cells. Consequently, the metabolically overactive nude mouse has higher demonstrable levels in their sera.

Blood pressure in nu/nu homozygotes of different background strains is normal and they do not develop spontaneous hypertension as do haired, euthymic mice of the BALB/c, C3H, and NZB strains.[34] The explanation may be looked for in the neuroendocrine peculiarities of nude mice in general (Chapter 10).

The increased metabolic level of nude mice is, however, reflected in the tissue porphyrins in mice older than 3 months.[35] Porphyrins in general are intermediate products or by-products of hemoprotein synthesis in all tissues, especially at the erythropoietic sites. Using high-performance liquid chromatography, equal levels of porphyrins in the liver and Harderian gland in *nu/nu*, *nu/+*, and *+/+* of BALB/c, B10.LP, and B10 ScSn backgrounds (SPF), aged 39 to 57 days were found; in the kidney, nude females had a lower porphyrin content than euthymic mice.[35] In BALB/c *nu/nu* mice aged 99 to 127 days, there was a significant increase of porphyrins in the liver; the increase was much higher in males. Griseofulvin induced high levels of porphyrins also in 30- to 40-day-old BALB/c and B10.LP nudes, as it did in euthymic controls. It was suggested that the effects of light on erythrohepatic protoporphyria may be studied in the nude mouse model.[35] Liver uptake of iron (^{59}Fe) was found similar in *nu/+* and *nu/nu* mice of the BALB/c background, aged 2 to 3 months, no measurements were done in older mice.[36] In the same material, iron uptake was five times greater in the *nu/nu* spleen than in *nu/+* spleen, this is obviously due to higher erythropoiesis. In the skeleton, iron uptake was markedly lower in *nu/nu* mice[36] which points again in the direction of the connective tissue defect mentioned in Chapter 6, Section II.

The reports that liver physiology may be affected by higher levels of alpha-fetoprotein in nudes up to the 4th week of life[37,38] could not be confirmed in our SPF BALB/c and C57B1 mice. Both liver hemopoiesis and alpha-fetoprotein demonstrable by immunofluorescence vanished simultaneously after the 20th postnatal day in *nu/nu*, *nu/+*, and *+/+* mice kept in undisturbed litters.[38a]

Also, the relation of some enzymatic changes in the nude mouse liver (amino acid decarboxylase,[39] histidinase[29]) to the endocrine disorders or to inapparent infections has to be resolved in a broader, well-controlled study and in mice of different ages. Glutamic acid and tyrosine decarboxylase activities were found to be higher in 10-day-old nude mice and to decline much more gradually than in euthymic controls;[39] about the same slower decrease was described for serum acid phosphatase, whereas serum nonspecific esterase falls only in the nudes.[40]

Changes may be found almost everywhere in the metabolic parameters, the problem is only where, when, and which one should be studied, i.e., which one may be essential or primary.

The *nu* gene-linked basic disorders are corrected by the coexistence of normal tissues, either completely or partially. Aggregated embryos (BALB/c-*nu/nu* × C3H/HeN) transferred to ICR females produced 39 adult mice, 17 of which were chimeric. Two of these had complete hair cover, 15 partial hair covering, with hairlessness in the albino (BALB/c) regions. In one of the chimeric mice, no thymus was found, 16 had thymuses "of normal size".[41] Allophenic mice may be, together with embryologic studies, the way to a deeper insight into the mechanism of nu mutation expression.

Hairlessness itself should not play a major pathogenic role (Chapter 10, Section II) except for the thermo-regulatory problems and their consequences. In a number of hairless mutants no alterations in the main immunological parameters were found.[42]

Microbial natural pathogens, among which protozoa must not be neglected,[43] obviously trigger the bulk of secondary disorders. In germ-free nude and control mice of the fourth backcross to C3H/He the longevity was 1042 days for nude females vs. 1059 days for euthymic controls and 1078 days for nude males compared to 1085 days for control males.[44] The odds ratio of risk for a lethal disease in the germ-free conditions was in athymic vs. normal mice 12.3 to 15.1 (female-male) for lymphatic tissue neoplasms (mainly reticulum cell sarcoma and lymphosarcoma), 0.6 to 2.0 for degenerative and dystrophic diseases, 2.4 (females) for sepsis and 2.3 to 1.9 for undetermined causes ("old age"). On the other hand, there was a significantly reduced risk for solid neoplasms (ovarian adenoma, hepatocellular adenoma, Harderian gland adenoma), with the exception of alveolar adenoma[44] (which may be closely related to the state of bronchus-associated lymphatic tissue).

The mortality started after 1 year of life, earlier in nude mice and in females and the overall survival rates were significantly reduced for nudes because of the lymphatic tissue malignancies.[44] Autoimmune phenomena as a cause of morbidity in these germ-free mice were unlikely[44] and thus the degenerative phenomena in the vasculature, renal glomeruli, and thyroids[44] were rather due to the same minor primary ontogenetic disorders. So were the lymphatic malignancies, obviously consequent to a major ontogenetic disorder leading to the thymus defect, follicular dendritic cell defect, and changed B-cell turnover.

An increased incidence of lymphomas in the nu/nu was observed also in an NIH(s) mouse colony where the nudes lived for 7 to 34 months.[45] Reconstitution by thymic grafts reversed the lymphoma incidence in C57Bl/6 *nu/nu* and +/+ mice.[46]

However, Stutman found in large numbers of mice (in perfect health and long living, CBA/H and BALB/c background), the incidence of spontaneous tumors, including lymphomas, comparable between nude and normal mice in observation periods up to 47 months.[47] Even the transfer of the viable yellow gene, a dominant gene increasing the incidence of tumors, provoked in mice 14 months old the same percentage of lung and liver tumors in *nu/nu* and +/+ mice and the incidence of lymphomas was 6 and 5% (males-females) in +/+, 10 and 13% in *nu*/+, and 5 and 10% in *nu/nu*.[47]

Spleen cells from 1-month-old nude mice which have been inoculated with Moloney murine leukemia virus after birth do develop lymphomas upon transfer to syngeneic recipients (400 R-irradiated and with opposite sex to permit identification of donor cells).[48] Spleen cells taken from euthymic donors (CBA, BALB/c) after the same leukemogenic treatment produce lymphomas in the recipients faster than *nu/nu* spleen cells and arise from at least two T-cell subsets, one terminal deoxynucleotidyl transferase positive, the other 20 β-hydroxysteroid dehydrogenase positive. The BALB/c *nu/nu* spleen cells were negative for these enzymes and had to mature into the enzyme-positive cells in the thymus-bearing recipient.[48]

On the whole we are left with the impression that there are no intrinsic reasons which would decisively discriminate the nude mouse in the viability and life span. In wild mouse populations, life expectation at birth is about 100 days in a stressful environment.[49]

REFERENCES

1. **Flanagan, S. P.,** 'Nude', a new hairless gene with pleiotropic effects in the mouse, *Genet. Res. (Cambridge),* 8, 295, 1966.
2. **Ryggard, J. and Friis, C. W.,** The husbandry of mice with congenitally absence of the thymus (nude mice), *Zschr. Versuchstierkunde,* 16, 1, 1974.
3. **Rigdon, R. H. and Packchanian, A. A.,** Histologic study of the skin of congenitally athymic "nude" mice, *Texas Rep. Biol. Med.,* 32, 711, 1974.
4. **Eaton, G. J.,** Hair growth cycles and wave patterns in "nude" mice, *Transplantation,* 22, 217, 1976.
5. **Yamakado, M. and Yohro, T.,** Subdivision of mouse vibrissae on an embryological basis, with descriptions of variations in the number and arrangement of sinus hairs and cortical barrels in BALB/c (*nu*/+; nude, *nu/nu*) and hairless (*hr/hr*) strains, *Am. J. Anat.,* 155, 153, 1979.
6. **David, L. T.,** The external expression and comparative dermal histology of hereditary hairlessness in mammals, *Z. Zellforsch. Mikrosk. Anat.,* 14(B), 616, 1931/32.
7. **Gordon, G.,** Variety of the common or house mouse *(Mus musculus),* *Zoologist,* 8, 2763, 1850.
8. **Pendry, A. and Alexander, P.,** Stimulation of hair growth on nude mice by Cyclosporin A, in *Cyclosporin A,* White, J. G., Ed., Elsevier, Amsterdam, 1982, 77.
8a. **Sawada, M., Terada, N., Taniguchi, H., Tateishi, R., and Mori, Y.,** Cyclosporin A stimulates hair growth in nude mice, *Lab. Invest.,* 56, 684, 1987.

9. **Tenenhouse, H. S., Gold, R. J. M., Kachra, Z., and Fraser, F. C.,** Biochemical marker in dominantly inherited ectodermal malformation, *Nature,* 251, 431, 1974.

9a. **Hattori, A., Kunz, H., Gill, T. J., III, and Shinozuka, H.,** Thymic and lymphoid changes and serum globulin abnormalities in mice receiving cyclosporine, *Am. J. Pathol.,* 128, 111, 1987.

10. **Kindred, B.,** Nude mice in immunology, *Prog. Allergy,* 26, 137, 1979.

11. **Wortis, H. H.,** Pleiotropic effects of the nude mutation, *Birth Defects Orig. Artic. Series,* XI, 528, 1975.

12. **Brysk, M. M., Miller, J., Chen, S., and Rajaraman, S.,** Modified distribution of epidermal glycoproteins in the nude mouse, *Exp. Cell Biol.,* 54, 163, 1986.

13. **Krueger, G. G., Chambers, D. A., and Shelby, J.,** Epidermal proliferation of nude mouse skin, pig skin, and pig skin grafts. Failure of nude mouse skin to respond to the tumor promoter 12-*O*-tetradecanoyl phorbol 13-acetate, *J. Exp. Med.,* 152, 1329, 1980.

13a. **Hoover, T. L., Morison, W. L., and Kripke, M. L.,** Ultraviolet carcinogenesis in athymic nude mice, *Transplantation,* 44, 693, 1987.

14. **Chambers, D. A., Cohen, R. L., and Heiss, M. A.,** Heterogeneity of epidermal cells detected by the presence of Thy-1 antigen in athymic (nude) and normal BALB/c mice, *Exp. Cell Biol.,* 52, 129, 1984.

15. **Iversen, O. H.,** Epidermal cell kinetics in the nude mouse, *Virchows Arch. B,* 28, 93, 1978.

16. **Pierpaoli, W. and Besedovsky, H. O.,** Role of the thymus in programming of neuroendocrine functions, *Clin. Exp. Immunol.,* 20, 323, 1975.

17. **Hunter, J. A. A., Fairley, D. J., Priestley, G. C., and Cubie, H. A.,** Langerhans cells in the epidermis of athymic mice, *Br. J. Dermatol.,* 94, 119, 1976.

18. **Silberberg-Sinakin, I., Baer, R. L., and Thorbecke, G. J.,** Langerhans cells, *Prog. Allergy,* 24, 268, 1978.

19. **Krueger, G. G., Daynes, R. A., Roberts, L. K., and Emam, M.,** Migration of Langerhans cells and the expression of Ia on epidermal cells following the grafting of normal skin to nude mice, *Exp. Cell Biol.,* 52, 97, 1984.

20. **Haynes, B. F.,** The human thymic microenvironment, *Adv. Immunol.,* 36, 87, 1984.

21. **Didierjean, L. and Saurat, J. H.,** Epidermis and thymus. Similar antigenic properties in Hassall's corpuscle and subsets of keratinocytes, *Clin. Exp. Dermatol.,* 5, 395, 1980.

22. **Viac, J., Schmitt, D., Staquet, M. J., and Thivolet, J.,** Epidermis-thymus antigenic relations with special reference to Hassall's corpuscles, *Thymus,* 1, 319, 1980.

23. **Streilein, J. W.,** Skin-associated lymphoid tissues (SALT): origins and functions, *J. Invest. Dermatol.,* 80, 12 s, 1983.

24. **Nicolas, J. F., Dardenne, M., Faure, M., Gaucherand, M., Gagneraut, M. C., Thivolet, J., and Bach, J. F.,** Production of a lymphocyte differentiating factor (ELDIF) by cultured human epidermal cells, *Immunol. Lett.,* 9, 65, 1985.

25. **Luger, T. A., Stadler, B. M., Katz, S. I., and Oppenheim, J. J.,** Epidermal cell (keratinocyte)-derived thymocyte-activating factor (ETAF), *J. Immunol.,* 127, 1493, 1981.

26. **Luger, T. A., Stadler, B. M., Luger, B. M., Mathieson, B. J., Mage, M., Schmidt, J. A., and Oppenheim, J. J.,** Murine epidermal cell-derived thymocyte-activating factors resembles murine interleukin 1, *J. Immunol.,* 128, 2147, 1982.

26a. **Stingl, G., Koning, F., Yamada, H., Yokoyama, W. M., Tschachler, E., Bluestone, J. A., Steiner, G., Samelson, L., Lew, A. M., Coligan, J. E., and Shevach, E. M.,** Thy-1$^+$ dendritic epidermal cells express T$_3$ antigen and the T-cell receptor γ chain, *Proc. Natl. Acad. Sci. U.S.A.,* 84, 4586, 1987.

27. **Burkhardt, A., Bos, I. R., Löning, T., Gebbers, J.-O., Otto, H. F., and Seifert, G.,** Interepithelial cells of the oral mucosa in mice, *Virchows Arch. A,* 384, 223, 1979.

27a. **Kuziel, W. A., Takashima, A., Bonyhadi, M., Bergstresser, P. R., Allison, J. P., Tigelaar, R. E., and Tucker, P. W.,** Regulation of T-cell receptor γ-chain RNA expression in murine Thy-1$^+$ dendritic epidermal cells, *Nature,* 328, 263, 1987.

28. **Ikenberry, R. D., Curtis, S. K., and Cowden, R. R.,** Ultrastructural and gas-chromatographic analysis of the preputial glands of male nude (*nu/nu*) mice, *Cell Tissue Res.,* 211, 78, 1980.

29. **Pantelouris, E. M. and Lintern-Moore, S.,** Physiological studies on the nude mouse, in *The Nude Mouse in Experimental and Clinical Research,* Fogh, J. and Giovanella, B. C., Eds., Academic Press, New York, 1978, 29.

30. **Weihe, W. H.,** The thermoregulation of the nude mouse, *Exp. Cell Biol.,* 52, 140, 1984.

31. **Møller Nielsen, I. and Heron, I.,** Diet and immune response in *nu/nu* BALB/c mice, *Exp. Cell. Biol.,* 52, 137, 1984.

32. **Kazdová, L., Vrána, A., and Holub, M.,** Serum lipid levels in nude mice, *Folia Biol. (Prague),* 1989, in press.

33. **Paigen, B., Morrow, A., Brandon, C., Mitchell, D., and Holmes, P.,** Variation in susceptibility to atherosclerosis among inbred strains of mice, *Atherosclerosis,* 57, 65, 1985.

34. **Svendsen, U. G.,** The level of blood pressure in nude and haired mice of five different strains of commercially available mice, *Folia Biol. (Praque),* 24, 440, 1978.

35. **Janoušek, V., Sanitrák, J., Krijt, J., and Holub, M.,** Tissue porphyrins in athymic nude mice, *Folia Biol. (Praque),* 1989, in press.
36. **Bamberger, E. G., Machado, E. A., and Lozzio, B. B.,** Hematopoiesis in hereditary athymic mice, *Lab. Animal Sci.,* 27, 43, 1977.
37. **Serova, I. A., Kaledin, V. I., Yunker, V. M., and Gruntenko, E. V.,** High alpha-fetoprotein (AFP) contents in liver and blood of nude mice in the early postnatal ontogenesis, *Folia Biol. (Prague),* 24, 437, 1978.
38. **Serova, I. A., Yunker, V. M., Kaledin, V. I., Alexeyeva, G. V., and Grutenko, E. V.,** Vliyanie mutacii nude na syntez alfa-fetoproteina i gemopoez v petcheni myshey v postnatalnom periode razvitiya, *Ontogenez,* 10, 483, 1979.
38a. **Větvička, V., Holub, M., Kovářů, H., Šiman, P., and Kovářů, F.,** Alpha-fetoprotein in athymic nude mice, *Immunol. Lett.,* 1988, in press.
40. **Pantelouris, E. M.,** Athymic development in the mouse, *Differentiation,* 1, 437, 1973.
41. **Ohsawa, N., Kojima, H., and Yokoyama, M.,** Phenotypes of chimeras between BALB/cA-*nu/nu* and C3H/HeN, *Exp. Cell Biol.,* 52, 111, 1984.
42. **Smith, S. M., Forbes, P. D., and Linna, T. J.,** Immune responses in nonhaired mice, *Int. Arch. Allergy Appl. Immunol.,* 67, 254, 1982.
43. **Boorman, G. A., Lina, P. H. C., Zurcher, C., and Nieuwerkerk, H. T. M.,** Hexamita and Giardia as a cause of mortality in congenitally thymusless (nude) mice, *Clin. Exp. Immunol.,* 15, 623, 1973.
44. **Holland, J. M., Mitchell, T. J., Gipson, L. C., and Whitaker, M. S.,** Survival and cause of death in aging germfree athymic nude and normal inbred C3Hf/He mice, *J. Natl. Cancer Inst.,* 61, 1357, 1978.
45. **Parker, J. W., Joyce, J., and Pattengale, P.,** Spontaneous neoplasms in aged athymic (nude) mice, in *Proc. 3rd Int. Workshop on Nude Mice,* Reed, N. D., Ed., G. Fischer, New York, 1982, 347.
46. **Eaton, G. J., Custer, R. P., and Crane, A. R.,** Spontaneous tumors of long-lived, reconstituted nude mice, in *Proc. 3rd Int. Workshop on Nude Mice,* Reed, N. D., Ed., G. Fischer, New York, 1982, 359.
47. **Stutman, O.,** Spontaneous, viral, and chemically induced tumors in the nude mouse, in *The Nude Mouse in Experimental and Clinical Research,* Fogh, J. and Giovanella, B. C., Eds., Academic Press, New York, 1978, 411.
48. **Asjö, B., Skoog, L., Palmiger, I., Wiener, F., Isaak, D., Černý, J., and Fenyö, E.-M.,** Influence of genotype and the organ of origin on the subtype of T-cell in Moloney lymphomas induced by transfer of preleukemic cells from athymic and thymus-bearing mice, *Cancer Res.,* 45, 1040, 1985.
49. **Berry, R. J.,** Genetical processes in wild mouse populations. Past myth and present knowledge, in *The Wild Mouse in Immunology,* Potter, M., Nadeau, J. H., and Cancro, M. P., Eds., Springer, Heidelberg, 1986, 86.

Chapter 10

NEUROENDOCRINE REGULATIONS

I. ENDOCRINE ORGANS AND FUNCTIONS

The state of endocrine organs and functions may be in part influenced by the absence of a normal lymphatic thymus, as shown in the case of female sexual functions in thymectomized or nude mice.[1] In this pioneer work on nude mouse endocrine abnormalities it was found that the effect of thymic dysgenesis is not mediated by infections; Nude BALB/c mice kept in germ-free conditions had the same delay in female sexual maturation.[1] The alteration of adrenal cortex was thought to be connected with this delay.[1,2]

However, neuroendocrine agents and neuropeptides also exert a clear-cut influence on the immune system;[3-6] therefore, some of the endocrine disorders which would eventually be found in the athymic mouse could be primary and affect in turn the thymus-dependent system. Such disorders may or may not be caused by the same basic alteration which induces thymic dysgenesis. In addition, they are likely to be influenced by other physiological abnormalities, in the first place by the thermoregulatory and consequent metabolic alterations. Nutritional and environmental conditions in single nude mouse colonies account for the variable results from different laboratories dealing with single endocrine functions.

A systematic study of the morphology of a series of endocrine organs in C57B1/10.LP mice (SPF, but housed in conventional conditions) revealed pituitary changes in nude males aged 6 and 12 weeks, no observable changes in females and in younger mice (animals older than 12 weeks were not included).[7] The difference noted in the *nu/nu* male adenohypophysis was a marked decrease of acidophilic cell size and the number of granules; this may be correlated with a lower somatotropin (STH, growth hormone) level in the pituitary of the nude mouse, compared to a *nu/+* control. Degranulation of STH-producing cells and enlargement of their rough endoplasmic reticulum (similar to the picture observed in neonatally thymectomized conventional or germ-free mice) was found electron microscopically in nude mice which were "senescent" or "wasting".[2,8,9] A thorough study of pituitary histology revealed a decrease of the nuclear volumes of acidophilic cells and hence the "signs of reduced activity" of these cells in nudes aged 3, 5, and 7 weeks and compared with haired controls.[10] Ohsawa and co-workers[11] have in fact observed a decrease of growth hormone in the nude mouse pituitary (radioimmunoassay, BALB/c mice SPF, 7 to 11 weeks old). The difference was present between *nu/nu* and +/+ mice of both sexes; the plasma levels of STH were somewhat higher in the younger nudes, lower in the 11-week group (males), but the body weight of the nude and control animals did not suggest any major alteration of STH function.[11] Using the same technique in BALB/c nudes we have found a decline of plasma growth hormone (0.69 ng/mℓ) at 14 weeks and the difference in the same parameter in *nu/+* vs. +/+ mice; at 30 weeks of life the mean value for *nu/+* was 3.24 ng/mℓ, and for +/+, 1.32 ng/mℓ. This is the only hint so far that the heterozygous mouse may also be different in the endocrine status.

An increased demand for somatotropin and somatomedin affecting proteosynthesis and blood glucose levels may arise in the athymic model which is influenced also by the thermoregulatory problems and possible liver enzymatic changes.[12] Also, some growth hormone effect on the growth and function of lymphatic tissues, counteraction on cortisol-induced immunosuppression and a small delay of wasting in thymectomized mice was described.[4,13] The supportive capacity for terminal differentiation of T cells and possibly other lymphoid cells[14] may influence somatotropin metabolism in the athymic animal. This may be mirrored by the cytological features of the pituitary especially in older, senescent, and wasting animals.

It is likely that there is a central, hypothalamic defect which would lead to the impairment of the hypothalamic control of the pituitary.[10,15-17] The hypothalamic programming may be influenced by the perinatal presence or absence of the endocrine thymus[1,15,16] or by other ontogenetically deeper factors.

In nude rats, however, no effect of implanted growth hormone-producing adenoma cells on maturation of T-cell functions and NK activity was obtained.[17a]

There may also be changes in other pituitary hormone secretions and metabolism in the nudes. A significant deficiency of basophilic cells was described;[10] the functional subtype of the deficient cells was not given, but it may have been mostly thyreotropin-producing cells. In another study, "very large numbers" of luteotropic hormone-producing cells were identified ultrastructurally in the nude pituitary,[18] together with high levels of luteotropic hormone and decreased levels of prolactin.[18] At the same time an antibody blockade of the adenohypophysis was found to prevent reconstitution of the allograft reaction in the nude mouse by thymus transfer.[18] In prepubertal nude females, diminished gonadotropin secretion was recorded.[18a] Thus, the pituitary and hypothalamic status of the nude mouse appears to be involved in its immune reactivity.

There is a concensus on decreased thyroxine levels in the sera of nude mice.[2,16,19,20] This was already observed in 6- and 14-day-old mice.[16] However, in SPF nude mice of the BALB/c background, the differences between *nu/nu* and +/+ mice were minimal.[11] In 6-, 8-, and 12-week-old B10.LP nudes histological changes in the thyroid could also be observed; both in males and females the follicles were smaller, the lining epithelia higher and vacuolated.[7] No changes were noted in another laboratory in the thyroids of SPF BALB/c nude mice aged 4 to 19 weeks.[21] In wasting and senescent nudes the thyroid follicles were extremely distended and the lining cells flattened;[2] these changes corresponded to those of normal 2- to 3-year-old mice.[2] The serum level differences were larger for triiodothyronine (T_3) than for free thyroxine (T_4) in 70-day-old NIMR mice.[19] The free T_4 level could be raised by 30% by increasing the ambient temperature from 21 to 32°C.[19] Wasting nude mice had a considerably reduced iodine-binding capacity compared to thriving nudes (NMRI background).[19]

Thermoregulatory problems of individual nudes affect T_4 deiodination markedly (Section II).

Pierpaoli and Besedovsky regard the low levels of thyroxine in adult nude mice as an expression of an altered hypothalamic function "for synthesis and secretion of thyrotropin-releasing factor".[16] This should be caused by the absence of thymic action on hypothalamus development in perinatal life.[16] The argument may also be reversed, since literary data are quoted[16] on the influence of thyroxine on the development of the entire brain early in fetal life. The thyroid precedes the thymus in embryonic development, in the mouse the thyroid diverticula appear on gestational day 9.5 and glandular cells may be found on day 10 to 11.[22,23] The analogy with the neonatally thymectomized mouse which also has low thyroxine levels may not be entirely correct; while thymus implantation does not alter the thyroxine level in the athymic mouse,[16] injection of thyrotropin does. This means that the alteration of the thyroid function occurs "primarily at the hypothalamic-pituitary level" and the "organization of the hypothalamus for thyroid function occurs earlier in ontogeny"[16] — possibly at the time when thyroxine affects the central nervous development.

Without embryological data pointing in another direction it is possible to conclude that the thyroid may also be affected during early ontogeny of the branchial region where thymic dysgenesis develops. Consequently, the thyroid alteration resulting in the low thyroxine output may be parallel, not secondary to the thymic mishap. The structure and function of the thyroid are obviously further affected by the microbiological status of the animal.

Cold acclimation of hypothyroid animals is dependent on the increased compensatory activity of the sympathetic nervous system; in hypothyroid rats the increase of noradrenalin

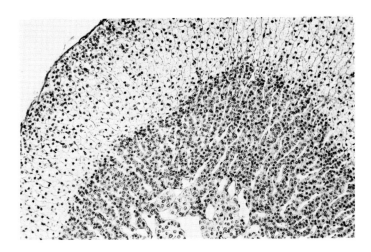

FIGURE 1. Adrenal gland of a CBA/J *nu/nu* male, aged 76 days: a normal histological structure. This mouse gave a high primary antibody response against xenogeneic erythrocytes. (Hem.-eos.; magnification × 120.)

excretion depends on the severity of cold stress imposed.[24] The mildly hypothyroid nude mouse obviously compensates during cold adaptation by noradrenalin secretion and turnover and the resulting nonshivering thermogenesis mainly in the brown adipose tissue (Section II).

The results of adrenal structure and function studies in nude mice can hardly be compared among single laboratories. No changes in male and female adrenals of *nu/nu* mice of the B10.LP background, aged 2 to 12 weeks, were seen.[7] The corticosterone levels of SPF nu/nu mice of the BALB/c background did not show significant changes at 7, 8, and 11 weeks of age, in the females a slight tendency to lower corticosterone levels compared with +/+ controls was reported.[11] In nondefined, originally SPF nudes, gross alterations of the adrenal cortex were found in another laboratory;[2] 50-day-old mice had a "severe enlargement" of the zona reticularis[2] (which may have been the fetal cortical zone[16]) whereas senescent or wasting nudes displayed a "shrunken cortex" and absence of the zona reticularis.[2] The same laboratory has found in BALB/c nudes a slight increase of serum corticosterone in comparison with *nu/+* controls and on days 14, 42, and 56, but not in 8-month-old males.[16] The persistence of the fetal cortical zone which disappears *de norma* by the 3rd to 4th week of life in males and with the first pregnancy in females was prolonged for different periods of time in male nudes;[25] another laboratory has described this prolongation only in females (BALB/c nudes, SPF).[21] Also a persisting activity of a z. reticularis enzyme (20 α-hydroxysteroid dehydrogenase) in adrenals of adult BALB/c nude mice was found;[26] this activity disappeared in *nu/+* controls by the 5th week.[26] We did not find any adrenal cortical alteration in adult CBA/J nudes in perfect health and with good immune reactivity in *nu/nu* standards (Figure 1).

Given the variability of adrenal structure in different mouse strains and the profound changes of adrenal cortical structure and function during stress, acclimation, inapparent infections, and exhaustive phenomena, it is almost impossible to arrive at any conclusion on a lack of a thymus-derived factor affecting the adrenals or on the derangement of the pituitary by missing interaction with the thymus in the athymic state.[2,16,27] However, since the adrenals of nude mice respond normally to ACTH in vitro[16] the possible alteration of the hypothalamic-pituitary regulation, reflected also in other *nu/nu* endocrine disorders, must be considered.[16]

Also, the effect of corticoids in the nude mouse tissues may differ from normal mice.

For instance, nude mice do not produce adequate amounts of a glucocorticoid-antagonizing factor and consequently, have an abnormal response to endotoxin poisoning.[28]

Gonadal alterations seem to be present to a variable degree in all nude mouse strains and colonies, but the literary data are again to be interpreted with utmost caution, since they come from a most heterogeneous material. The comprehensive study of ovaries by Sprumont was performed on conventionally reared NMRI nudes and +/+ controls in a low ambient temperature and without special lighting.[29-31] It was found that the ovaries of 15-day-old nudes were more mature in terms of follicle size[29,30] and cell differentiation;[31] this may suggest an earlier surge of the follicle-stimulating hormone (FSH).[30,31] Pheromonal influences were excluded as a cause of this difference between *nu/nu* and +/+ ovaries.[30] This appears contradictory to the finding that 10-day-old nudes in less specified conditions of housing had more small follicles and fewer medium and large follicles than their littermates; this could be corrected by a luteinizing gonadotrophin.[32] Also, diminished gonadotropin secretion was found in young females in another mouse colony.[18a]

The difference recorded by Sprumont[30] was overcompensated in his nudes by a slower growth of follicles and ovaries; from 21 days on, the normal NMRI mice had more large follicles. This period corresponds to the end of FSH surge with progressive elevation of luteinizing hormone.[30] At 28 days, nude females had more massive follicular atresia than the +/+ NMRI females. This corresponds to the observation on BALB/c *nu/nu* vs. *nu/+* mice in the third postnatal week.[33] Sprumont hypothesized that this could be the result of negative feedback of estrogens on the gonadotrophin release.[30] The main finding in oocytes were virus-like particles;[31] this reiterates the possibility of infects as one of the factors; nude mouse fertility is directly related to the epidemiological status of the colony.[34,35] However, Sprumont's results are compatible with the primary alteration of the hypothalamo-pituitary-gonadal axis.[30]

In our experience, nude females have a different breeding history from *nu/+* and +/+ controls. They have smaller litters with higher early mortality and their third and later pregnancies are usually unsuccessful due to increasing lactation problems. There are, of course, individual exceptions as Fortmeyer's nude female with 32 offspring within 6 months.[36]

In any case, the result of an altered hormonal balance is a delay in the sexual maturity in nude females; the delay is present also in germ-free BALB/c nudes,[1] if we may regard the germ-free nude mouse as hormonally more ''normal'' and viable than the SPF nude mouse or, ideally, the nude with a controlled gut microflora.[36,37]

The first ovulation was recorded in outbred nudes in conventional epidemiological conditions at 2.5 months of age[38] and by 4 months a reduction of the overall follicle population was found and ovulation ceased.[38] For BALB/c nudes, the presence of only occasional corpora lutea was recorded up to the 7th week of life, many corpora lutea were found in nudes between 9 and 12 weeks of life.[33] The same was recorded for B10.LP nudes.[7] In a well-controlled SPF colony of BALB/c nudes 42% of nude females had corpora lutea at 8 weeks, compared to 84% of *nu/+* or +/+ females.[21] In our BALB/c nudes, corpora lutea were found at 16 weeks.[39] In any single colony, animals with almost normal ovaries can be found concomitantly with animals with immature ovaries and ovaries with an increased breakdown of follicles and increased mass of secondary interstitial tissue.[33,39] The fertility of the nudes may be hampered also by uterine infections.[33]

Since thymectomy of normal mice also interfers with ovarian development, and thymus implantation results in athymic nude mice with partial normalization of sexual functions (normalization of the blood estradiol level[16] and of the onset of the estrus cycle[37]), it is likely that the thymic dysgenesis is one of the factors of the ovarian alterations of the nude females.[16,37] The nude mouse ovaries can be restored to normal morphology by gonadotrophin injections[40] and the lack of cyclic ovulatory gonadotrophin release is due to a defective hypothalamic control, possibly the secretion of gonadotrophin-releasing hormone.[17] It was inferred that a perinatal androgenic influence may further change the programming of nude mouse neural centers.[17] This influence has been shown in rats to be abolished by the injection of thymocytes;[41] in mice thymocytes appear to be the source of progesterone-metabolizing enzymes.[42] Thus, an ontogenetically earlier alteration of the hypothalamus may be aggravated in the perinatal period by the lack of a lymphatic thymus, not necessarily by the thymic endocrine intervention. However, thymic peptidic hormones may be at play, too, since it has been shown that they have a triggering effect on the secretion of the gonadotropin-releasing hormone.[43]

Little differences in testicular structure and testosterone levels have been found. In mice of different backgrounds a lower serum testosterone level was established (in nude males and females aged 6 days and males aged 14 days)[16] retardation of spermatogenesis was noted only in 1-month-old nudes,[7] and almost no differences in the testosterone content were found in the testes after gonadotropin injection at 7 to 11 weeks of life.[11] SPF BALB/c nudes between 8 and 19 weeks of life had a normal plasma testosterone level; they had mature spermatozoa in the testes by 8 weeks of life just as the controls.[21] The male structural characteristics were present in the submaxillary glands and kidneys of mature nudes in an SPF environment.[21] Sexual dimorphism was not found in submaxillary glands of nudes housed in conventional conditions.[7,25] There is a consensus of a normal male fertility of nude mice.

There is no systematic knowledge on Langerhans' islets and insulin. Even blood sugar levels of nude mice have not been consistently studied. Fortmeyer gives lower blood glucose levels for nude nonfasting females compared to heterozygous females of the same age.[36] We have used blood sugar levels as an indicator of the general condition of experimental mice considering levels over 190 mg/100 mℓ as a signal of incipient wasting in CBA/J and BALB/c nude mice. Healthy nude BALB/c males had lower glycemia at 8 weeks than $+/+$ males (mean values 106.9 mg/100 mℓ vs. 169.3 mg/100 mℓ). There was an increase in blood glucose levels in fasting BALB/c nude females between 6 weeks (mean value 142.8 mg/100 mℓ) and 8-week-old nude females (182.2 mg/100 mℓ) compared to $nu/+$ females (160.7 mg/100 mℓ at 8 weeks), but there was no decline of immunoreactive insulin which would be comparable to the values recorded for a diabetogenic colony of BALB/c nude mice.[44] We did not see any histological changes in pancreatic islets in nude females or males aged 1 to 4 months.

Nude mice have been applied in the study of insulinitis induced by repeated subdiabetogenic doses of streptozocin.[45] As in other immunocompromised models, hyperglycemia and mononuclear cell infiltration of islets could not be induced in nude mice (CD1 background), except in individuals grafted with thymus.[45] In BALB/c AJCL mice which are not susceptible to insulinitis induced by streptozocin, no differences between nu/nu and thymus-grafted nu/nu were found in plasma glucose levels.[45]

It was confirmed in this study that plasma testosterone levels in nude mice of both backgrounds were not different from $nu/+$ testosterone levels.[45]

The lack of information on the insulin-linked variations in the ontogeny and physiology of nude mice is surprising. Insulin emerges as an important agent enhancing the energy metabolism of stimulated lymphocytes and increasing the overall rates of protein synthesis.[14]

In general, endocrine and neuroendocrine systems may affect the deficient immune system even more decisively than a normal one. Also, mouse splenic cells produce ACTH, endorphins and, possibly, also the growth hormone, thyrotrophin and gonadotrophic hormones and they do so not only after immunologic stimuli, but also in response to ''cognitive stimuli via hypothalamic cortico-releasing factor''[46] in the case of ACTH.

In the search for one clear target of the primary endocrine alteration ''consequent to thymic aplasia'', for one central, well-defined hormonal defect, an entirely new mechanism was suggested by Maestroni and Pierpaoli — the pineal body and its control of the circadian periodicity by cyclic release of neurohormones of the whole neuroendocrine system.[47] Nude mice were found to have a significantly lower level of melatonin, one of the main pineal messengers, during the day and normal levels during the night.[47] Properly timed inoculation of melatonin in nude mice reconstituted with neonatal T cells induced the ability to reject skin allografts which the T cells alone did not.[48] Circadian release of melatonin was believed to promote the differentiation of the T cells transferred.[47] This opens another vast area of possibilities of a neuroimmunological approach to the mutation and its general consequences.

The nude mouse presents a good, but so far almost virgin, model for this new branch of immunology. At present, it can only be stated that some deviations of the nude endocrine functions start at the hypothalamic level, that they may be influenced by thymic dysgenesis or by a mechanism related to the cause of thymic dysgenesis and that they are less marked in nude mice kept in a strict SPF or germ-free environment.[11,21]

At the same time, the compensatory mechanisms of the T-deficient mouse may contribute to some endocrine peculiarities. Interleukin 1 has been shown, for instance, to be a potent stimulator of the adrenocorticotropic hormone and glucocorticoid levels in the nude mice, acting as a feedback circuit with glucocorticoids inhibiting IL 1 production and action.[49]

II. THERMOGENESIS AND NEUROTRANSMITTERS

In the mouse, hairlessness poses a greater problem than in the larger mammals because of the relatively extensive surface area in relation to body volume; even the homeothermy of the normal laboratory mouse is questionable.[36] There is a tendency to decrease the body temperature/skin temperature/ambient temperature gradients by resetting the thermoregulatory centers. The loss of fur which is evolutionally the main thermoregulatory device has been, in the long history of observations of hairless mammals, linked with ''general weakness'', low fertility, and low viability.[50] The nu/nu mouse is in this respect an outstanding exception since it survives for some time even in free nature in Denmark (J. Rygaard, personal communication) and in laboratory conditions at temperatures which are considerably under the thermoneutrality zone. This zone is for the nude mouse at 30 to 32°C and already at 28°C the heat balance of the nudes becomes negative.[19]

Hairless animals cope with the increased heat loss due to the lack of hair insulation by higher metabolic rates. In unspecified hairless mice (probably *hr/hr* which have an almost normal thymus) there was a nearly twofold metabolic intensity, compared to haired albino (H) mice at 4 weeks of age and at an ambient temperature of 23°C; the metabolic intensity remained higher in the hairless mutant during the whole observation period (up to 22 weeks of life); the rectal temperatures of the hairless mice were lower at all ages.[51] It was established that the heat insulation equivalent of the hairless skin was about one half to two thirds that of the haired skin.[51] The same differences between hairless and haired mice were found in other studies[52] and the possible contribution of an increased ''bodily activity'' suggested as a cause of additional heat loss in the hairless model.[52]

In the nude mutant (*nu/nu*), the behavioral activity is definitely not higher than in haired littermates[20] and should not affect its heat balance.

There is of course a behavioral component in the thermoregulatory repertoire of the nude mouse; haired littermates huddling together with nudes can provide an auxiliary source of heat in environments up to 28°C. At 32°C, the behavior of haired littermates and of haired mothers is disturbed and they neglect their littermates and litters, as suggested by our observations both on BALB/c and C57B1 mice. The possible difference in the thermal balance between white and black nudes has not been tested so far. It has been shown that the effect of social aggregation is more pronounced in hairless than in furred mice and that the formation of pairs is relatively the most important improvement of the thermal balance.[53]

In white nude mice isolated during measurements in experimental chambers, the metabolic rates are almost twice as high as the rates of haired control mice at the environmental temperature of 18°C, significantly higher at 25°C, and equal to haired mice at 35°C.[54] At ambient temperatures of 21 or 25°C, the deep colonic temperature and the skin temperature in the interscapular region and over the left loin was markedly lower in NMRI nude mice than in NMRI *nu/+* mice of both sexes, aged 70 days or 3 months.[19] In healthy individuals this can be interpreted as an adaptive trait, an energy-saving device reducing the heat flow to the environment. Also, the body/skin temperature gradients are different over the trunk of nude mice, while the fur insulation in *nu/+* mice assures a uniform gradient.[19] The body and skin temperature decreases further within days in wasting nude mice which lose weight at the same time.[19] Even wasting mice can increase their body temperature if brought to a 32°C ambient temperature and fed an ''easily consumable'' diet.[19]

The nude mouse also experiences an increased water loss through the hairless skin and a high relative humidity of 40 to 60%[37,55,56] or even 65%[36] is recommended for nude mouse colonies. Weihe found a difference in the water intake between *nu/nu* and *nu/+* NMRI mice even larger than the difference in food intake. For 70-day-old mice at 25°C, the food (Altromin diet 1414) intake was 18.7 g/100 g body weight (BW) for the nudes and 8.4 g for *nu/+*, the water intake 40.2 mℓ/100 g BW for nudes and 16.0 mℓ for nu/+.[19] Only at 32°C the *nu/nu* food intake per 100 g BW was about equal to the intake of the heterozygotes.[19] The high water/food quotient of the *nu/nu* mice indicates a high evaporative loss by transepidermal perspiration.[19,57] Transepidermal perspiration obviously contributes to the thermal disbalance of the nudes.

Metabolic heat production is increased by stimulation of the adrenergic systems and by thyroid hyperfunction.[58,59] The thyroid of the nude homozygote is all but hyperfunctional (see Section I), but thyroxine (T_4) production is obviously sufficient. Nonshivering thermogenesis during all kinds of cold adaptation of the nude mouse is based on catecholamine-mediated metabolic changes in the brown adipose tissue depots.

The development of interscapular brown adipose tissue (IBAT) is clearly influenced by social thermoregulation; single hairless mice were found to develop during cold adaptation more BAT than hairless mice living in pairs or groups with normal littermates.[53] Consequently, the quantitative estimates of IBAT in nude mice have only a limited value, unless the individual behavioral history of the animals is monitored and recorded. Weihe[19] has found at an ambient temperature of 25°C the mean IBAT weight per 1 g body weight to be 3.99 mg for *nu/+* and 3.66 mg for *nu/nu* of the NMRI background, with considerable individual variations (SE).

We have measured the IBAT weight in fetuses finding no difference or even a smaller IBAT in *nu/nu* (Table 1); in postnatal mice, the relative weight of IBAT was clearly higher in *nu/nu* mice caged individually at 22°C (in some experiments even at 28°C) at least for 3 weeks (Table 1), compared to haired controls. White adipose tissue was replaced by brown fat at the periphery of IBAT and also in the dysgenetic thymus area.[60]

The essential question is, then, the possibility of a metabolic difference in BAT of nude and normal mice, specifically the uncoupling of oxidation and phosphorylation in the mitochondrial membrane and the conversion of the energy of the proton gradient formed in oxidative processes into heat. Preliminary experiments with IBAT from 42- to 60-day-old mice of BALB/c and C57B1/10.LP backgrounds housed in the described conditions showed no difference between nude and haired individuals in the specific enzymatic equipment of IBAT mitochondria.[60]

The quantities of the uncoupling protein (UP or GDP protein) — which ensures the essential BAT function, direct generation of heat from the energy of oxidated free fatty acids by means of conversion of the oxidation-generated proton electrochemical gradient of the mitochondrial membrane — were analyzed immunochemically and found to be 5 to 15 times higher in *nu/nu* held in 22°C than in haired control mice [60] (Figure 2). Also, *nu/nu* caged

Table 1
**INTERSCAPULAR BROWN ADIPOSE TISSUE WEIGHTS
mg/g BODY WEIGHT IN PRENATAL, POSTNATAL,
AND DIFFERENT AMBIENT TEMPERATURE EXPOSED
NUDE MICE**

	nu/nu	*nu/+*	*+/+*
Fetuses BALB/c			
GD[a]16	3.6 ± 0.75	5.0 ± 0.51	
GDa17	7.5 ± 0.4	8.0 ± 0.3	
GD[a]19	10.8 ± 0.58	9.3 ± 0.34	
Fetuses B10.LP			
GD[a]19	5.1 ± 0.3	9.1 ± 0.5	7.1 ± 0.4
Postnatal B10.LP			
Day 15	3.2 ± 0.3		5.5 ± 0.5

Mice exposed individually to 22 or 28°C at 30 days of age, for time span indicated

	nu/nu-22°	*nu/nu-28°*	*nu/+* and *+/+*
21—28-day exposure			
BALB/c	3.07 ± 0.13[b]	2.09 ± 0.32	2.55 ± 0.11
B10.LP	2.71 ± 0.11[c]	2.01 ± 0.26	1.38 ± 0.30
45—60 day exposure			
B10.ScSn	3.54 ± 0.26[b]	1.31 ± 0.08[c]	1.13 ± 0.12
B10.LP	2.04 ± 0.19[b]	1.25 ± 0.09[c]	0.91 ± 0.12

Note: Means from four to six mice of both sexes, ± SEM.

[a] Gestation day.
[b] Significant difference from *nu/nu-28°* and euthymic mice, $p > 0.05$.
[c] Significant difference from euthymic mice, $p > 0.05$.

individually at 28°C had a significantly increased content of UP. This was clearly due to mitochondrial membranes where the UP increment exceeded in *nu/nu* — 22°C nearly three times the parallel increase of oxidative capacity. The capacity to phosphorylate ATP decreased (lower content of F_1-ATPase in *nu/nu* — 22°C).

The up-regulation of the thermogenic potential of the nude mouse was connected with a significantly increased level of serum T_3[60] (Section I); it was almost three times higher in *nu/nu* exposed to 22°C for 2 months than in haired mice, whereas T_4 further decreased in cold-exposed nudes. The serum and liver content of triglycerides was much lower in *nu/nu* at 22°C.[60]

Interesting changes of the immune status resulted from the exposure of isolated nude mice to 22°C: phagocytic uptake in blood professional phagocytes further increased (exceeding also the uptake in *nu/nu* at 28°C), and natural killer cell activity in *nu/nu* at 22°C was 8 times higher after 3 weeks of exposure[60] and 14 times higher after 8 weeks of exposure than that of haired mice. Complement activity in the alternative pathway descreased in *nu/nu* at 22°C, suggesting an increased consumption.[60] The proportion of Thy 1[+] cells in the spleen and lymph nodes was lower in *nu/nu* mice at 22°C than at 28°C; the primary response to xenogeneic erythrocytes (plaque forming cells in the spleen) was, however not significantly changed after 3 weeks of exposure of nude mice to 22°C, there were only smaller individual variations among the 22°C-exposed nudes.[60] The dysgenetic thymus itself displayed reduced cellularity with total loss of the subepithelial tissue of the cystic portion and reduction of acinar cells.[60]

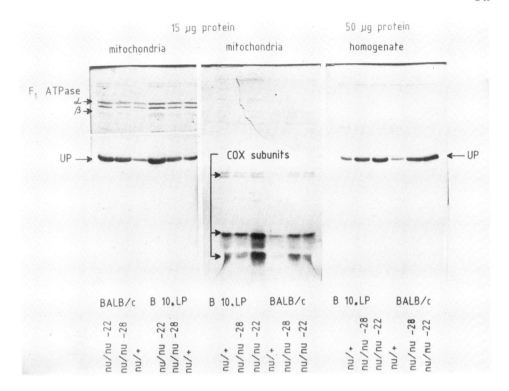

FIGURE 2. Immunoblotting of the uncoupling protein (UP) content, cytochrome oxidase (COX) content and f_1 ATPase content in interscapular brown adipose tissue of *nu/nu* mice reared individually for 3 weeks after weaning in ambient temperature of 22°C (*nu/nu*-22), or 28°C. Haired heterozygote littermates were kept at 28°C.[60]

It follows that the nude mouse can cope for some time with the metabolic consequences of high nonshivering thermogenesis mainly by paraimmunological mechanisms. However, it is evident how important is the physiological state of nude mice also in immunological studies.

Hypothyroid rats caged individually undergo cold acclimation without deleterious effects and adapt with only a slight increase of IBAT and with a considerable increase of the activity of the sympathetic nervous system and noradrenaline excretion.[24] Cold-adapted animals have permanent hyperactivity of the sympathetic nervous system.[61] It can be suggested that higher sympathetic activity and noradrenaline levels may play some role in the nude mouse. In an occasional observation, the infusion of noradrenaline (6 ng/g/min) did increase the metabolic rate by only 33% in the BALB/c nude mouse at 30°C; this was a smaller increase than in an equally treated euthymic mouse. One of the possible interpretations is a hyperadrenergic state with a decreased number of available adrenergic receptors in the young adult nude mouse.

In fact, noradrenaline content was more than twice as high in nude mouse spleens compared to the spleens of *nu/+* mice at 7 to 21 days of age.[62] This difference is abrogated in the nudes by thymus implantation at birth, but the reconstitution may lead at the spleen T lymphocyte-recirculation sites to prolonged graft-vs.-host and host-vs.-graft reactions causing phasic decreases of sympathetic nerve endings-released noradrenaline.[63] The sympathetic fibers branch off from a dense plexus around the spleen white pulp central artery and among the lymphocytes in the periarterial zone.[64] No differences of noradrenalin content were found in the kidney,[62] but no data are available on the sympathetic innervation and catecholamine turnover elsewhere. The local immune response may as well increase the noradrenaline turnover. There is, however, strong evidence for the restraining sympathetic influences on the immune responses and for the inhibition of hypothalamic noradrenaline synthesis during the immune response.[63] After sympathetic ablation, beta adrenergic receptor density increases on splenic T and B lymphocytes, together with the increase of Thy 1[+] cells; among them, the proportion of Lyt 2[+] suppressor cytotoxic lymphocytes decreases after neonatal sympathectomy.[65]

It may be speculated that the low T-dependent mitogen and antigen reactivity of the young nude mice and a developmentally predisposed hypothalamic alteration (Section I) could result in a circular interplay of high noradrenaline-low immune reactivity, with an inhibitory influence of noradrenaline on hypothalamic neurons[63] and on lymphoid cells and their recirculation in sympathetically innervated areas of lymphatic organs.

An additional influence on the nude immune reactivity may result from the alterations of thyroid functions (Section I), taking into account also the ontogenetic influence of T3 on the development and function of catecholamine receptors.

Studying the nude and control mouse phrenic nerve-diaphragm preparations, no difference was established in the numbers, distribution, and affinity of acetylcholine receptors in the diaphragm;[54,66] the nude mouse end plate had, however, fewer acetylcholine-carrying synaptic vesicles which were twice as large as the vesicles in control mice. The amplitude of miniature end-plate potentials was twice as high in the nude mouse.[54] This difference was attributed to the smaller diameter of the nude mouse muscle fibers.[54] The total reserve of the transmitter in the nude preparation was about half that of the control, but sufficient to give rise — upon stimulation — to normal muscle twitches and evoked end-plate potentials. No explanation for the subtle differences has been offered; they could be corrected by protracted administration of a thymic hormone (thymopoietin) to the nudes.[54]

The vast area of interrelations of neurotransmitters, neuropeptides, and the immune system is so far a black box in the nude mouse with its basic immune defect and possible central nervous system alterations (Section III). Any further accomplished definitions of the thermoregulatory solutions of the nude mouse await some more light to be shed on its neuroimmunology. It seems that these solutions are relatively so successful that additional factors should be considered, such as interleukin 1 (IL 1) and other activated macrophage-released hormones. In addition to the well-known IL-1-induced, prostaglandin-mediated pyrogenic action on specialized neurons in the preoptic region of the anterior hypothalamus[67] the local metabolic effects of the IL 1 activation of membrane phospholipases and release of arachidonic acid may have some relevance in a model which is so very dependent on the mononuclear phagocyte system as the nude mouse (Chapter 7). Dinarello[67] proposes a four-step cascade of (1) IL 1 release from stimulated macrophages, (2) IL 1 induction of neuropeptides secreted in the CNS and cells of the immune system, (3) neuropeptide regulation of the febrile response directly or via other mediators in the hypothalamus, and (4) neuropeptide control of the immune response, directly or via certain hormones. In such an intricate network there is plenty of room for one to consider local effects of some of the factors.

III. CENTRAL NERVOUS SYSTEM AND BEHAVIOR

Hypothalamus was the first central structure which was implicated in the athymic nude mouse ontogenic sequence of deviations[1,68] (Chapter 10, Section I). Under the assumption that in an "athymic" animal everything must come from the missing thymus, the deviations were interpreted as "reflecting the absence of thymic contribution to hypothalamic programming"[69] which occurs in the perinatal period and involves a broad spectrum of hormonal influences.[70] Thymic involvement, more exactly the involvement of thymic hormones is, of course, possible but no firm conclusions can be drawn before we know exactly what the secretory function of the thymic rudiment, the polycystic organ of the nude mouse, is (Chapter 3, Section V).

The development and condition of other central nervous structures is even more difficult to relate to the athymic state. It is a little daring to blame the thymus for something which differentiates both in structural and functional terms before the thymic anlage appears.

In 1981, it could be stated by right that "one aspect almost totally ignored so far is a comparison of the nervous system of normal and nude mice";[69] the first contribution came from the Pantelouris laboratory: Purkinje cells of the cerebellum were reduced in number and size in nude mice of an unspecified background, from the 17th day of life onwards.[69] Purkinje cells seemed to have fewer dendrites and were spindle shaped, the length of the boundary line between the molecular and granular layers in the lobulus centralis and lingula cerebelli was 56 to 59% of the same parameter in the cerebellum of normal mice; the nude mouse cerebellum was smaller.[69]

No neurotransmitter-synthesizing enzyme differences were found in an earlier study in nonspecified germ-free nude and $nu/+$ mice; identical activities of tyrosine hydroxylase have been found in the midbrain ventral tegmentum, the olfactory tubercle, the striatum, and the frontal cortex corners and of glutamic acid decarboxalase in the midbrain tegmentum[71] testifying that there are no demonstrable changes in dopaminergic and GABA-ergic neurons in the nudes. At the same time it was established that the axonal injury has identical consequences in the euthymic and athymic mouse, that there is no axonal regeneration or any motor recovery in mice after forebrain and spinal cord hemisections.[71] This, of course, should not be taken as a proof of noninvolvement of the "cellular part of the immune response" in preventing axonal regeneration[71] without any attempt to state the age-dependent T-cell differentiation and function (Chapter 4) in the actual experimental animals.

Some alterations in both the neuronal and the glial populations were substantiated in the nude mice.

In BALB/c mice aged about 10 weeks and kept in an SPF state, differences between nu/nu and $nu/+$ mice were described in the glia of lumbar spinal cord ventral horns. There was no difference in the number of neurons and in the total neuroglial cell count, but in the nudes oligodendrocytes decreased by 28% and astrocytes increased by 51%, while microglia was unchanged.[72] The possible explanations included activation of oligodendrocytes into cells indistinguishable from astrocytes or a retardation of overall development which would favor astrocytes over oligodendrocytes developing later.[72] Some relation to the presence of Thy 1 antigens which occur on neurons and astrocytes[73,74] and may be reduced in the nude mouse brain[27] was mentioned.[72]

BALB/c nude cerebral cortices were compared to $+/+$ brains in 4-month-old females — the thickness of the lateral frontal lobe and lateral somatosensory cortex was reduced and the left hemisphere, in general, thinner than the right one in the nudes.[75] In the left occipital cortical area 18 there were slightly fewer neurones and considerably fewer oligo-dendrocytes in the nudes.[76] In view of the data on the influence of lesions in the lateral and dorsal left cortex on the T-cell populations and functions (a 50% reduction in Thy 1^+ cells in the spleen) in mice,[76] or on the influence of T-cell factors on the proliferation and maturation of astrocytes and oligodendrocytes,[77] it is hard to exclude some rational link between the alterations of the cerebral cortex and the immune system of the nude mouse. Cortical input to the hypothalamus must also be considered.[75]

We have found a constant deficit in the brain wet weight of BALB/c and C57B1/10 ScSn nude mice compared to $nu/+$ or $+/+$ mice of the same age and sex.[78] The deficit was smaller than the deficit in body weight, in BALB/c the deficit of brain weight was -5% up to the 10th day of life, -10 to -21% in 2-month-old animals (Figure 3). There was considerable variation in the development of the frontal lobes of the forebrain hemispheres and olfactory lobes of the nude mice. In some 2-month-old BALB/c nude females a decrease of the anterio-posterior (-20%), in others a decrease of the latero-lateral (-15 to -20%) hemisphere dimension was found. A marked asymmetry of the hemispheres occurred in

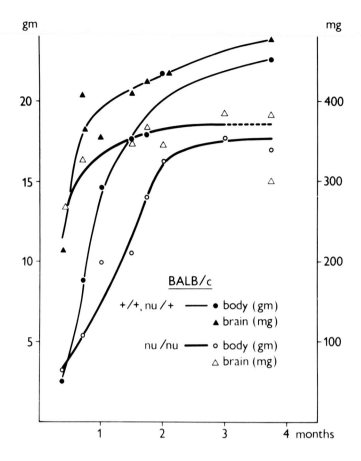

FIGURE 3.   Body weights and brain weights in BALB/c mice.

some young adult BALB/c mice of either sex and genotype, a decrease of cerebellum size was present in some nude females. In 6-month-old B10 Sn nude males the olfactory lobes were much smaller than the lobes of +/+ controls. In general, some defect in brain development appeared to affect different structures in different nude mice.[78]

No difference was established in the numbers of dividing (DNA-synthesizing) glial and endothelial cells in the periventricular layer of the forebrain of 6-month-old B10 Sn nudes and +/+ mice (13.1 and 12.0%, respectively, by 3H thymidine incorporation); a marked difference between these groups of mice was found in the hippocampus area (1.75 labeled cells per unit area in the nudes vs. 3.25 in controls).[78]

It may be suggested that the variations of brain development found in different colonies of nude mice in different laboratories may have a common denominator in a factor or factors which would affect both the structural and the functional development of the central nervous system and would be linked with the mechanism causing the thymic dysgenesis. Thy 1 glycoprotein antigens are present in small amounts in the brain of neonatal mice and rats; they increase and reach adult values by about 20 days of age.[79-82] This is coincident with important developmental events, e.g., formation of synaptic junctions, onset of bioelectric activity, and elaboration of behavioral patterns.[83,84] Also, nerve growth factor was found in tissue cultures to augment rapidly Thy 1 expression with a kinetics similar to neurite regeneration.[84a] Brain Thy 1 is antigenically indistinguishable from thymic Thy 1 and has an identical protein moiety.[85,86] Assuming that Thy 1 molecules may represent one of the key factors resulting from the nude mutation, we analyzed the nude mouse central nervous

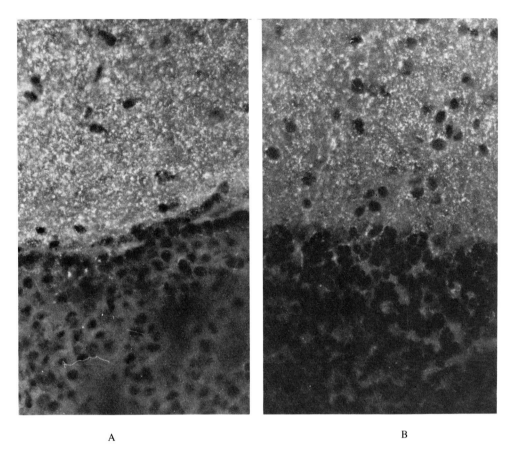

A   B

FIGURE 4. Thy 1.2 positivity in the molecular layer of the cerebellum in C57Bl/10 Sc males: (A) +/+ (B) *nu/nu*. Monoclonal antimouse Thy 1.2. (SWAM-FITC; magnification × 200.)

structures by enzyme-linked immune assay for the amount of Thy 1.2 extractable by Tween® 40.[78] In 57-day-old BALB/c *nu/nu* males, compared to +/+ males, the deficit was 16.4% in the cerebellum and 24% in the olfactorial bulbs; in 131-day-old B10.LP females the deficit in the nudes was 12% in the cerebellum and 20% in the olfactorial bulbs; little differences were found in the hemispheres and in the brain stem.[78] In the hemispheres the Thy-1 content was even higher in some nude mice which have been physiologically altered (ambient temperature, diet).[78] Anti-nude brain sera prepared in rabbits were found to be completely comparable to antisera of normal mouse brains,[86a] so that the deficit of Thy 1 is not general in the nude brain.

A decreased content of Thy 1.2 was revealed also by immunofluorescence in the molecular layer of the cerebellum and in submitral layers of olfactory bulbs in 1- to 3-month-old nu/nu mice of the BALB/c or B10 Sn background compared to +/+ animals of the respective age and sex; in the nudes, there was also a less uniform distribution of the antigen[78] (Figure 4).

Also, the behavioral traits observed in nude males (BALB/c, 5 to 6 weeks old) correspond to some cerebral deficit, especially in the olfactorial area, and in connection with the endocrine peculiarities.[20] The experimental mice were housed in heterosexual pairs at 22°C environmental temperature which could have increased the sociability of the nude test animals; *nu/nu* and *nu/*+ males were successively tested in four variants of social interactions

Table 2
BEHAVIORAL ACTIVITY OF NUDE AND HETEROZYGOUS BALB/c
MICE ON SOCIAL ENCOUNTERS (GROUPS OF 7 MICE)

Encounter variant	Mice tested	Acts or postures — mean frequency in 10 min			
		Aggressive	Timid	Sociable	Locomotor
Neutral cage, test animal introduced 30 min before encounter, stimulus animal —	*nu/nu*	2.0	4.4	23.0	35.6[b]
male of the same genotype	*nu/+*	2.7	6.7	28.7	73.7
Neutral cage, test animal introduced immediately before encounter, stimulus animal — male of the same	*nu/nu*	0.0	4.6	10.6[b]	38.1[a]
genotype	*nu/+*	2.1	7.3	27.7	70.3
Home cage, stimulus animal	*nu/nu*	3.7	4.4	16.0[a]	38.7
— male *nu/+*	*nu/+*	0.1	6.7	26.4	43.0
Home cage, stimulus animal	*nu/nu*	0.0	1.1	20.1[b]	31.7
— female *nu/+*	*nu/+*	0.3	4.4	38.3	36.6

[a]   Significant difference from *nu/+* $p < 0.05$.
[b]   Significant difference from *nu/+* $p < 0.01$.

in a randomized order. Social encounters between one tested animal and one "stimulus" animal took place in the home cages of the tested animal or in a neutral cage and were videotaped for 10 min. Eleven acts and postures classified in four categories were recorded by a keyboard punch-tape system and the records processed by a computer. It was clearly shown that the nude male mice had in all situations a lower social activity, with the possible exception of aggressive behavior of nudes in their home cages interacting with male *nu/+* stimulus animals (Table 2).[20] The lower locomotor activity of the nudes may have been influenced also by the need to prevent heat losses, but the general behavioral pattern was compatible with some neurophysiological alterations. It was noted, too, that the heterozygous control males differed from the highly aggressive BALB/c ($+/+$) behavioral pattern, so that some influence of the *nu* gene may be expected in wider areas than the immune response and the myeloid stem cell potential; the behavior of *nu/nu* may differ even more from the normal BALB/c type and at least some of the neurophysiological parameters are obviously not caused by the "athymic" state.

Social factors have been shown to have a greater influence on female sexual maturation in mice than dietary factors;[87] therefore, social factors such as presence of male pheromones must be considered in nude mice breeding systems.

Also, the most interesting experiment linking major histocompatibility complex not only to lymphocyte behavior, but also to mating choices of male mice[88,89] may have some bearing on the nude mouse breeding, behavior, and prospects, especially in view of the possibility of altered olfactory areas in the brain.[78]

The behavioral patterns of athymic nude mice are a vast open area awaiting future progress of the nude mice studies.

REFERENCES

1. **Besedowsky, H. O. and Sorkin, E.,** Thymus involvement in female sexual maturation, *Nature,* 249, 356, 1974.
2. **Pierpaoli, W. and Sorkin, E.,** Alterations of adrenal cortex and thyroid in mice with congenital absence of the thymus, *Nature New Biol.,* 238, 282, 1972.
3. **Pierpaoli, W. and Sorkin, E.,** Hormones and immunologic capacity. I. Effect of heterologous antigrowth hormone (ASTH) antisera on thymus and peripheral lymphatic tissue in mice. Induction of a wasting syndrome, *J. Immunol.,* 101, 1036, 1968.
4. **Fabris, N., Pierpaoli, W., and Sorkin, E.,** Hormones and the immunological capacity. IV. Restorative effects of developmental hormones or of lymphocytes on the immunodeficiency syndrome on the dwarf mouse, *Clin. Exp. Immunol.,* 9, 227, 1971.
5. **Gillis, S., Crabtree, G. R., and Smith, K.,** Glucocorticoid-induced inhibition of T cell growth factor production. I. The effect on mitogen-induced lymphocyte proliferation, *J. Immunol.,* 123, 1624, 1979.
6. **Snyder, D. S. and Unanue, E. R.,** Corticosteroids inhibit murine macrophage Ia expression and interleukin I production, *J. Immunol.,* 129, 1803, 1982.
7. **Ruitenberg, E. J. and Berkvens, J. M.,** The morphology of the endocrine system in congenitally athymic (nude) mice, *J. Pathol.,* 121, 225, 1977.
8. **Bianchi, E., Pierpaoli, W., and Sorkin, E.,** Cytological changes in the mouse anterior pituitary after neonatal thymectomy: a light and electron microscopical study, *J. Endocrinol.,* 51, 1, 1971.
9. **Pierpaoli, W., Bianchi, E., and Sorkin, E.,** Hormones and the immunological capacity. V. Modification of growth-hormone-producing cells in the adenohypophysis of neonatally thymectomized germfree mice: an electron microscopical study, *Clin. Exp. Immunol.,* 9, 889, 1971.
10. **Henderson, R. S., McEwan, B., and Pantelouris, E. M.,** Pituitary and cerebellum of nude mice, *Thymus,* 3, 359, 1981.
11. **Ohsawa, N., Matsuzaki, F., Esaki, K., and Nomura, T.,** Endocrine functions of the nude mouse, in *Proc. 1st Int. Workshop on Nude Mice,* Rygaard, J. and Povlsen, C. O., Eds., G. Fischer, Stuttgart, 1975, 221.
12. **Pantelouris, E. M. and Macmenamin, P. N.,** Amino acid decarboxylase activity in "nude" mouse liver, *Comp. Biochem. Physiol.,* 45B, 967, 1973.
13. **Fabris, N., Pierpaoli, W., and Sorkin, E.,** Hormones and the immune response, in *Developmental Aspects of Antibody Formation and Structure,* Šterzl, J. and Říha, I., Eds., Academia, Prague, 1970, 79.
14. **Snow, E. C.,** Insulin and growth hormone function as minor growth factors that potentiate lymphocyte activation, *J. Immunol.,* 135, 776s, 1985.
15. **Pantelouris, E. M.,** Effects of athymia on development, in *The Early Development of Mammals, 2nd Symp. Br. Soc. Dev. Biol.,* Balls, M. and Wilds, E. A., Eds., Cambridge University Press, London, 1975, 373.
16. **Pierpaoli, W. and Besedowsky, H. O.,** Role of the thymus in programming of neuroendocrine functions, *Clin. Exp. Immunol.,* 20, 323, 1975.
17. **Weinstein, Y.,** Impairment of the hypothalamo-pituitary-ovarian axis of the athymic "nude" mouse, *Mech. Ageing Dev.,* 8, 63, 1978.
17a. **Davila, D. R., Brief, S., Simon, J., Hammer, R. E., Brinster, R. L., and Kelley, K. W.,** Role of growth hormone in regulating T-dependent immune events in aged, nude and transgenic rodents, *J. Neurosci. Res.,* 18, 108, 1987.
18. **Pierpaoli, W., Kopp, H. G., and Bianchi, E.,** Interdependence of thymic and neuroendocrine functions in ontogeny, *Clin. Exp. Immunol.,* 24, 501, 1976.
18a. **Rebar, R. W., Morandini, I. C., Ericson, G. F., and Petze, J. E.,** The hormonal basis of reproductive defects in athymic mice. I. Diminished gonadotropin secretion in prepubertal females, *Endocrinology,* 108, 120, 1981.
19. **Weihe, W. H.,** The thermoregulation of the nude mouse, *Exp. Cell Biol.,* 52, 140, 1984.
20. **Kršiak, M., Holub, M., and Karasová, L.,** A lower behavioural activity of nude mice on social encounters, *Act. Nerv. Super.,* 29, 117, 1987.
21. **Davidson, K. A., Holland, J. M., Hall, J. W., and Gipson, L. C.,** Endocrine morphology and reproductive function in athymic nude mice, in *Proc. 3rd Int. Workshop on Nude Mice,* Reed, N. D., Ed., G. Fischer, New York, 1982, 197.
22. **Rugh, R.,** *The Mouse: Its Reproduction and Development,* Burgess, Minneapolis, 1972.
23. **Rømert, P. and Gauguin, J.,** The early development of the median thyroid gland of the mouse, *Z. Anat. Entwicklungsgesch.,* 139, 319, 1973.
24. **Sellers, E. A., Flattery, K. V., and Steiner, G.,** Cold acclimation of hypothyroid rats, *Am. J. Physiol.,* 226, 290, 1974.
25. **Shire, J. G. M. and Pantelouris, E. M.,** Comparison of endocrine function in normal and genetically athymic mice, *Comp. Biochem. Physiol.,* 47(A), 93, 1974.

26. **Müller, E.,** Histochemical studies of 3β- and 20α-hydroxysteroid-dehydrogenase in the adrenals and ovaries of the nu/nu mouse, *Histochemistry*, 43, 51, 1975.

27. **Pantelouris, E. M.,** Athymic development in the mouse, *Differentiation*, 1, 437, 1973.

28. **Moore, R. N., Goodrum, K. J., Berry, L. J., and McGhee, J. R.,** An abnormal response of nude mice to endotoxin, *J. RES Soc.*, 21, 271, 1977.

29. **Sprumont, P.,** Ovarian follicles of normal NMRI mice and homozygous "nude" mice. I. Quantitative methodological study in the pubescent "nude" mouse, *Cell Tissue Res.*, 170, 341, 1976.

30. **Sprumont, P.,** Ovarian follicles of normal NMRI mice and homozygous "nude" mice. II. Morphometric comparison before puberty and after puberty in various environments, *Cell Tissue Res.*, 188, 389, 1978.

31. **Sprumont, P.,** Ovarian follicles of normal NMRI mice and homozygous "nude" mice. III. Ultrastructural comparison, *Cell Tissue Res.*, 188, 409, 1978.

32. **Lintern-Moore, S. and Pantelouris, E. M.,** Ovarian development in athymic nude mice. V. The effect of PMSG upon the numbers and growth of follicles in the early juvenile ovary, *Mech. Ageing Dev.*, 5, 259, 1976.

33. **Alten, H.-E. and Groscurth, P.,** The postnatal development of the ovary in the "nude" mouse, *Anat. Embryol.*, 148, 35, 1975.

34. **Poiley, S. M., Overeja, A. A., Otis, A. P., and Reeser, C. R.,** Reproductive behavior of athymic nude (*nu/nu*-BALB/c(A) BomCr) mice in a variety of environments, in *Proc. 1st Int. Workshop on Nude Mice*, Rygaard, J. and Povlsen, C. O., Eds., G. Fischer, Stuttgart, 1974, 189.

35. **Eaton, G. J., Outzen, H. C., Custer, R. P., and Johnson, F. N.,** Husbandry of the "nude" mouse in conventional and germfree environments, *Lab. Anim. Sci.*, 25, 309, 1975.

36. **Fortmeyer, H. P.,** Thymusaplastische Maus (*nu/nu*). Thymusaplastische Ratte (*rnu/rnu*), Paul Parey, Berlin, 1981.

37. **Ediger, R. and Giovanella, B. C.,** Current knowledge of breeding and mass production of the nude mouse, in *The Nude Mouse in Experimental and Clinical Research*, Fogh, J. and Giovanella, B. C., Eds., Academic Press, New York, 1978, 15.

38. **Lintern-Moore, S. and Pantelouris, E. M.,** Ovarian development in athymic nude mice. I. The size and composition of the follicle population, *Mech. Ageing Dev.*, 4, 385, 1975.

39. **Bukovský, A., Presl, J., and Holub, M.,** Ovarian morphology in congenitally athymic mice, *Folia Biol. (Prague)*, 24, 442, 1978.

40. **Lintern-Moore, S. and Pantelouris, E. M.,** Ovarian development in athymic nude mice. III. The effect of PMSG and oestradiol upon the size and composition of the ovarian follicle population, *Mech. Ageing Dev.*, 5, 33, 1976.

41. **Kincl, F. A., Oriol, A., Folch Pi, A., and Maqueo, M.,** Prevention of steroid induced sterility in neonatal rats with thymic cell suspension, *Proc. Soc. Exp. Biol. Med.*, 120, 252, 1965.

42. **Weinstein, Y., Lindner, H. R., and Eckstein, B.,** Thymus metabolises progesterone — possible enzymatic marker for T lymphocytes, *Nature*, 226, 632, 1977.

43. **Rebar, R. W.,** The thymus gland and reproduction: do thymic peptides influence the reproductive lifespan of females?, *J. Am. Geriatr. Soc.*, 30, 603, 1982.

44. **Zeidler, A., Kumar, D., Johnson, C., and Parker, J.,** Development of a diabetes-like syndrome in an athymic nude BALB/c mouse colony, *Exp. Cell Biol.*, 52, 145, 1984.

45. **Nakamura, M., Nagafuchi, S., Yamaguchi, K., and Takaki, R.,** The role of thymic immunity and insulinitis in the development of streptozocin-induced diabetes in mice, *Diabetes*, 33, 894, 1984.

46. **Blalock, J. E., Harbour-McMenamin, D., and Smith, E. M.,** Peptide hormones shared by the neuroendocrine and immunologic systems, *J. Immunol.*, 135, 858s, 1985.

47. **Maestroni, G. J. M. and Pierpaoli, W.,** Pharmacologic control of the hormonally mediated immune response, in *Psychoneuroimmunology*, Ader, R., Ed., Academic Press, New York, 1981, 405.

48. **Pierpaoli, W.,** Inability of thymus cells from newborn donors to restore transplantation immunity in athymic mice, *Immunology*, 29, 465, 1975.

49. **Besedovsky, H., Del Rey, A., Sorkin, E., and Dinarello, C. A.,** Immunoregulatory feedback between interleukin-1 and glucocorticoid hormones, *Science*, 233, 652, 1986.

50. **David, L. T.,** The external expression and comparative dermal histology of hereditary hairlessness in mammals, *Z. Zellforsch. Mikrosk. Anat.*, 14(Part B), 616, 1931/32.

51. **Hošek, B., Chlumecký, J., and Mišustová, J.,** A comparison of energy exchange and thermal insulation in hairless and normal mice, *Physiol. Bohemoslov.*, 14, 476, 1965.

52. **Mount, L. E.,** Metabolic rate and thermal insulation in albino and hairless mice, *J. Physiol.*, 217, 315, 1971.

53. **Heldmaier, G.,** The influence of the social thermoregulation on the cold-adaptive growth of BAT in hairless and furred mice, *Pflügers Arch.*, 355, 261, 1975.

54. **Pantelouris, E. M. and Lintern-Moore, S.,** Physiological studies on the nude mouse, in *The Nude Mouse in Experimental and Clinical Research*, Fogh, J. and Giovanella, B. C., Eds., Academic Press, New York, 1978, 29.

55. **Rygaard, J. and Friis, C. W.,** The husbandry of mice with congenital absence of the thymus (nude mice), *Z. Versuchstierkd.,* 16, 1, 1974.

56. **Poiley, S. M., Ovejera, A. A., Otis, A. P., and Reeder, C. R.,** Reproductive behavior of athymic nude (*nu/nu*)-BALB/c/A/BOM Cr) mice in a variety of environments, in *Proc. 1st Int. Workshop on Nude Mice,* Rygard, J. and Poulsen, C. O., Eds., G. Fischer, Stuttgart, 1975, 189.

57. **Hattingh, J.,** The correlation between transepidermal water loss and the thickness of epidermal components, *Comp. Biochem. Physiol.,* 43A, 719, 1972.

58. **Héroux, O., Johnson, G. E., and Flattery, K. V.,** Seasonal changes in catecholamine content and composition of interscapular brown fat in rats fed a commercial chow or a semipurified diet, *Can. J. Physiol. Pharmacol.,* 50, 30, 1972.

59. **Nicholls, D. G.,** Brown adipose tissue mitochondira, *Biochem. Biophys. Acta,* 549, 1, 1979.

60. **Holub, M., Hoyštěk, J., Janíková, D., Rychter, Z., Větvička, V., Vrána, A., and Kazdová, L.,** Influence of ambient temperature on nude mouse metabolic and immune status, in *Immune-deficient Animals in Biomedical Research, Proc. 6th IWIDA,* Wu, Bing-quan and Zheng, Jie, Eds., S. Karger, Basel, 1989, in press.

61. **Steiner, G.,** Neural and humoral regulation of BAT metabolism, in *Temperature Regulation and Drug Action, Proc. Symp.,* Lomax, P., Schönbaum, E., and Jacob, J., Eds., S. Karger, Basel, 1975, 150.

62. **Besedovsky, H. O., del Rey, A. E., Sorkin, E., Burri, R., Honegger, C. G., Schlumpf, M., and Lichtensteiger, W.,** T lymphocytes affect the development of sympathetic innervation of mouse spleen, *Brain, Behavior and Immununity,* in press.

63. **Besedovsky, H. O., del Rey, A. E., and Sorkin, E.,** Immune-neuroendocrine interactions, *J. Immunol.,* 135, 750s, 1985.

64. **Felten, D. L., Felten, S. Y., Carlson, S. L., Olschowka, J. A., and Livnat, S.,** Noradrenergic and peptidergic innervation of lymphoid tissue, *J. Immunol.,* 135, 755s, 1985.

65. **Miles, K., Chemicka-Schorr, E., Atweh, S., Otten, G., and Arnason, B. G. W.,** Sympathetic ablation alters lymphocyte membrane properties, *J. Immunol.,* 135, 797s, 1985.

66. **Wolfe, A. F. R., Dryden, W. F., Marshall, I. G., and Pantelouris, E. M.,** Pharmacological aspects of neuromuscular transmission in the thymus deficient (*nu/nu*) mouse, *Exp. Neurol.,* 51, 503, 1976.

67. **Dinarello, C. A.,** Interleukin-1, *Rev. Infect. Dis.,* 6, 51, 1984.

68. **Pantelouris, E. M.,** Effects of genetic athymia on development, in *Early Development of Mammals,* Balls, M. and Wild, A., Eds., Cambridge University Press, London, 1974, 373.

69. **Henderson, R. S., McEwan, B., and Pantelouris, E. M.,** Pituitary and cerebellum of nude mice, *Thymus,* 3, 359, 1981.

70. **Gorski, R. A., Harlan, R. E., and Christensen, L. W.,** Perinatal hormonal exposure and the development of neuroendocrine regulatory processes, *J. Toxicol. Environ. Health,* 3, 97, 1977.

71. **Gilad, G. M., Gilad, V. H., and Kopin, I. J.,** Reaction of the mutant mouse nude to axonal injuries of the central nervous system, *Exp. Neurol.,* 65, 87, 1979.

72. **Kerns, J. M. and Frank, M. J.,** Non-neuronal cells in the spinal cord of nude and heterozygous mice. I. Ventral horn neuroglia, *J. Neurocytol.,* 10, 805, 1981.

73. **Mirsky, R. and Thompson, E. J.,** Thy-1-(theta)-antigen on the surface of morphologically distinct brain cell types, *Cell,* 4, 95, 1975.

74. **Pruss, R.,** Thy-1 antigen on astrocytes in long-term cultures of rat central nervous system, *Nature,* 280, 688, 1979.

75. **Diamond, M. C., Rainbolt, R. D., Guzman, R., Greer, E. R., and Teitelbaum, S.,** Regional cerebral cortical deficits in the immune-deficient nude mouse: a preliminary study, *Exp. Neurol.,* 92, 311, 1986.

76. **Bardos, P., Degenne, D., Lebranchu, Y., Biziere, K., and Renoux, G.,** Neocortical lateralization of NK activity in mice, *Scand. J. Immunol.,* 13, 609, 1981.

77. **Merril, J. E., Kutsumai, S., Mohlstrom, C., Hofman, F., Groopman, J., and Golde, D. W.,** Human T lymphocytes promoted proliferation and maturation of oligodendroglial and astroglial cells, *Science,* 224, 1428, 1984.

78. **Mareš, V., Holub, M., and Píša, P.,** Thy 1.2 expression and DNA synthesis in the brain of nude mice, *Histochem. J.,* 20, 620, 1988.

79. **Reif, A. E. and Allen, J. M. V.,** Mouse thymic iso-antigens, *Nature,* 209, 521, 1966.

80. **Douglas, T. C.,** Occurrence of theta-like antigen in rats, *J. Exp. Med.,* 136, 1054, 1972.

81. **Acton, R. T., Morris, R. J., and Williams, A. F.,** Estimation of the amount and tissue distribution of rat Thy-1.1 antigen, *Eur. J. Immunol.,* 4, 598, 1974.

82. **Morris, R. J. and Williams, A. F.,** Antigens on mouse and rat lymphocytes recognised by rabbit antiserum to rat brain: the quantitative analysis of a xenogeneic serum, *Eur. J. Immunol.,* 5, 274, 1975.

83. **Aghajanian, G. K. and Bloom, F. E.,** The formation of synaptic junctions in developing rat brain: a quantitative electron microscopic study, *Brain Res.,* 6, 716, 1967.

84. **Deza, L. and Eidelberg, E.,** Development of cortical electrical activity in the rat, *Exp. Neurol.,* 17, 425, 1967.

84a. **Doherty, P. and Walsh, F. S.,** Control of Thy-1 glycoprotein expression in cultures of PC 12 cells, *J. Neurochem.,* 49, 610, 1987.

85. **Barclay, A. N., Letarte-Muirhead, M., and Williams, A. F.,** Purification of the Thy-1 molecule from rat brain, *Biochem. J.,* 151, 699, 1975.

86. **Williams, A. F. and Gagnon, J.,** Neuronal cell Thy-1 glycoprotein: homology with immunoglobulin, *Science,* 216, 696, 1982.

86a. **Kraal, G., Boden, D., and Van 'T Hull, E.,** The specificity of heterologous antiserum against brain of nude mice, *Immunology,* 36, 799, 1979.

87. **Vanderbergh, J. G., Drickhamer, L. C., and Colby, D. R.,** Social and dietary factors in the sexual maturation of female mice, *J. Reprod. Fertil.,* 28, 397, 1972.

88. **Yamazaki, K., Boyse, E. A., Mike, V., Thaler, H. T., Mathieson, B. J., Abbott, J., Boyse, J., Zayas, Z. A., and Thomas, L.,** Control of mating preferences in mice by genes in the major histocompatibility complex, *J. Exp. Med.,* 144, 1324, 1976.

89. **Yamaguchi, M., Yamazaki, K., Beauchamp, G. K., Bard, J., Thomas, L., and Boyse, E. A.,** Distinctive urinary odors governed by the major histocompatibility locus of the mouse, *Proc. Natl. Acad. Sci. U.S.A.,* 78, 5817, 1981.

Chapter 11

NUDE GENE TRANSFER AND REMUTATION

The *nu* gene was successfully transferred into a number of mouse strains bearing other important physiological or immunological defects. Fortmeyer et al. succeeded in breeding mice homozygous for the nude and for the *ob* gene, derived from the obese strain C57B1(6J-*ob*).[1] The viability and life span of these nude obese mice was astonishingly good, the diabetic syndrome and obesity developed later than in the original obese mice; the obesity reached extreme values (50 g body weight).[1]

Also, the viability of the athymic-asplenic mouse (lasat) was surprisingly good in SPF conditions and using outbred mice of the N:NIH(s) background.[2,3] Hereditary asplenic mice (*Dh/+*) manifest a decrease in the numbers of B cells in all lymphatic tissues and a retardation of T-cell maturation[4,5] caused by the absence of spleen. Also, major abnormality of the hind legs, hemimelia, is caused by the *Dh* gene. Athymic-asplenic mice survived up to 9 months without any increased risk for spontaneous tumors. IgA levels in sera were increased compared to nu/nu; also IgG$_1$ and IgG$_2$ levels were elevated whereas IgM was considerably lower than in *nu/nu*.[5] Thy 1.2$^+$ cells were reduced compared to *nu/+* or *Dh/+* littermates, however significantly higher than in *nu/nu*, especially in Peyer's patches and lymph nodes. On the other hand, the bone marrow content of CFU-C, i.e., monocyte and granulocyte precursors, was elevated in athymic-asplenic mice compared to *Dh/+* and equal to the *nu/nu* figures. Leukopenia was similar to the *nu/nu* counts. The antibody response to sheep red blood cells and the mitogenic action of PHA were reduced as in the *nu/nu* mouse.[5]

The nude mutation was transferred also to the backgrounds of the autoimmune models, New Zealand black (NZB) and New Zealand white (NZW) mice by repetitive selective backcrossing.[6] NZB nude mice did not survive beyond weaning. NZW nudes had a good survival time comparable to BALB/c nudes. The autoimmune phenomena developed very early in NZB nudes and a "dramatic absence of T cell progenitor population" was noted.[6] These nudes had almost no detectable Thy 1.2-bearing cells in the spleen. NZW nudes did not show comparable alterations.

With the exception of NZB nudes, most other transfers of the nude gene to different immunologically compromised backgrounds show a good viability and the nude mouse mononuclear phagocyte system seems to be one of the important factors transferred with athymia.

Particularly interesting is, however, the remutation at the nude locus described by Schultz et al. in 1978.[7] It occurred in the inbred strain of the AKR/J and consequently it had no residual genetic contamination which remained after backcrossing.[8] It is really congeneic. It was called streaker (*nu^{str}*), occurred in 1974 as a spontaneous recessive autosomal mutation and linkage tests have shown that the new mutation allelic with nude, mapped on chromosome 11, 20.6 ± 4.9 recombination units from Rex.[9] It may or may not be identical to nude.[8,10] The survival time of the streaker mutant was about 240 days in conventional conditions and it was refractory to thymoma incidence which is almost 100% in AKR/J mice. Streaker mice have the same depletion of lymphocytes in the T areas (Chapter 8, Section I). Thy 1.1$^+$ cells were slightly less numerous in the streaker than in the *nu/nu* lymphatic tissues.[10]

Interestingly, streaker mice do not share the leukopenia with *nu/nu*, only the percentage of lymphocytes seems to be depressed in 10-week-old *nu^{str}/nu^{str}* individuals. Also, the normal or supranormal levels of serum IgM found in *nu/nu* could not be ascertained in *nu^{str}/nu^{str}*, although the IgM levels were the least affected compared to +/+ AKR mice. IgG$_1$ was most severely affected in 10-week-old mice.[10]

Streaker mice did not reject skin allografts and displayed a marked decrease of antibody responses to thymus-dependent antigens. The reduction of IgM antibodies to sheep red blood cells was 20-fold, compared to AKR/J controls. The responses of blood lymphocytes to T-cell mitogens, concanavalin A and PHA, were depressed — like in *nu/nu* mice.[10]

Streaker mutation seemed to show no significant difference from AKR/J mice in the expression of ecotropic C-type virus of murine leukemia, however the expression of the xenotropic virus was markedly decreased in spleens of nu^{str}/nu^{str} compared to normal AKR/J,[11] reminiscent of the conditions in *nu/nu*.

While thymoma incidence was nil in nu^{str}/nu^{str}, as mentioned, several reticulum cell sarcomas of type A or B were found in aging streaker mice. Thymus reconstitution results in an increased incidence of lymphomas.[10]

Streaker mice provide a unique and so far not fully exploited model for analyses of lymphoma development, leukemia virus expression, and thymic dysgenesis and, if available, they should be used in parallel studies with the original *nu/nu* model.

REFERENCES

1. **Fortmeyer, H. P., Schwedes, U., Obert, I., and Usadel, K. H.,** Introduction of the mutant "nude" in a strain of obese mice, *Folia Biol. (Prague),* 24, 445, 1978.
2. **Lozzio, B. B. and Wargon, B. B.,** Immune competence of hereditary asplenic mice, *Immunology,* 27, 167, 1974.
3. **Lozzio, B. B., Machado, E. A., Lozzio C. B., and Lair, S.,** Hereditary asplenic-athymic mice: transplantation of human myelogenous leukemic cells, *J. Exp. Med.,* 143, 225, 1976.
4. **Fletcher, M. P., Ikeda, R. I., and Gershwin, M. E.,** T-cell maturation in the mouse: immunobiology of the hereditarily asplenic (Dh/ +) mouse, *J. Immunol.,* 119, 110, 1977.
5. **Gershwin, M. E., Ahmed, A., Ikeda, R. M., Shifrine, M., and Wilson, F.,** Immunobiology of congenitally athymic-asplenic mice, *Immunology,* 34, 631, 1978.
6. **Gershwin, M. E. and Ohsugi, Y.,** The immunopathology of congenitally athymic (nude) New Zealand mice, in *Proc. 3rd Int. Workshop on Nude Mice,* Reed, N. D., Ed., G. Fischer, New York, 1982, 263.
7. **Schultz, L. D., Heiniger, H. J., and Eicher, E. M.,** Immunopathology of streaker mice: a remutation to nude in the AKR/J strain, in *Comparative and Developmental Aspects of Immunity and Disease,* Gershwin, M. E. and Cooper, E. L., Eds., Pergamon Press, New York, 1978, 211.
8. **Kindred, B.,** Deficient and sufficient immune systems in the nude mouse, in *Immunologic Defects in Laboratory Animals,* Vol. 1, Gershwin, M. E. and Merchant, B., Eds., Plenum Press, New York, 1981, 215.
9. **Eicher, E. M.,** Remutations, *Mouse News Lett.,* 54, 90, 1976.
10. **Shultz, L. D., Bedigian, H. G., Heiniger, H.-J., and Eicher, E. M.,** The congenitally athymic streaker mouse, in *Proc. 3rd Int. Workshop on Nude Mice,* Reed, N. D., Ed., G. Fischer, New York, 1982, 33.
11. **Bedigian, H. G., Shultz, L. D., and Meier, H.,** Expression of endogenous murine leukemia viruses in AKR/J streaker mice, *Nature,* 279, 434, 1979.

Chapter 12

CONCLUSIONS

1. The immunological and physiological profile of the nude mouse may change with time, due also to improving breeding conditions.
2. The nude mutation may be one of the large numbers of spontaneous, natural mutants which are neutral in natural selection processes. Its so far unique association of the hair and thymus defect may not be so unique if the numbers of hairless mouse mutants were adequately analyzed.
3. Thymic dysgenesis results in the nude mouse from a yet unidentified defect which may be both ectodermal and mesenchymal. Failure of the anlage to receive appropriate innervation may play some role in early or later organogenesis of the dysgenetic thymus. The dysgenetic thymus is, however, not a meaningless remnant but provides under certain conditions some rudimentary inductive environment for T-cell subpopulations and secretes some factors which may have some important function, such as stimulation of mononuclear phagocyte progenitor cells. The thymus of the $nu/+$ heterozygote is compared to the thymus of the $+/+$ homozygote, hypoplastic.
4. The nude mouse has a small, but slowly expanding population of T cells, in addition to the prethymic cells which make up the bulk of the nude mouse T-cell populations. Nude mice of some backgrounds may develop a quantitatively and qualitatively almost normal T-cell system. The T-cell repertoire appears to be oligoclonal. Natural killer cells and analogous paraimmunological cell systems are abundant in the nude mouse and affect cell-mediated reactions of all kinds, perhaps including the control of hematopoiesis.
5. The B-cell turnover and differentiation is affected not only by a more or less altered T-cell regulation, but also by homing conditions and, possibly, even by a defect in one of the B-cell lineages. While antibody responses to T-independent antigens are normal or enhanced as a consequence of defective suppressive mechanisms, responses to T-dependent antigens are low and confined to the IgM class. There are no secondary responses in most situations. The responses of the $nu/+$ heterozygote are different from those of the $+/+$ homozygote; the presence of the nu gene has some codominant traits. To be sure, $nu/+$ heterozygotes cannot serve as normal controls in most experimental situations. Tolerance induction in nude mice follows different patterns from that in the euthymic mice. B-cell polyclonal activators give better responses in vitro than in vivo. IgM and IgM-containing cells are normal and supranormal in nude mice in general, depending on the microbiological status; the levels of IgG subclasses increase with age. IgA is also detectable in most situation and may be associated with an altered distribution of the gut-associated lymphatic tissue. So far, this seems to be more defective than any other lymphatic tissue of the nude mouse.
6. Bone marrow stem cells are depressed in all nu gene-bearing mice. However, direct progenitors of mononuclear phagocytes and granulocytes appear to be abundant in the periphery. It is suggested that the central stem cell defect results from a basic mesenchymal disorder which affects the embryogenesis of the nude mouse in general. The stem cell defect is reflected by white blood cell counts in the nu gene-bearing mice and also by the altered development of connective tissue components in the nu/nu homozygotes.
7. Phagocytic systems and monokines secreted by mononuclear phagocytes are the main compensatory measure for the T deficiency. Mononuclear phagocytes are already stimulated prenatally and, in the postnatal period, the gut microflora provides an additional and steady activating effect on the mononuclear and, through it, on polymorphonuclear phagocyte systems.

8. Lymphatic tissues of nude mice are preconditioned by a somewhat deficient development of the follicular (B-cell area) reticulum and sufficient or overshooting development of the interdigitating cell reticulum of T-cell areas. T-cell-mediated immune reactions are defective in most nude mice, however a general tolerant state to malignant or normal allotransplants and xenotransplants does not exist. The nude mouse may serve as a test system of human tumors only in some specific cases.

9. Hairlessness is caused by imperfect keratinization of hair which grows in waves more frequently than in normal haired mice. The loss of body insulation and the resultant heat losses are compensated, as in all hairless mutants, by a considerably increased food and water intake at temperatures below 28°C. An increased cholesterol level results and, especially in mice over 3 month of age, other minor metabolic alterations occur. The life-span of nude mice is not shortened in a germ-free environment. They die of degenerative processes and — according to some studies — of an increased incidence of lymphomas.

10. During their short history, a number of endocrine disorders have been described in the nude mice, in many cases dependent on their microbiological status. A general developmental alteration may be the hypothalamic programming in early life, a hypothyroid state, and a delay of female sexual maturation. Thermoregulatory strains are compensated by increased noradrenalin levels which may negatively affect the immune reactions. Nonshivering thermogenesis triggered at all ambient temperatures below the thermoneutrality zone is connected with the development of thermogenic mitochondria in the brown adipose tissue, deiodination of thyroxine and a conspicuous increase of phagocytic and natural killer cell activity. Social behavior seems, however, to be one of the principal solutions of thermoregulatory problems.

    There is a growing body of evidence of variable reductions of different components of the central nervous system connected with a decreased Thy 1.2 glycoprotein content. The nude mutant emerges as an interesting neurophysiological model. The label "athymic" may not be completely fair; there is an altered thymus and there are numbers of minor secondary or primary alterations which in combination contribute to the immunological peculiarities of the mutant, but do not basically endanger its viability and existence.

11. Athymic-asplenic mice and the streaker remutation at the nude locus provide new possibilities for basic studies of immune defects and their solutions.

INDEX